D1720628

With compliments of the

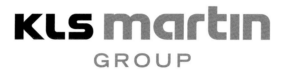

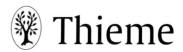

Atlas of Craniomaxillofacial Osteosynthesis

Microplates, Miniplates, and Screws

Franz Haerle, MD, DMD
Professor Emeritus and Former Director
Oral and Maxillofacial Surgery
Christian Albrechts University of Kiel
Germany

Maxime Champy, MD, DMD
Professor Emeritus and Former Director
Oral and Maxillofacial Surgery
University Hospital Strasbourg
France

Bill C. Terry, DDS
Professor Emeritus and Former Director
Oral and Maxillofacial Surgery
School of Dentistry
University of North Carolina
Chapel Hill
USA

With illustrations by Andreas Reinhardt, Kiel, Germany

With contributions by
P. Blez, R. R. M. Bos, J. I. Cawood, G. C. Chotkowski, U. Eckelt, K. L. Gerlach, H. Gropp, W. Heidemann, J. Hidding, B. Hoffmeister, T. Iizuka, U. Joos, C. Krenkel, W. Kretschmer, C. Lindqvist, G. Lauer, C. Meyer, S. Mokros, A. Neff, F. Neukam, E. Nkenke, H.-D. Pape, M. Rasse, J. Reuther, H. F. Sailer, O. Scheunemann, R. Schmelzeisen, I. Springer, P. J. W. Stoelinga, H. Terheyden, K. Wangerin, P. Ward Booth, L. M. de Zeeuw, W. Zoder, J. E. Zoeller

2nd edition

414 illustrations

Thieme
Stuttgart · New York

Library of Congress Cataloging-in-Publication Data is available from the publisher.

Library of Congress Cataloging-in-Publication Data
Atlas of craniomaxillofacial osteosynthesis : microplates, miniplates, and screws / [edited by] Franz Haerle, Maxime Champy, Bill Terry ; with illustrations by Andreas Reinhardt. -- 2nd ed.
   p. ; cm.
   Rev. ed. of: Atlas of craniomaxillofacial osteosynthesis / Franz Härle, Maxime Champy, Bill C. Terry. 1999.
   Includes bibliographical references and index.
   ISBN 978-3-13-116492-6 (alk. paper)
  1. Facial bones--Surgery--Atlases. 2. Internal fixation in fractures--Atlases. I. Champy, Maxime. II. Terry, Bill C., 1930- III. Härle, Franz. IV. Härle, Franz. Atlas of craniomaxillofacial osteosynthesis.
   [DNLM: 1. Maxillofacial Injuries--therapy--Atlases. 2. Bone Plates--Atlases. 3. Bone Screws--Atlases. 4. Facial Bones--surgery--Atlases. 5. Fracture Fixation, Internal--instrumentation--Atlases. 6. Fracture Fixation, Internal--methods--Atlases. WU 600.7 A8805 2009]
   RD523.H378 2009
   617.5'2059--dc22
          2009002211

Important note: Medicine is an ever-changing science undergoing continual development. Research and clinical experience are continually expanding our knowledge, in particular our knowledge of proper treatment and drug therapy. Insofar as this book mentions any dosage or application, readers may rest assured that the authors, editors, and publishers have made every effort to ensure that such references are in accordance with **the state of knowledge at the time of production of the book.**

Nevertheless, this does not involve, imply, or express any guarantee or responsibility on the part of the publishers in respect to any dosage instructions and forms of applications stated in the book. **Every user is requested to examine carefully** the manufacturers' leaflets accompanying each drug and to check, if necessary in consultation with a physician or specialist, whether the dosage schedules mentioned therein or the contraindications stated by the manufacturers differ from the statements made in the present book. Such examination is particularly important with drugs that are either rarely used or have been newly released on the market. Every dosage schedule or every form of application used is entirely at the user's own risk and responsibility. The authors and publishers request every user to report to the publishers any discrepancies or inaccuracies noticed. If errors in this work are found after publication, errata will be posted at www.thieme.com on the product description page.

© 2009 Georg Thieme Verlag,
Rüdigerstrasse 14, 70469 Stuttgart, Germany
http://www.thieme.de
Thieme New York, 333 Seventh Avenue,
New York, NY 10001, USA
http://www.thieme.com

Cover design: Thieme Publishing Group
Typesetting by Primustype Hurler, Notzingen, Germany
Printed in Germany by APPL, aprinta druck, Wemding

ISBN 978-3-13-116492-6   1 2 3 4 5 6

List of Contributors

Patrick Blez, MD, DMD
Oral and Maxillofacial Surgery
University Hospital Strasbourg
France

Rudolf R. M. Bos, DDS, PhD
Professor
Oral and Maxillofacial Surgery
Academisch Ziekenhuis Groningen
The Netherlands

John I. Cawood, BDS, FDSRCS
Oral and Maxillofacial Surgery
Grosvenor Nuffield Hospital
Chester
Great Britain

Maxime Champy, MD, DMD
Professor Emeritus and Former Director
Oral and Maxillofacial Surgery
University Hospital Strasbourg
France

Gregory C. Chotkowski, DMD
Oral and Maxillofacial Surgery
Mount Sinai School of Medicine
New York
USA

Uwe Eckelt, MD, DMD
Professor
Oral and Maxillofacial Surgery
University Hospital Dresden
Germany

Klaus Louis Gerlach, MD, DMD
Professor
Oral and Maxillofacial Surgery
University Hospital Magdeburg
Germany

Henning Gropp, MD, DMD
Oral and Maxillofacial Surgery
Bremen
Germany

Franz Haerle, MD, DMD
Professor Emeritus and Former Director
Oral and Maxillofacial Surgery
Christian Albrechts University of Kiel
Germany

Wolfgang Heidemann, MD, DMD
Oral and Maxillofacial Surgery
Stendal
Germany

Johannes Hidding, MD, DMD
Professor
Bethesda Hospital
Oral and Maxillofacial Surgery
Mönchengladbach
Germany

Bodo Hoffmeister, MD, DMD
Professor
Oral and Maxillofacial Surgery
Charité University Hospital
Berlin
Germany

Tateyuki Iizuka, MD, DMD
Professor
Cranio-Maxillofacial Surgery
University Hospital Bern
Switzerland

Ulrich Joos, MD, DMD
Professor
Oral and Maxillofacial Surgery
University Hospital Münster
Germany

Christian Krenkel, MD, DMD
Professor
Oral and Maxillofacial Surgery
University Hospital Salzburg
Austria

Winfried Kretschmer, MD, DMD
Oral and Maxillofacial Surgery
Marienhospital Stuttgart
Germany

Christian Lindqvist, MD, DMD
Professor
Oral and Maxillofacial Surgery
Helsinki University Central Hospital
Finland

Guenter Lauer, MD, DMD
Professor
Oral and Maxillofacial Surgery
University Hospital Dresden
Germany

Christophe Meyer, MD, DMD
Professor
Oral and Maxillofacial Surgery
Jean Minjoz University Hospital
Besancon
France

Steffen Mokros, MD, DMD
Oral and Maxillofacial Surgery
Ameos Salvator Hospital
Halberstadt
Germany

Andreas Neff, MD, DMD
Professor
Oral and Maxillofacial Surgery
University Hospital Marburg
Germany

Friedrich Neukam, MD, DMD
Professor
Oral and Maxillofacial Surgery
University Hospital Erlangen
Germany

Emeka Nkenke, MD, DMD
Associate Professor
Oral and Maxillofacial Surgery
University Hospital Erlangen
Germany

Hans-Dieter Pape, MD, DMD
Professor Emeritus
Oral and Maxillofacial Surgery
University Hospital Cologne
Germany

Michael Rasse, MD, DMD
Professor
Oral and Maxillofacial Surgery
University Hospital Innsbruck
Austria

Juergen Reuther, MD, DMD
Professor Emeritus
Oral and Maxillofacial Surgery
University Hospital Würzburg
Germany

Herman F. Sailer, MD, DMD
Professor
Aesthetic Oral and Maxillofacial Surgery
Bethanien Private Hospital
Zürich
Switzerland

Oliver Scheunemann
KLS Martin Group
Tuttlingen
Germany

Rainer Schmelzeisen, MD, DMD
Professor
Oral and Maxillofacial Surgery
University Hospital Freiburg
Germany

Ingo Springer, MD, DMD
Professor
Oral and Maxillofacial Surgery
Aesthetic Clinic Oslo
Norway

Paul J. W. Stoelinga, MD, DMD
Professor Emeritus
Oral and Maxillofacial Surgery
University Hospital Nijmegen
The Netherlands

Hendrik Terheyden, MD, DMD
Professor
Oral and Maxillofacial Surgery
Red Cross Hospital
Kassel
Germany

Bill C. Terry, DDS
Professor Emeritus and Former Director
Oral and Maxillofacial Surgery
School of Dentistry
University of North Carolina
Chapel Hill
USA

Konrad Wangerin, MD, DMD
Professor
Oral and Maxillofacial Surgery
Marienhospital Stuttgart
Germany

Peter Ward Booth, MD, DMD
Consultant, Oral
and Maxillofacial Surgery
Queen Victoria Hospital
East Grinstead
Great Britain

Leen M. de Zeeuw †
KLS Martin Group
Tuttlingen
Germany

Werner Zoder, MD, DMD
Oral and Maxillofacial Surgery
Marienhospital Stuttgart
Germany

Joachim E. Zoeller, MD, DMD
Professor
Oral and Maxillofacial Surgery
University Hospital Cologne
Germany

Preface

Miniplate osteosynthesis without interfragmentary compression is now considered the best treatment for fractures of the mandible. The experimental and clinical investigations that allowed the advantages of this technique to be demonstrated were carried out in Strasbourg by a team drawn from the Department of Maxillofacial Surgery of the Faculty of Medicine, the Higher National School of Arts and Industries, and the Research Group in Bone and Joint Biomechanics of Strasbourg.

This research was purposely limited to the biomechanical study of osteosynthesis of the horizontal body and mandibular angle. It was concluded that the best method of surgical treatment in mandibular fractures was inevitably the result of a compromise in which all the constraints under which the operator works should be taken into account. These include anatomical and physiological conditions, biological requirements with regard to the equipment used, mechanical properties of the mandible and mechanical characteristics of miniaturized equipment set against the forces which are exerted on the bone, surgical imperatives.

The choice of osteosynthesis by small plates in other sectors of facial surgery (such as mandibular condyles, midfacial surgery, and orthopedic surgery) arises in part from the therapeutic orientation of the surgeon, based on nonexperimental but logical deductions from investigations carried out on the mandible, partly from the convenience that the plates offer, and is finally confirmed by the results obtained.

The improvements in quality of treatment of facial injuries far exceed the expectations that we had following the results of the first biomechanical research in the early 1970s.

The essential objectives of our biomechanical and clinical research were to apply the rigorous principles of modern orthopedic surgery to maxillofacial surgery and to reduce the empiricism which all too often guides the choice of therapy.

I should like to extend my thanks to the engineering students A. Boyoud, J. Patti, B. Sustrac, and J. P. Villebrun as well as to engineering professors Schmidt and Freund from ENSAIS; to Prof. I. Kempf and Dr. J. H. Jaeger, founder and chief manager, respectively, of the research group at the Centre de Traumatologie, and to Dr. J. P. Loddé, the surgeon responsible for maxillofacial surgery in this team; to Dr. J. M. Schnebelen, a faithful and committed colleague during the long and difficult phase of preparation; and finally to all those young colleagues who enthusiastically accepted and reviewed the technique as well as the new biomechanical drafts, Dr. A. Mariano, Dr. L. G. Gastello, Dr. P. Mercks, and Dr. M. J. Rauscher.

Many thanks are owed to all oral and maxillofacial surgeons who have disseminated the concept of miniplate osteosynthesis internationally, both by their convictions and by the quality of their work. They are too numerous for me to name them all individually. Some of them are coauthors of this book, including in particular Prof. Dieter Pape and Prof. Klaus Gerlach, with whom I have enjoyed a prolific scientific cooperation.

Maxime Champy

Introduction to the First Edition

In the past intermaxillary fixation has been the traditional method for supporting bone ends in close apposition to allow undisturbed bone healing of fractures of the facial skeleton and also of osteotomies after orthognathic surgical procedures. Although techniques of fracture immobilization utilizing bone plates and screws were described by Lambotte (1913), Warnekros (1917), and Wassmund (1927), it was not until the late 1960s and early 1970s that Hans Luhr (1968), Bernd Spiessl (1969), Wilfried Schilli (1969), and Rüdiger Becker (1973) popularized this technique and introduced methods of bicortical compression utilizing maxiplates and screws for the fixation of mandibular fractures. Such techniques are often utilized in an extraoral approach and open reduction. The basic principles require anatomical reduction, stable internal fixation, and a surgical technique causing minimal trauma to achieve early, pain-free mobilization. To allow bicortical screw fixation of the mandible bone, plates have to be positioned at the lower border to avoid damage to the dental roots and also to the inferior alveolar canal. Application of compression plates at the site of compression at the lower border is biomechanically unfavorable resulting in distraction at the area of tension, namely the upper border of the mandible, and also causing distraction in the dental arch. In addition, application of compression to the convex buccal surface of the mandible results in distraction of the fracture on the lingual side, which is very difficult to overcome.

Maxime Champy and coworkers (1975) developed the technique of Francois Michelet and A. Moll (1971). He described a method of monocortical fixation using miniaturized plates applied to the narrow surface of the mandible via an intraoral approach. He studied the tension and compression forces of fractured mandibles and found that miniplate application on the tension side of the mandible produced adequate stability to render inter-maxillary fixation unnecessary. The technical advantages of miniplate osteosynthesis are as follows: plates are small and easily adapted, they are applied monocortically, the approach is intraoral and they provide functional stability since the system is biomechanically balanced. Subsequently the method has been accepted worldwide.

As a tribute to his home town, Champy founded the Strasbourg Osteosynthesis Research Group (SORG), together with Dieter Pape. SORG comprises an international group of surgeons with a clinical and scientific interest in osteosynthesis techniques. The aims of SORG are to foster scientific development at all levels by controlled clinical studies and research, individual and collaborative publications, continuing educational courses and by the development of new techniques and improved instrumentation to further develop the principle of osteosynthesis in the fields of oral and craniomaxillofacial surgery.

Although miniplate osteosynthesis is directed to the management of mandibular fractures, the principles of osteosynthesis have now been applied to orthognathic surgery, craniofacial surgery, treatment of midfacial fractures, reconstructive bone surgery, and to reconstructive preprosthetic surgery including dental implantology. Although there are many different designs of miniplates and screws used throughout the world, these variants are all based on the original concept developed by Maxime Champy.

This book is written by many surgeons who have extensive experience in osteosynthesis techniques utilizing plates and screws with different systems. For this reason different techniques appear in the text, using different systems devised by Champy. It is for the reader to decide which technique is preferable. This book serves as an atlas of surgical procedures and offers clinical guidelines for using mini and microplate osteosynthesis in the craniomaxillofacial region.

We thank the editorial staff at Thieme International for their professionalism and attention to detail, John Cawood and Peter Ward Booth for checking the English, Andreas Reinhardt for the illustrations, and Verena Hinz for typing the manuscript.

Franz Haerle
Bill C. Terry

Introduction to the Second Edition

The *Atlas of Craniomaxillofacial Osteosynthesis* has been a topical work for almost 10 years. It has been reprinted twice, and has even been published in the Korean language.

Owing to continuous demand, we gladly complied with the wishes of Thieme Publishers and—together with the authors—have systematically revised the text, corrected the illustrations, and have overseen the completion of many new and revised chapters with new authors, in order to update them in line with current developments in osteosynthesis.

We thank the editorial staff of Thieme Publishers for their professional cooperation, Andreas Reinhardt for the illustrations, and Verena Hinz for typing the manuscript.

Franz Haerle
Bill C. Terry

Table of Contents

1 Anatomical Aspects and Biomechanical Considerations for the Body of the Mandible, the Midface, and the Cranium

Maxime Champy and Patrick Blez

Monocortical miniplate osteosynthesis is based on precise anatomical considerations and extensive biological and mechanical experiments that have led to the development of specific instruments and hardware.

Anatomical Considerations

The Mandible

Following innovative intraoral miniplate osteosynthesis (Michelet, Deymes, and Dessus, 1973), experimental work and clinical application have demonstrated that monocortical fixation by miniplates is strong enough to withstand the different strains created by masticatory forces (Champy et al., 1975; Champy et al., 1976a, b; Champy et al., 1977; Champy et al., 1978a, b; Champy and Lodde, 1976; Champy and Lodde, 1977; Jaeger, 1978). Because fixation is accomplished by anchoring the miniplates to the bone by means of screws, it is important to know both:

- the regions where the bone provides the screws with a firm anchorage
- the topography of the dental apices and inferior alveolar nerve, to avoid damaging them when inserting the screws

The outer cortex of the body of the mandible has an average thickness of 3.3 mm; it is particularly strong and offers a good anchorage for the osteosynthesis screws. The cortical bone is thicker in the chin region and is reinforced laterally by the oblique line, which runs from the coronoid process to the molar region. In the symphysis region cross-sections of the mandible show the thickest cortex to be at the lower border; behind the third molar it is stronger at the upper border (**Fig. 1.1**).

Near the alveolar process the thickness of the bone is variable; the anatomy of the tooth roots and the structure of the bone do not allow screw fixation in this region (Gerber, 1975). To avoid damaging the root apices, it is safe to place the screws away from the occlusal plane by a distance of at least three times the length of the crown of the tooth.

The inferior alveolar nerve runs in the mandibular canal, from the lingula to the mental foramen, on a concave course. Measurements show that, from back to front, it runs ever closer to the outer cortex and to the lower

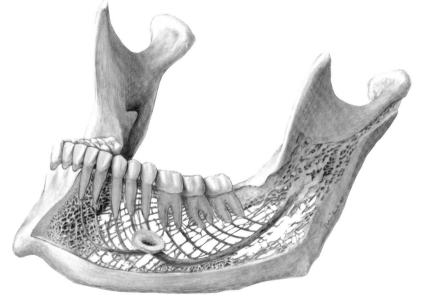

Fig. 1.1 Lateral view of a mandible.
The lateral and inner cortex of the body of the mandible is taken out.

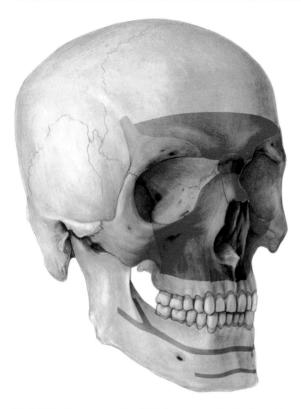

Fig. 1.2 Elective zones of miniplate osteosynthesis. Favorable regions are colored blue. The red zone is a region where microplates can be used. The green zone is a region where microplates or miniplates can be used.

border. At its lowest point it is 8–10 mm away from the basilar border of the mandible. Although the average thickness of the cortex in that region is 5 mm, it may be less than 3 mm in some cases. About 1 cm before the mental foramen, the canal turns upward and forward (Härle, 1977). The foramen lies approximately midway between the alveolar crest and the lower border of the mandible on a vertical line corresponding to the first or second premolar. It is important to remember that the mental foramen sometimes lies higher than the canine apex. Therefore, osteosynthesis in this region involves a certain risk of apical injury.

In most cases the mandibular canal surrounds the neurovascular bundle as a bony tunnel, but sometimes its bony structure is poorly developed. Repeated tests in freshly prepared mandibles have shown that the intrusion of a screw into the canal does not usually cause nerve injury, because the nerve moves away from the instrument (Gerber, 1975). Drilling the holes appears to be more dangerous to the nerve than inserting the screws.

It should be noted that, with aging, the alveolar bone atrophies and the structure of the mandible is reduced to the two cortical layers. In edentulous patients the flat upper border of the mandible is composed of sclerous bone, giving poor anchorage for the screws.

One should keep in mind that in children the mandibular body is occupied by dental germs.

The alveolar bone is covered with attached mucosa. When a fracture occurs, the gum is often lacerated, exposing the mandibular bone to the risk of infection from the oral cavity if treatment is not instituted within 12 hours.

During the first years of life, the blood supply of the mandible depends on the inferior dental artery (Cohen, 1960). Later, periosteal vascularization increasingly takes over. In the adult subject, as demonstrated by Bradley (1975), the blood supply relies entirely on the periosteum of the basilar process. This area should therefore be treated with care. Extensive periosteal stripping should be avoided to preserve the blood supply. For this reason a transmucosal rather than a transcutaneous approach is preferred.

The Midface and the Cranial Bones

In the facial and cranial skeleton the thickness of cortical bone is variable. The use of miniplate osteosynthesis in cranial and midface surgery has been advocated by Loddé and Champy (1976), and Champy, Loddé, and Grasset (1977). Short miniscrews of 3 mm or 5 mm in length should be used in cranial surgery. Those areas where the cortical bone is thick and therefore suitable for osteosynthesis include the cranium, the nasal bone, the zygomatic bone, the orbital rim, the marginal rim of the piriform aperture and the zygomatic buttress (Mariano, 1978). Elsewhere the cortical bone that constitutes the walls of the various cavities is thin and does not provide a very solid anchorage for osteosynthesis screws, and is only suitable for fixation with microscrews and microplates (**Fig. 1.2**).

The frontal bone ranges from 4 to 9 mm in thickness. The upper orbital margins are particularly well-suited for plate placement, but care should be taken to localize the contours of the frontal sinus. Bone thickness allows placement of 5 mm long screws without risking dural penetration. The parietal bone also provides adequate thickness for fixation with screws of 3 mm in length.

The frontozygomatic process, which resembles a triangular prism, is made of compact cortical bone and provides an excellent area for fixation of cortical screws. It is covered with a periosteum that is easily elevated, except at the frontomalar suture.

The lateral orbital rim extending to the zygomatic arch provides sufficient bone for screw fixation. The eye should be protected during the operation by using an appropriate retractor. After Champy et al., 1975, the anterior cerebral fossa can be avoided; its deepest point is located 16–20 mm above the frontomalar suture, or 5 mm above a horizontal line tangential to the upper orbital margin (**Fig. 1.3**).

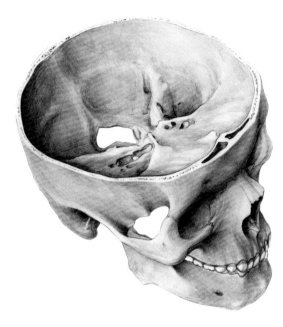

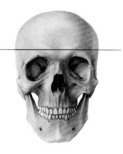

Fig. 1.3 Localization of the anterior cerebral fossa. Its deepest point lies 16–20 mm above the frontomalar suture, 5 mm over the tangential line of the upper orbital margin.

The lower orbital rim is also an area of thick cortical bone. However, because neither muscular force nor any strain is exerted on it, its fixation with a plate seems unwarranted. If isolated fragments require immobilization, absorbable ligatures or microplates are mechanically sufficient.

The maxilla has only two buttresses made of compact and strong bone: the lateral inferior aspect of the piriform aperture (medial or nasomaxillary buttress), and the lateral or zygomatic or maxillary buttress. The importance of these pillars or buttresses was described in 1928 by Sicher and Tandler, by de Brul (1970) and more recently by Manson, Hooper, and Su, 1980. The anterior wall of the maxillary sinus is thin and less suitable as a support for miniplates.

Finally, remember that many cavities exist in this area, some of which contain organs that must be preserved, such as the dura, the eyes, and the dental roots. The walls of the frontal, maxillary, and ethmoid sinuses, the nasal fossae, and the buccal cavity are generally thin and fragile. Protrusion of screws into these cavities should be avoided, as there is a risk of causing infection, particularly in the frontal sinus and the nasal cavity.

Biomechanical Principles

Physiology is the scientific study of the properties and functions of tissues in living beings.

Mechanics is the scientific study of the equilibrium of forces and the movements that generate them.

Biomechanics is the study of biological phenomena with the objective of proposing explanations or therapeutic solutions for such phenomena (e.g., fractures). In practice it consists of an amalgamation of knowledge from engineers and biologists.

The biomechanical principles of monocortical miniplate osteosynthesis are based on mathematical and experimental studies performed in Strasbourg, France, by the Groupe dEtudes en Biomecanique Osseuse et Articulaire de Strasbourg. The objective of this biomechanical research is to reduce as much as possible the empiricism that too often guides the surgeon's choice of treatment, and to obviate the need for experimental human research—or even illegal human and animal experiments. This research work, which concerned the mandible only, resulted in the development of a stable, elastic, dynamic osteosynthesis system that is able to guarantee fracture healing without either maxillomandibular fixation or interfragmental compression (Champy in Huckel, 1996). This has been achieved as a result of the following considerations and experiments.

Goals

The ideal method of treating mandibular fractures is one that establishes a functional therapy by movement. Therefore, it should aim for:
- re-establishment of previous occlusion
- perfect anatomical reduction
- complete and stable fixation, allowing painless mobilization of the injured region
- maintenance of the blood supply of the fragments, of the fracture surfaces, and of the surrounding tissues

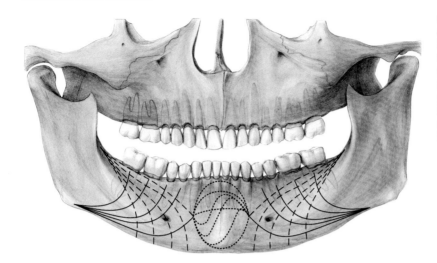

Fig. 1.4 Forces exerted on the mandible from the angle of the mandible to the incisor region. Throughout the body of the mandible, biting forces produce tension forces (dashed lines) at the upper border and compressive forces (solid lines) at the lower border. Torsion forces are produced anterior to the canines (dotted lines).

The biomechanical requirements for optimal osteosynthesis are that:

- the plates and screws must withstand the various stresses due to those tensile and torsional forces to which the mandibular bone is typically subject
- the plates have to be malleable for easy adaptation to the bone surface, especially in the curved symphysis and molar region, to secure anatomical reduction and to restore perfect dental occlusion
- the dimensions of the plates should ensure minimal periosteal elevation and fracture site exposure; furthermore, the oral mucosa must be able to cover the plate without any difficulty, without any dead space around the plate and the head of the screws
- the size of the screws has to be appropriate for the thickness of the cortex

Masticatory Stress Distribution in the Mandible

Knowledge of masticatory stresses exerted on the mandible is fundamental, because these stresses determine the rational design and positioning of osteosynthesis plates and their mechanical characteristics.

The activity of the muscles of mastication can be divided into temporalis forces, masseter forces, and reactive biting forces. The latter have the most adverse effects on immobilization of the fracture. These forces vary from patient to patient. By means of strain gauges connected to a Wheatstone bridge, maximal biting forces in young men with healthy teeth were measured. The following values were obtained:

- incisor region: 290 N (Champy–Loddé) 265 N (Meyer)
- canine region: 300 N (Champy-Loddé) 300 N (Meyer)
- premolar region: 480 N (Champy-Loddé) 480 N (Meyer)
- molar region: 660 N (Champy-Loddé) 506 N (Meyer)

The interaction of these forces varies from patient to patient and affects the degree of fracture displacement that must be overcome by treatment.

It is important to understand the distribution of strains created within the mandible as a result of these external forces. Physiologically coordinated muscle function produces tension forces at the upper border of the mandible and compressive forces at the lower border (Weigele, 1921; Winkler, 1922; Motsch, 1968; Küppers, 1971; Boyoud and Paty, 1975; Champy and Lodde, 1976; Tillmann, Härle and Schleicher, 1983). In addition, Sustrac and Villebrun (1976) and Weigele (1921) demonstrated that torsion forces are produced anterior to the canines (**Fig. 1.4**).

In every mandibular fracture these forces cause distraction at the alveolar crest region, accentuated by the degree of trauma and by contraction of the muscles of the floor of the mouth, which can lead to displacement of the fragments. The compressive force at the lower border is a dynamic and physiological force, which is exerted permanently on the fractured fragments along their basilar border (Boyoud and Paty, 1975; Champy and Lodde, 1976; Ewers and Härle, 1985a). This compression is due to muscular tonus and increases during masticatory function. When the osteosynthesis is adequately performed, and provided there is no defect in the fracture site, this dynamic compression exactly equals the physiological strains that are exerted on an intact mandible (Champy and Lodde, 1976; Tillmann, Härle and Schleicher, 1983).

The momentums of compression, tension, and torsion have been established using a mathematical model of the mandible using the formula $E = F \times L/d$, where E is the state of constraints, F the masticatory forces, L the distance from chin to the fracture line, and d the distance from the plate to the lower border of the mandible.

In any method of fixation of a fractured bone, friction forces controlling shearing and torsion stresses are a very important factor of stability. These forces between fracture surfaces exist due to interdigitation and are enhanced by compression forces. With interdigitation of poor quality, friction forces are reduced or even nonexistent. A double plate fixation is then necessary. This is the case in surgical interruptive osteotomy, fractured atrophic mandible, infected fracture, pseudoarthrosis, and reconstructive surgery (Champy and Lodde, 1975).

Definition of an Ideal Osteosynthesis Line on the Mandible

Given the unique anatomy of the mandible, this biomechanical study defines an ideal osteosynthesis line for the mandibular body (**Fig. 1.5**). It corresponds to the course of a tension line at the base of the alveolar process inferior to the root apices. In that region a plate can be fixed with monocortical screws, as follows:

- behind the mental foramina the plate is applied immediately below the dental roots and above the inferior alveolar nerve
- at the angle of the jaw the plate is placed ideally on the inner broad surface of the external oblique line; if this has been destroyed, the plate is fixed on the external cortex as high as possible (**Fig. 1.5**)
- in the anterior region, between the mental foramina, in addition to the subapical plate, another plate near the lower border of the mandible is necessary to neutralize the torsion forces

The result of such a monocortical stable–elastic–dynamic osteosynthesis is the neutralization of the distraction and torsion strains exerted on the fracture site, while physiological self-compression strains are restored. Interfragmentary compression by means of rigid plate and bicortical screws does not permit this effect. In cases of comminuted fractures it is necessary to apply additional plates to re-establish the physiological strains and to neutralize torsion strains (**Fig. 1.6**).

Other Therapeutic Applications

- An osteotomy of the mandible with a saw corresponds to a loss of substance of 1–2 mm. Therefore, neither interdigitation nor friction forces occur between the two separated surfaces of the fragments. Bringing the fragments close together will have bad consequences for dental occlusion. A double plate fixation is necessary to maintain the preoperative position of the fragments and to re-establish a correct occlusion (Champy and Lodde, 1975).
- In the edentulous mandible the correct position of the plate is on the outer cortex of the mandible, where the biting forces produce tension forces at the upper border of the mandible. The plate should never be fixed on the upper flat surface where the bone is sclerous (**Fig. 1.7**).

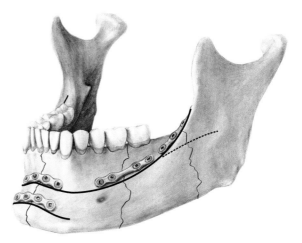

Fig. 1.5 The ideal osteosynthesis position and ideal osteosynthesis line on the mandibular body.

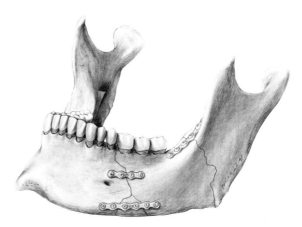

Fig. 1.6 Osteosynthesis position on the mandibular body with a comminuted fracture and a displaced basal triangle segment. The small fragment may be replaced in anatomical position between larger mandibular segments, so that the compressive forces at the lower border can re-establish the physiological strains when the miniplate neutralizes the distraction forces at the upper border. The fracture on the mandibular angle is fixed on the inner surface of the external oblique line.

- In the case of an advanced atrophy of the mandible, tension and compression strains are concentrated in a narrow bundle. Fracture surfaces are very narrow and friction forces between them are small. These small surfaces do not offer the miniplate an adequate support for the compressive forces, thus even the reduced masticatory forces entail the risk of deformation or rupture of the plate. The mathematical formula $E = F \times L/d$, defined above, demonstrates that the strains exerted on the plate are inversely proportional to the distance between the plate and the lower border. A double plate fixation is then necessary, with a distance of at least 2 mm in between.

Where the vertical dimension of the buccal cortex is less than 1 cm, a reinforced plate has to be used.

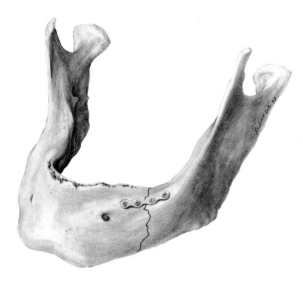

Fig. 1.7 Fractured edentulous mandible. A miniplate has been applied on the upper border of the mandible on the outer cortex. It should not be placed on the superior flat surface of the mandible consisting of sclerous bone (see also **Fig. 7.19**).

In any case, bone being sometimes brittle in elderly patients, fixation of the plates has to be done on each side of the fracture line with at least three screws (Champy et al., 1978a).

More recent clinical experience in this particular case showed that the use of reinforced six-hole miniplates is preferable to standard miniplates (A. Wilk, 2007, personal communication).

- In reconstructive surgery of the mandible, a subsequent study using the finite elements method corroborated the solidity of the mandibular reconstruction using a free bone graft fixed by two reinforced plates (see Chapter 27; Boutemy, 1994; Rousseau and Ségard, 1994; Dalsanto et al., 1995; Champy in Huckel, 1996 pp. 47–48).

Discussion: The fixation of a fractured mandible performed following these biomechanical principles is a **stable–elastic–dynamic osteosynthesis** (SED) (Champy in Huckel, 1996 pp. 52–53).

Stable
An osteosynthesis is stable when:
- no movement of distraction is visible between the fragments
- it neutralizes the harmful distraction strains
- with precise repositioning of fragments it provides the compressive muscular forces with a solid support at the basilar border and ensures interdigitation and friction forces between the contacting fracture surfaces
- it allows early mobilization of the mandible but not complete loading

- it has been demonstrated through computer-assisted calculation (Rousseau and Segard, 1994; Dal Santo et al., 1995)

Elastic
The osteosynthesis plate has an adequate degree of elasticity adapted to that of the bone and is fixed at a high position.

Rigid immobilization of the fractured bone ends can disrupt the process of natural bone repair by inhibition of the inflammatory phase of bone healing (Sarmiento et al., 1984; Sarmiento, Sobol et al., 1984).

Both complete inhibition of limb function and rigid fixation of fracture fragments are deleterious to natural healing (Cornell, 1992). Micro motion between the fracture surfaces enhances the healing process (Cornell, 1992).

Dynamic
Because of the adequate elasticity of the plate, masticatory muscles activity creates compression strains at the lower border. The interdigitation between the fracture surfaces creates friction, enhancing the stability of the osteosynthesis.

The produced compression is dynamic and physiological. The strains are transferred from one fragment to the other, eventually to a bone graft. This leads to a perfect contact between bone surfaces due to the adequate elasticity of the plate and, simultaneously, to a stimulus for bone healing.

Using the finite elements method (Dalsanto, 1995), we proved the existence of micro motion between the contacting surfaces of a bone graft and the reconstructed mandible. This is the case in the technique of reconstructive surgery according to Pape and Gerlach (1993) where the free bone graft is fixed by double miniplate osteosynthesis.

The value of micro motion is of 0.5 μm. The dimension of the osteon is of 60 μm. It is generally accepted that motion inferior to the dimensions of the osteon is not deleterious for the healing process. If this mobility is impaired or abolished by a rigid plate, the normal inflammatory period of bone repair is shortened and even suppressed. The degree of motion is key.

Appropriate stimulus and blood supply are crucial (Cornell, 1992). Controlled motion at a micro mechanical level appears to optimize the chemical and electrical conditions that govern fracture repair.

Biomechanics and Principles of Surgical Repair in the Midface and Cranium by Microplates or Miniplates (Traumatology and Deformities)

The use of monocortical miniplate osteosynthesis in the cranium and midface, although not based on experimental work, can be considered as a logical extension of this method and is supported by excellent clinical results. The forces exerted on the cranium and facial bones are complex, three-dimensional, and difficult to evaluate. They produce various strains on osteosynthesis plates, in every direction, with a preponderance of bending and torsion stresses as opposed to compression forces. The first source of strain is the result of the masticatory forces, lingual pressure, and action of masseter and lateral pterygoid muscles. This strain is certainly less important and easier to neutralize than that on the mandible, as demonstrated in 1976 by Champy and Lodde (**Fig. 1.8**).

The technique for midface surgery has evolved directly from orthopedic and reconstructive craniofacial surgery, utilizing direct fixation and immediate bone grafting (Tessier, 1967).

- In midface traumatology (and in orthopedic surgery), after occlusion has been re-established, the principles of repair involve four important concepts. First, reconstruction of the anterior maxillary buttresses is the key to maxillary repair. Second, direct exposure and fixation of these buttresses provide exact anatomical reconstruction. Third, reinforcement of unstable buttresses with miniplates or replacement of comminuted or damaged buttresses with immediate bone grafting will allow reconstruction and stabilization of even the most severe injuries without the need for internal cranial suspension or external fixation devices. Finally, buttress reconstruction will prevent late midfacial collapse or elongation and secondary deformity. Monocortical miniplate osteosynthesis has proved to be strong enough to withstand all the detrimental forces and to ensure bone healing without interfragmentary compression.

- In craniofacial surgery the use of osteosynthesis by miniplates has been advocated by Champy and Loddé (1977, 1978) and has been considered by Tessier as a major contribution for the treatment of fractures or congenital deformities. The advantage of fixation by plate over wire fixation is to provide a three-dimensional immobilization of the bone fragments in the desired position, rendering useless all devices of fixation like halo-frame, etc.

- For the anesthetist, all procedures being done without intermaxillary fixation (IMF), osteosynthesis represents remarkable and much appreciated progress (Rauscher, 1978):
  - tracheostomy more frequently avoidable in many cases
  - better airway protection during the operation and in the recovery phase (reducing the postoperative agitation, especially in polytrauma, psychiatric, or alcoholic patients)

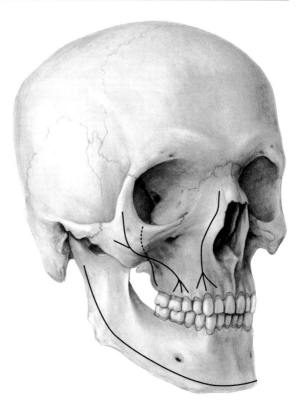

Fig. 1.8 Maxillary and mandibular buttresses. This figure shows the two anterior buttresses (medial or nasomaxillary and lateral or zygomaticomaxillary) and the posterior buttress (pterygomaxillary). The relationship of these buttresses to the cranial base and the orbit above, the mandible below and the correct occlusion is seen. Torsion forces (dotted line) are produced by muscle activity anterior to the canines of the mandible (see **Figs. 1.4, 2.1, and 21.1**).

  - reduction of the risk of asphyxia
  - easy control of vomiting (gastric intubation not necessary)
  - possible reintubation in case of respiratory distress
  - comfort for the patient (Williams and Cawood, 1990)

The use of submandibular tracheal intubation (Altemir, 1986) makes all bimaxillary procedures and the cranial approach safer.

In intensive care the miniplate osteosynthesis, eventually associated to submandibular tracheal intubation (Altemir, 1986), is a very important and determinant factor, often making possible, for the patient's benefit, a global, unique and definitive treatment.

2 Biomechanics of Fractures of the Condylar Region and Principles of Repair

Christophe Meyer

The anatomical feature of the ascending branches of the mandible is of great importance for the osteosynthesis of fractures of the condylar region. In the frontal plane, the ascending branch has a more or less pronounced S-shape, and the amount of spongy bone lying between the inner and outer cortices is very variable (Härle, 1980; Schneider et al., 2005), depending on the age and gender of the patient and on anatomical variation among individuals. This may sometimes hinder the insertion of an intramedullar axial lag screw. At the level of a typical condylar neck fracture, which is at the level of the sigmoid notch, cross-sections show that the thickest cortical bone is located dorsally and laterally at the outer cortex of the condylar neck (Härle, 1980; Tillmann et al., 1983; Krenkel, 1994). Ventrally, the outer and inner cortices merge in a thin blade-shaped ridge at the level of the sigmoid notch. This may explain why, historically, osteosynthesis plates have been placed vertically in the axis of the condylar neck.

The mandibular stresses during mastication are mainly related to the contraction forces of the masticatory muscles: temporalis, masseter muscles, medial and lateral pterygoid muscles, and lowering muscles. These muscular forces induce, in turn, two more external forces, namely the reactive biting force exerted on the teeth and the intra-articular reactive force exerted on the intra-articular point of contact. The muscular contraction forces producing these biting forces were also calculated indirectly by measuring the cross-section of these muscles and by registering their electromyographical activity during a given chewing exercise (Meyer et al., 1998, Meyer, 2008a). As an example, the values obtained for a biting exercise at maximal intensity performed between the first molars were as follows:

- anterior part of the temporal muscle: 412 N per side
- posterior part of the temporal muscle: 169 N per side
- masseter muscle: 475 N per side
- lateral pterygoid muscle: 418 N per side
- medial pterygoid muscle: 382 N per side
- lowering muscles (considered as a whole): 83 N per side

For the same exercise, the intra-articular force, calculated by solving the static equilibrium equations, was 676 N per side, which implies that the temporomandibular joint is a heavily loaded joint—at least, for this exercise.

Concerning the ascending branch of the mandible, these external forces were found to produce compressive forces at the posterior border of the ramus, running vertically and parallel to the condylar neck axis, and also tension forces running perpendicular to the compression forces mentioned above (**Fig. 2.1**) as demonstrated by Meyer et al., 2002, and Meyer, 2008a.

In case of condylar fracture, the physiological masticatory forces, therefore, tend to produce a gap in the ventral part of the fracture line (**Fig. 2.1**).

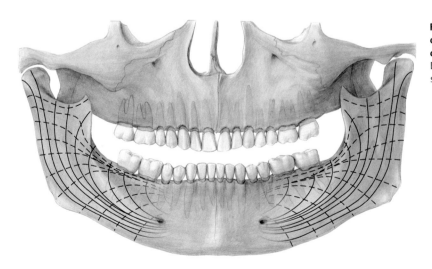

Fig. 2.1 Simplified representation of the stress distribution in the ascending branch of the mandible. Dotted lines: compression strains, solid lines: tension strains.

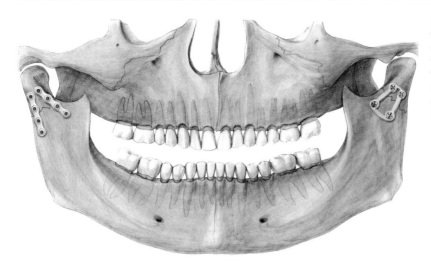

Fig. 2.2 Optimal osteosynthesis techniques for the stabilization of subcondylar fractures. Left: use of two straight miniplates. Right: use of a trapezoidal plate. The upper arm superimposes perfectly over the tensile strain lines running under the sigmoid notch.

In the condylar region, ideal osteosynthesis lines may be defined (**Fig. 2.1**). The superior one, which runs parallel under the sigmoid notch, is intended to restore the tension forces located in this area, similar to the line located in the mandibular body, The inferior one, located vertically in the axis of the condylar neck, is intended for maintaining the reduction out of the sagittal plane as rotation strains (in the axial plane) and bending strains (in the frontal plane) which may occur during function, leading to a secondary displacement of the fracture. That is why an increasing number of authors nowadays recommend the use of two straight miniplates, or the use of a three-dimensional trapezoidal plate (**Fig. 2.2**), as demonstrated by Meyer et al. (2006, 2007) and Meyer (2008a, b).

3 Sublingual Hematoma: Pathognomic of Fracture of the Mandible

Ingo N. Springer and Franz Haerle

Diagnostic radiology has made tremendous strides over the past 25 years. Today, we are able to image the entire human body within minutes, depicting both soft tissues and hard tissues in the same image. Computer-assisted three-dimensional reconstruction of radiological data provides images that are impressive and quite reliable, but at the same time they tempt us to forget the living correlate: the patient. In most cases this may even be admissible; however, it still appears to be beneficial to keep our set of clinical tools complete and begin our investigation with a thorough examination of the patient, prior to deciding a course of action.

After trauma, certain clinical signs are suggestive of a fractured mandible: for example, a disturbance of occlusion, mouth opening, and sensitivity of the lower lip. Other less specific indications include pain, swelling, and facial bruising. All of these, however, can also be associated with, or caused by, conditions other than fracture. The two most specific signs of a fracture are abnormal mobility of mandibular fragments and crepitation. Here, we would like to focus attention on the sublingual hematoma, which Frank Coleman (1910, 1912) found, almost 100 years ago, to be very useful when the usual signs of fracture of a jaw were either absent or difficult to detect. Of course, this was during a time when radiology was in its earliest stages of development, and not yet widely available.

Coleman described the sublingual hematoma in association with trauma as an effusion of blood into the floor of the mouth with elevation of the mucous membranes and a "characteristic bluish, tense swelling under the tongue." He suggested that the presence of a sublingual hematoma alone could differentiate between an external bruise from one that was additionally associated with disunion of the jaw. He considered a sublingual haematoma as "almost pathognomonic of fracture of the mandible" (Coleman 1910, 1912), a finding he based on over 50 observations. This discovery is often forgotten, and for this reason we would like to emphasize it again here.

During the past 25 years, the senior author has seen around ten patients, each of whom presented with a hematoma on the lingual side of the mandible and no other obvious signs of fracture. In all of these instances, the dislocation was so mild that the fragments were not evident on panoramic radiographs, but only on special dental (occlusal) projections.

In many cases the dislocation of mandibular fragments is so severe that, in addition to hematoma formation, a rupture of both the nonelastic periosteum and the elastic superficial mucosa will occur on the lingual and/or buccal side of the mandible. This rupture will be obvious even to the not-so-observant doctor, owing to a pooling of blood in the floor of the mouth. There are also cases in which the sublingual hematoma is more obvious and may cause extreme swelling in the floor of the mouth, leading to airway obstruction. This complication, although infrequent (and rarely associated with trauma), is serious and may necessitate emergency tracheotomy (Ferrari et al., 1962; Teichgräber, Rappaport, and Harris, 1991). It occurs most frequently with the iatrogenic laceration of arteries in the floor of the mouth during implant placement, when the lingual cortical bone of the mandible is accidently perforated. In these cases a rupture of the sublingual mucosa is often not present, thus when heavy bleeding occurs into the confined sublingual space, there is no pressure release for the rapidly increasing volume.

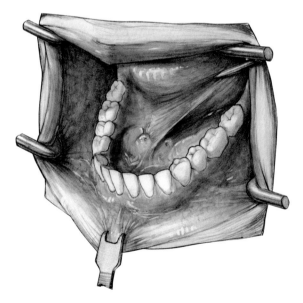

Fig. 3.1 A sublingual hematoma in the right premolar region with no other obvious signs of fracture of the mandible. The fracture line is so subtle that it is not evident on panoramic radiographs, but only on dental occlusal projection.

Our experience combined with the findings of others leads us strongly to suggest that if a hematoma (or even the slightest blueish tinge with no swelling or marginal bleeding) develops post-trauma on the lingual side of the mandible, then a fracture is also present. No matter how small the fracture or how mild the dislocation, the formation of the hematoma is the harbinger of an injury that will eventually become evident (**Fig. 3.1**).

4 Bone Repair and Fracture Healing

Franz Haerle

Structure of Facial Bone

The structure of facial bone is determined by its material properties and by its mechanical role. The bone marrow cavity, the cortex, and the spongiosa of the mandible and the midface are similar in their material composition. Their major difference is in the geometric distribution of the bone. The midfacial skeleton consists of thin laminae that provide an increased surface-area to bone-volume ratio as compared with the mandible. Consequently, the closer proximity of blood vessels provides a superior supply of nutrients and thus promotes an increased healing rate of the midfacial bones.

Bone is a dynamic tissue, constantly undergoing resorption and remodeling (Schenk, 1992). The cell types of which it is composed consist of osteoblasts, osteocytes, and osteoclasts (**Fig. 4.1**).

Osteoblasts are derived from pluripotential precursor cells. They produce osteoid, the organic matrix of bone, which is transformed into calcified bone. A layer of 1 μm of osteoid may be produced per day, followed by a maturation phase of 10 days before calcification.

The microscopic structure of osteoid is different in woven and lamellar bone. In woven bone the collagen fibrils are randomly orientated and have a felted texture. In lamellar bone they are arranged in parallel bundles. Woven bone mineralizes immediately after osteoid deposition. In fracture healing, woven bone is transformed into lamellar bone.

Fig. 4.1 Normal bone structure.

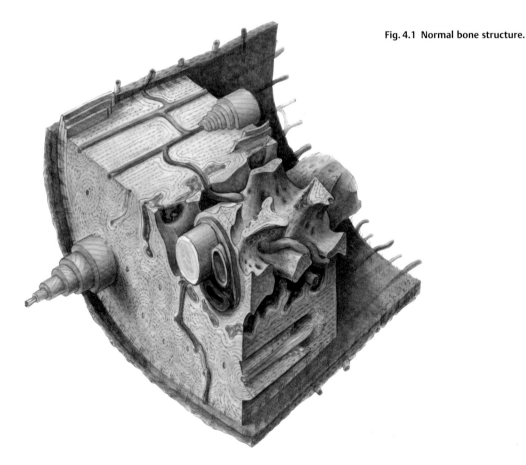

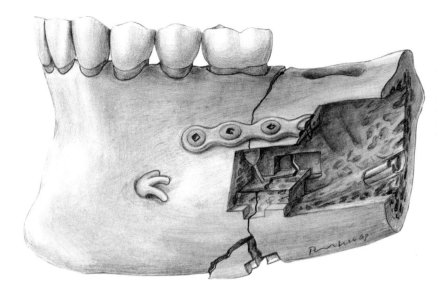

Fig. 4.2 Three windows in a mandibular fracture with miniplate osteosynthesis on the tension side. This shows indirect bone healing in the window on the inferior border of the mandible with the mobile fragment; direct bone healing in the window of the lateral cortex of the mandible by contact healing after perfect and anatomical reduction; direct bone healing in the window of the inner cortex of the mandible by gap healing.

Osteocytes are derived from osteoblasts. Sometimes osteoblasts can stop producing osteoid. They transform into osteocytes, which are connected with the deeper osteocyte cell layers. The osteocytes lie between the concentric lamellae.

Osteoclasts are multinucleate giant cells derived from mononuclear macrophages. Osteoclasts have a specialized role of bone breakdown. This activity is limited to Howship lacunae, which are small subcellular chambers with a low pH. The pH is maintained by hydrochloric acid, which dissolves the mineral. The organic matrix is degraded by proteases and collagenases. Osteoclasts are able to resorb 50–100 μm of bone per day.

Osteons are cylindrical vascular tunnels formed by an osteoclast-rich tissue (haversian canal). They contain pluripotential precursor cells and endosteum known as the cutting cone. The bone removed by the cutting cone is replaced by osteoblast-rich tissue, known as the closing cone. This forms concentric layers of lamellar bone which surround the vascular haversian canal. Volkmann canals also contain nutritional vessels arising from the periosteal and endosteal bone surface, which connect with the haversian vessels within the osteons (Schenk and Willenegger, 1964). The size of the osteonal transport system is 100 μm, which limits the width of an osteon to approximately 200 μm. The mean width of a lamella is 3–7 μm (see **Fig. 4.1**).

The three most important conditions necessary for bone formation and bone mineralization are pluripotential precursor cells, ample blood supply, and mechanical rest (Pauwels, 1940).

Fracture Healing

There are two types of fracture healing, namely indirect and direct bone healing. Direct bone healing is a synergism between contact and gap healing. Indirect bone healing occurs via the pluripotential cells located within the cortical and cancellous bone periosteum and associated soft tissue. Indirect bone healing results from the mechanical instability of the fracture, caused by resorption of fracture ends and callus formation.

In the case of direct bone healing, the close apposition of the fracture segments provides mechanical stability. Consequently, the osteons of the fracture end are in direct contact, allowing transverse bridging of the haversian system with no intervening callus formation (**Fig. 4.2**).

Indirect Bone Healing (Secondary Osseous and Soft-Tissue Healing)

Bone fracture leads to the rupture of blood vessels with hematoma formation in the surrounding soft tissue and localized avascularity of the fragment ends. Further complications are thrombosis of the vessels within the haversian and Volkmann canals a few millimeters from the ends of fragments (**Fig. 4.3**). Indirect bone healing occurs via callus formation, as seen in some cases of spontaneous bone healing, with or without direct fixation of the fracture site.

Several stages of callus formation can be distinguished. Initially, the formation of periosteal callus leads to a decrease in interfragmentary strain, which is followed by interfragmentary and endosteal callus formation. Invading granulation tissue replaces the initial hematoma and is transformed into interfragmentary connective tissue (**Fig. 4.4**). The ends of the fragments are resorbed by osteoclasts (**Figs. 4.4, 4.5**). The more interfragmentary con-

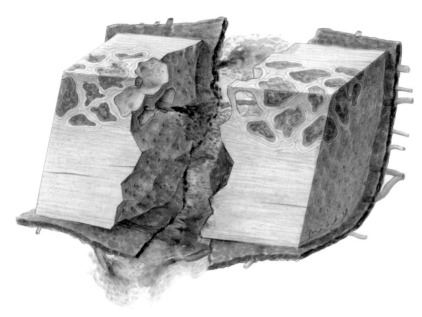

Fig. 4.3 Bone fracture with rupture of blood vessels and hematoma in surrounding soft tissues.

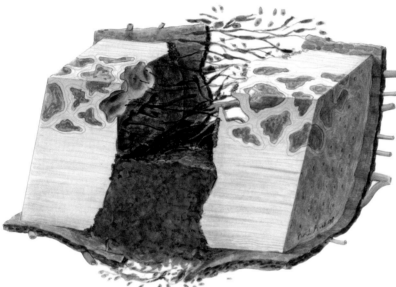

Fig. 4.4 Granulation tissue replaces the initial hematoma in the bone fracture, and the ends of the fragments will be resorbed by osteoclasts. Hematoma is shown only in the inferior part of the bone fracture.

nective tissue is remodeled into fibrocartilage (**Fig. 4.6**). Since fibrocartilage is more rigid than fibrous tissue, the interfragmentary tissue becomes stiffer and increases the resistance to motion of the fragments. Subsequently the fibrocartilage undergoes mineralization. Vascular invasion of fibrocartilage is combined with resorption of mineralized matrix. Calcified fibrocartilage must undergo resorption before osteoblasts can start to produce osteoid as a base for new bone deposition (**Fig. 4.7**). Initially the calcified fibrocartilage is replaced by woven bone. After the fracture is bridged by woven bone, stability is obtained and function is possible (Philipps and Rahn, 1992). Haversian remodeling proceeds, replacing woven bone with lamellar bone (**Fig. 4.8**).

Direct Bone Healing (Primary Osseous Healing)

Direct bone healing was first described in radiographs after perfect anatomical repositioning and stable fixation. Its features are lack of callus formation and disappearance of the fracture lines. Danis (1949) described this as *soudure autogène* (autogenous welding). Callus-free, direct bone healing requires what is often called "stability by interfragmentary compression" (Steinemann, 1983). In the craniomaxillofacial skeleton, interfragmentary compression for direct bone healing is not necessary—as demonstrated by Ikemura et al. (1984), Ewers and Härle (1983, 1985) experimentally, and by Champy and Lodde (1977) and Kahn and Khouri (1992) clinically. Schenk and

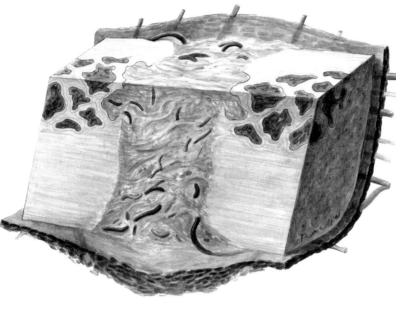

Fig. 4.5 Granulation tissue will be remodeled into interfragmentary connective tissue.

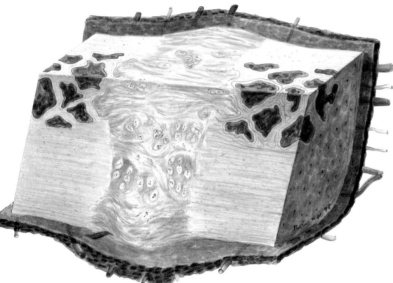

Fig. 4.6 Interfragmentary connective tissue will be remodeled into fibrocartilage.

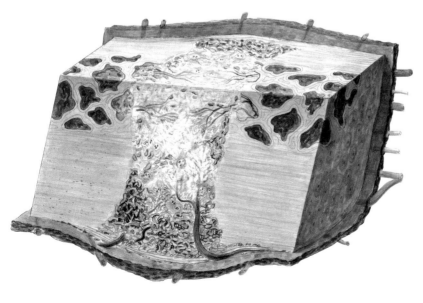

Fig. 4.7 Calcified fibrocartilage must be partially resorbed before osteoblasts can begin to produce osteoid.

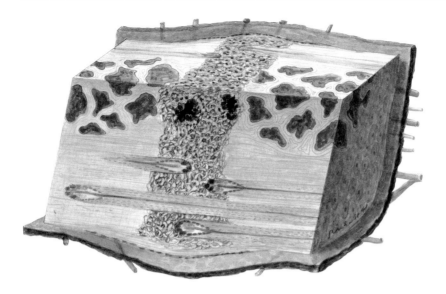

Fig. 4.8 Haversian remodeling begins to reconstruct the lamellar direction of the bone.

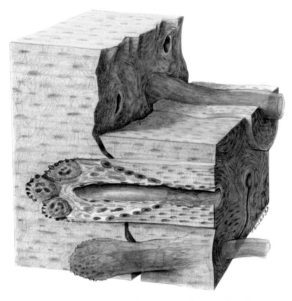

Fig. 4.9 Cutting cones are able to cross the interface from one fragment to the other by remodeling the haversian canal.

Willenegger (1963, 1964) described two different forms of direct bone healing, contact healing and gap healing.

Contact healing of the bone means healing of the fracture line after stable anatomical repositioning, with perfect interfragmentary contact and without the possibility for any cellular or vascular ingrowth. Cutting cones are able to cross this interface from one fragment to the other by remodeling the haversian canal. Haversian canal remodeling is the main mechanism for restoration of the internal architecture of compact bone (**Fig. 4.9**). Contact healing takes place over the whole fracture line after perfect anatomical reduction, osteosynthesis, and mechanical rest (**Fig. 4.10**). Contact healing is only seen directly beneath the miniplate (see **Fig. 4.2**).

Gap healing takes place in stable or "quiet" gaps with a width greater than the 200-μm osteonal diameter. Ingrowth of vessels and mesenchymal cells starts after surgery. Osteoblasts deposit osteoid on the fragment ends without osteoclastic resorption. The gaps are filled exclusively with primarily formed, transversely oriented lamellar bone. Replacement is usually completed within 4 to 6

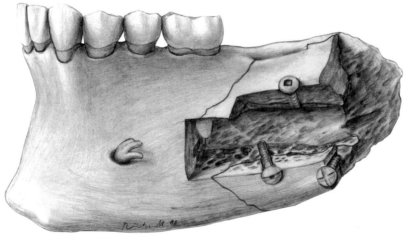

Fig. 4.10 Perfect anatomical repositioning of a mandibular fracture by lag screw osteosynthesis.

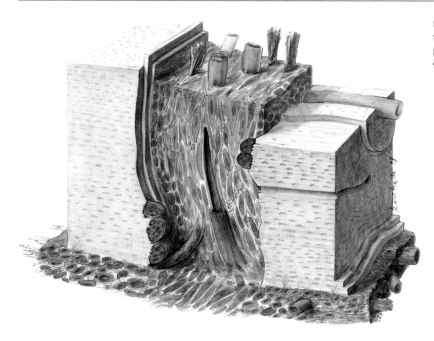

Fig. 4.11 Osteoblasts deposit osteoid, and the gaps are filled with primary formation of transversely orientated lamellar bone.

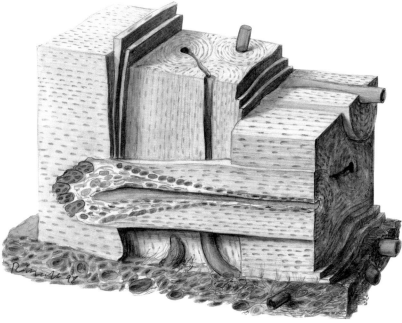

Fig. 4.12 Haversian remodeling. Transversely oriented bone lamellae are replaced by axially orientated osteons.

weeks (**Fig. 4.11**). In the second stage, the transversely oriented bone lamellae are replaced by axially orientated osteons, a process which is referred to as haversian remodeling (**Fig. 4.12**). After 10 weeks the fracture is replaced by newly reconstructed cortical bone. Gap healing is seen, for example, on the inner side of the mandible after miniplate osteosynthesis. Gap healing plays an important role in direct bone healing. Gaps are far more extensive than contact areas. Contact areas, on the other hand, are essential for stabilization by interfragmentary

friction. Contact areas protect the gaps against deformation. Gap healing is seen far from the plate (see **Fig. 4.2**).

Pseudoarthrosis

Pseudoarthrosis describes the nonunion caused by the failure of tissues to differentiate. Tissue differentiation is not possible if, for example, there is movement of the fracture ends due to excessive external forces. In these cases stabilization is required. When interfragmentary resorption has progressed so far that bony union is not possible, then bone grafting is necessary.

Craniomaxillofacial Bone Healing

Bone repair and fracture healing to restore original integrity (*restitutio ad integrum*) can be achieved with the use of miniplates and screw fixation to provide direct healing. In the mandible, the plate must be placed at the biomechanically most favorable site to neutralize the tension forces and torsional moments that cause fracture distraction. Bone plate fixation provides both contact and gap healing. Contact healing is seen adjacent to the plate and between lag-screw osteosynthesis. Gap healing occurs remotely from the plates. A combination of direct and indirect healing also occurs in the maxilla, zygoma, naso-ethmoid and cranium regions following the principles of miniplate osteosynthesis.

5 Surgical Approaches

Franz Haerle

Biomechanical Principles

The surgeon is encouraged to regain the maximum function of injured skin or mucosa with the least possible deformity and scarring. The ultimate appearance and function of a scar can be predicted by the static and dynamic skin tensions on the surrounding skin (Thacker et al., 1975). Static tension lines exist within the skin and are oriented in specific but variable directions throughout the body. This was first recognized by Dupuytren in 1834. He examined a suicide victim who had sustained three self-inflicted puncture wounds made by an awl. He noted that the skin incisions either gaped apart or remained closed in a consistent way, depending on the direction of the incision and their site on the body.

In 1861 Langer examined the skin of cadavers which were lying in a normal anatomical position. He inserted an awl to depths of 2 mm and 2.5 mm and so identified the direction of predominant tension. These static lines of maximal skin tension are now known as Langer lines (**Fig. 5.1**).

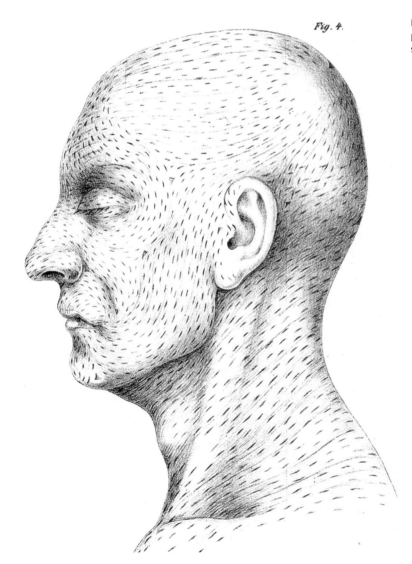

Fig. 4.

Fig. 5.1 Langer lines were noted after puncturing the skin of cadavers with a sharp awl. (Langer, 1861, Fig. 4.)

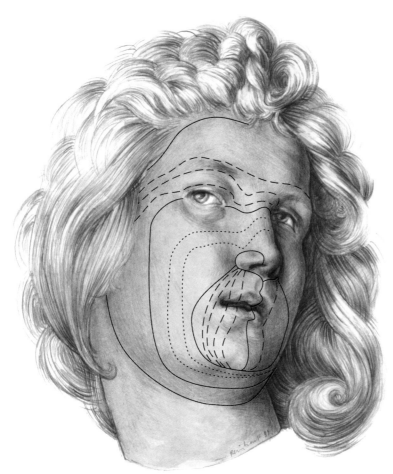

Fig. 5.2 Borges and Alexander "relaxed skin tension lines" indicate the directional pull that exists in relaxed skin. They can be determined by noting the "furrows and ridges" which are formed by pinching the skin (after Albrecht Dürer, *Angel Head*, 1506, Albertina, Vienna).

Extraoral Incision

Kocher was the first surgeon to recognize the surgical significance of Langer lines in 1892. He recommended that surgical incisions should be made in such a way as to follow the direction of Langer lines to obtain the best postoperative scars. This recommendation was reinforced by Kraissl (1951). However, Borges and Alexander (1962), while recognizing the importance of Langer lines, disputed their biological relevance, since they represented the lines of skin tension following rigor mortis. They observed that in the living body in a relaxed state, skin tension occurred in one specific direction (**Fig. 5.2**). They called this phenomenon "relaxed skin tension lines" (RSTL). On the face, Borges, Alexander, and Block (1965) distinguished four principal relaxed skin tension line directions:

- the facial median line
- the nasolabial line
- the palpebral line
- the marginal facial line

Borges (1973) recommended that to obtain optimal healing of scars the surgical incision should follow the relaxed skin tension line direction within these areas (**Fig. 5.3**). Skin tension lines are usually oriented perpendicularly to the underlying muscles (**Fig. 5.4**).

Today, it is generally recognized that the best aesthetic results in the face are obtained if the long axis of the scar lies in the direction of the maximal skin tension (Remmert et al., 1994). The more closely a wound follows the relaxed skin tension lines, the better the cosmetic result.

An extraoral approach for mini- or microplate and screw application is rarely used. However, in some cases an extraoral approach (such as the classical submandibular, lower eyelid, upper lid blepharoplasty, brow and coronal approaches) is required (**Fig. 5.5**). When such an approach is used, the facial nerve is potentially at risk and therefore the surgeon must be aware of, and consider, the relevant anatomy (**Fig. 5.6**).

Intraoral Incisions

The typical intraoral incision lines for exposure of either the maxilla or the mandible are made within the unattached mucosa 4–5 mm below the level of the attached gingiva (**Figs. 5.7, 5.8**).

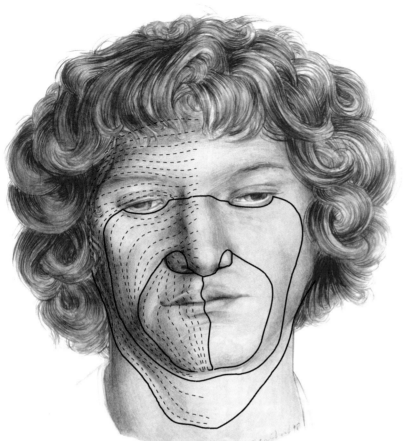

Fig. 5.3 The four principal relaxed skin tension lines. The facial median line, the nasolabial line, the palpebral line, and the marginal facial line (after Albrecht Dürer, *Portrait of an 18 year old lad*, 1503, Bibliothek der Akademie der Künste, Vienna).

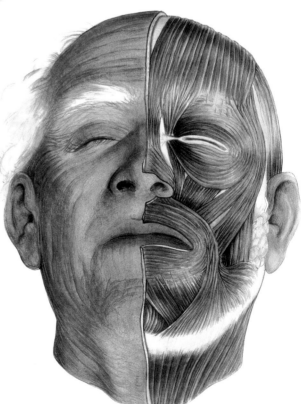

Fig. 5.4 Facial skin tension lines and facial muscle lines are usually oriented perpendicularly to muscles.

Alternatively, to reduce scar tissue formation and minimize the risk of infection, the marginal rim incision can be used (see **Figs. 5.7, 5.8**). To expose the posterior part of the mandible, the incision line is placed directly over the ascending ramus of the mandible. For the edentulous patient the incision line for exposure of the maxilla and the mandible is usually on the crest of the alveolar ridge (**Figs. 5.9, 5.10**).

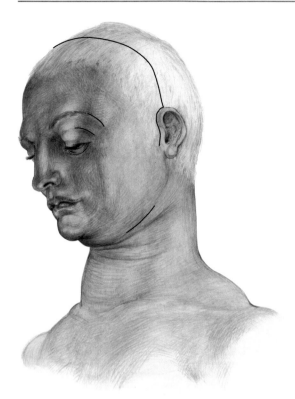

Fig. 5.5 Preferred surgical approaches to the facial skeleton (after Albrecht Dürer, *St. Apollonia*, 1521, Kupferstichkabinett, Berlin).

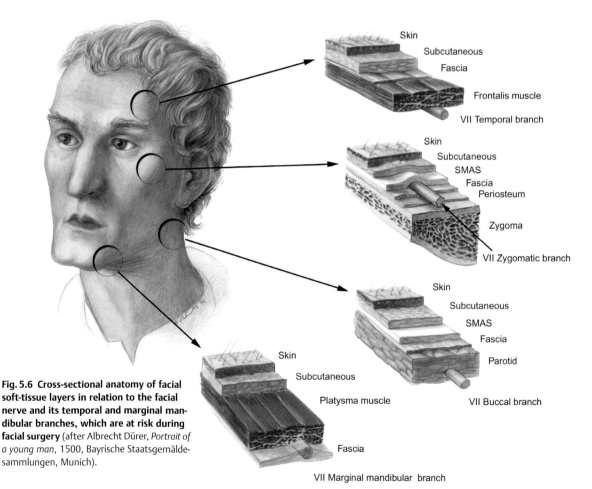

Fig. 5.6 Cross-sectional anatomy of facial soft-tissue layers in relation to the facial nerve and its temporal and marginal mandibular branches, which are at risk during facial surgery (after Albrecht Dürer, *Portrait of a young man*, 1500, Bayrische Staatsgemälde-sammlungen, Munich).

Skin
Subcutaneous
Fascia
Frontalis muscle
VII Temporal branch

Skin
Subcutaneous
SMAS
Fascia
Periosteum
Zygoma
VII Zygomatic branch

Skin
Subcutaneous
SMAS
Fascia
Parotid
VII Buccal branch

Skin
Subcutaneous
Platysma muscle
Fascia
VII Marginal mandibular branch

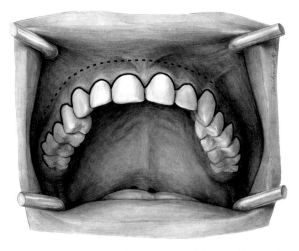

Fig. 5.7 Intraoral incision for exposure of the maxilla. Usually, this is made in the unattached mucosa 4–5 mm below the level of the attached gingiva (dashed line). Alternatively, the marginal rim incision (solid line) can be used.

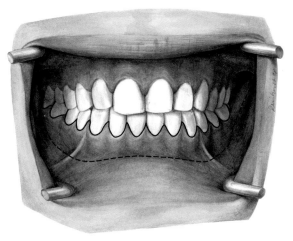

Fig. 5.8 Intraoral incision for exposure of the mandible. Details as in **Fig. 5.7**.

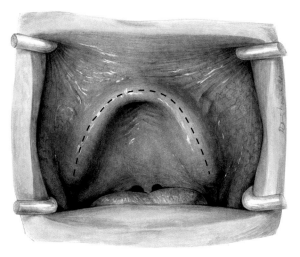

Fig. 5.9 Intraoral incision for exposure of the edentulous maxilla is made on the crest of the alveolar ridge.

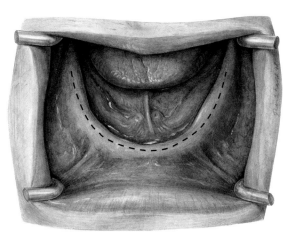

Fig. 5.10 Intraoral incision for the exposure of the edentulous mandible is made on the crest of the alveolar ridge.

Mandible

Mandible Intraoral Vestibular Approach

Depending on the fracture line, an incision is made following the oblique line and is continued forward, 4–5 mm below the attachment of the mucosa and gingiva. The incision is only carried through the mucosa. The following, second incision is made at right angles to the underlying bone and carried down through the submucosa, muscles, and periosteum (**Fig. 5.11**). Care must be taken to avoid injury to the mental nerve. The nerve has to be identified during the subperiosteal dissection. If exposure of the neurovascular bundle is necessary, an incision has to be made through the periosteum over the mental nerve (**Fig. 5.12**). After dissection of the neurovascular bundle the mandible can be exposed. The dissection must be performed inferiorly enough to allow adequate application of the fixation system. The periosteum should be handled with care and should not be elevated excessively. The extension of the incision should not be so small as to prevent wound dehiscences caused by local trauma. The wound can be closed in two layers. The first layer is usually a resorbable, horizontally running mattress suture. The second layer is closed in a simple, continuous fashion. When only one suture layer is preferred, the closure should be performed by placing the suture through mucosa, muscles, and periosteum.

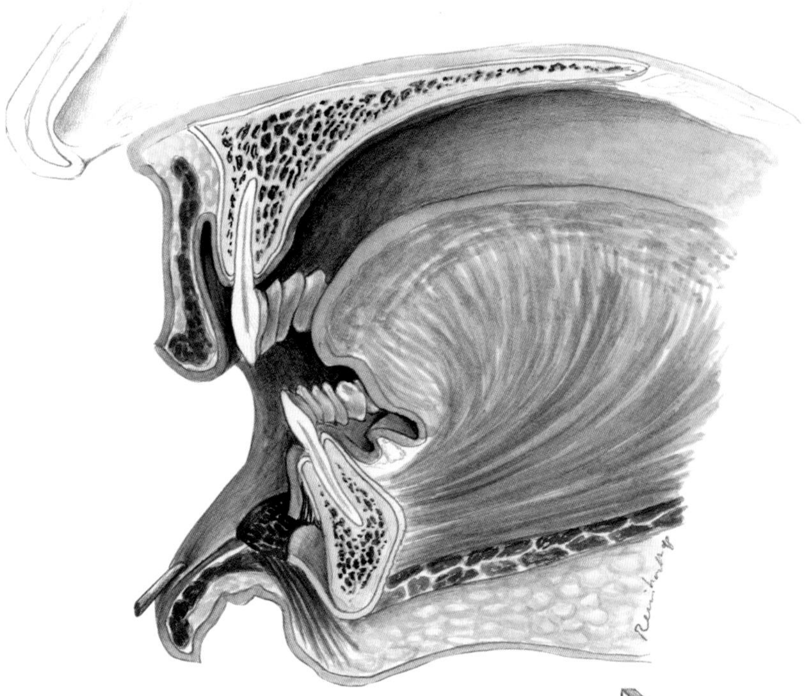

Fig. 5.11 Cross-sectional view of the vestibular approach to the mandible. Mucosa, submucosa, muscles, and periosteum are incised.

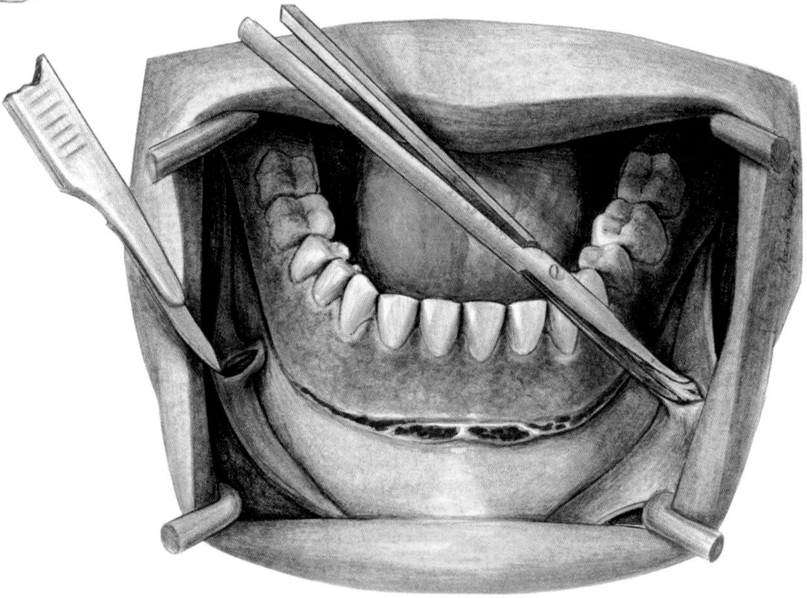

Fig. 5.12 Frontal view of the vestibular mandibular approach. Exposure of the mental nerve by an incision through the periosteum over the mental nerve and dissection of the neurovascular bundle.

Mandible Intraoral Marginal Rim Incision

For exposure of the alveolar crest or treatment of traumatized teeth, protection of lacerated mucosa is preferred. This can be achieved by using the marginal rim incision, which allows direct elevation of the underlying periosteum without involving incisions into the overlying mucosa, submucosa, muscle, and periosteal layers (**Figs. 5.13, 5.14**). Wound healing is excellent, without visible scarring

(Kreusch, Fleiner, and Steinmann, 1993; Kerscher, Soofizadeh, and Kreusch, 1995).

Mandible Combined Intraoral–Transbuccal Approach

For fixation of screws or plates at the angle of the mandible it may be necessary to expose the mandible by an intraoral–transbuccal approach. First, the mandible is ex-

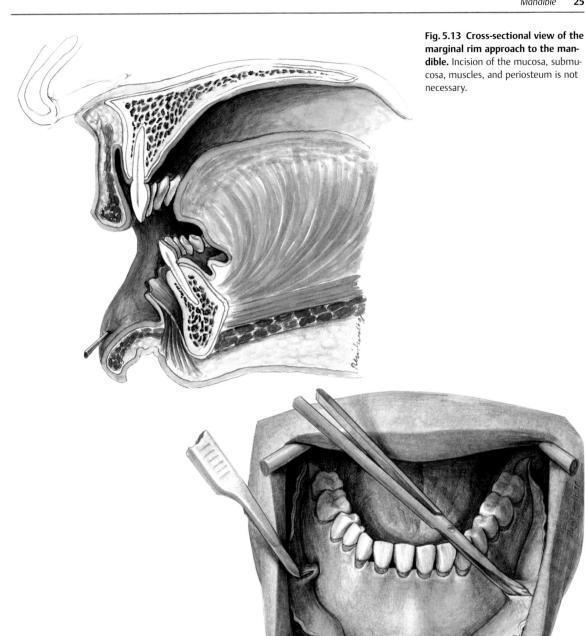

Fig. 5.13 Cross-sectional view of the marginal rim approach to the mandible. Incision of the mucosa, submucosa, muscles, and periosteum is not necessary.

Fig. 5.14 Frontal view of the marginal rim approach to the mandible.

posed by an intraoral approach. For transbuccal drilling, tapping, and screw insertion, a stab incision is made through the skin overlying the plate. The incision should follow the RSTL. Next, the transbuccal trocar is inserted and a transbuccal tunnel is established. The trocar is removed and a cheek retractor is inserted.

Mandible Extraoral Submandibular Approach

This incision should be made in a natural skin crease at a level approximately two finger widths below the inferior border of the mandible. Skin and subcutaneous tissue is incised to the level of the platysma muscle, which is incised at right angles to the muscle fibers. The dissection continues superiorly toward the inferior border of the mandible. The marginal mandibular branch of the facial nerve is closely related and must be identified immediately beneath the platysma muscle. Alternatively, the dissection can be developed through the deep cervical fascia at the level of the submandibular gland. The capsule of the gland is identified and the overlying facial vein and artery are ligated. The marginal branch of the facial nerve lies superior to these vessels and is therefore not endangered by this approach (**Figs. 5.15, 5.16**).

Eckelt (1991) developed a technique for lag-screw osteosynthesis of condylar fractures. A skin incision is made 1 cm inferior to the inferior border of the mandible and extended to the level of the platysma muscle. The facial nerve is then identified using a nerve stimulator. The masseter is incised superior to the facial nerve and reflected inferiorly, which avoids risk of damage to the facial nerve (**Figs. 5.17, 5.18**).

Wilk (1997) developed a technique for rectangular and trapezoidal plates for osteosynthesis of condylar fractures. A skin incision is made 1 cm inferior to the inferior border of the mandible and extended to the level of the platysma

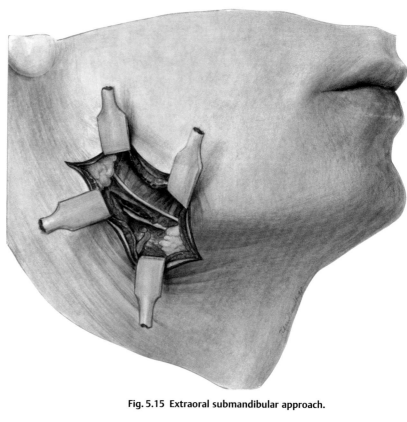

Fig. 5.15 Extraoral submandibular approach.

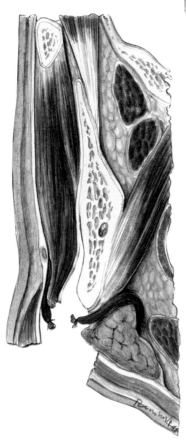

Fig. 5.16 Cross-sectional view of extraoral submandibular approach. The facial artery is ligated and turned up for preservation of the marginal branch of the facial nerve.

muscle. The facial nerve is then identified using a nerve stimulator. The masseter is incised superior to the facial nerve and reflected superiorly for exposure of the condylar fracture (**Figs. 5.19, 5.20**).

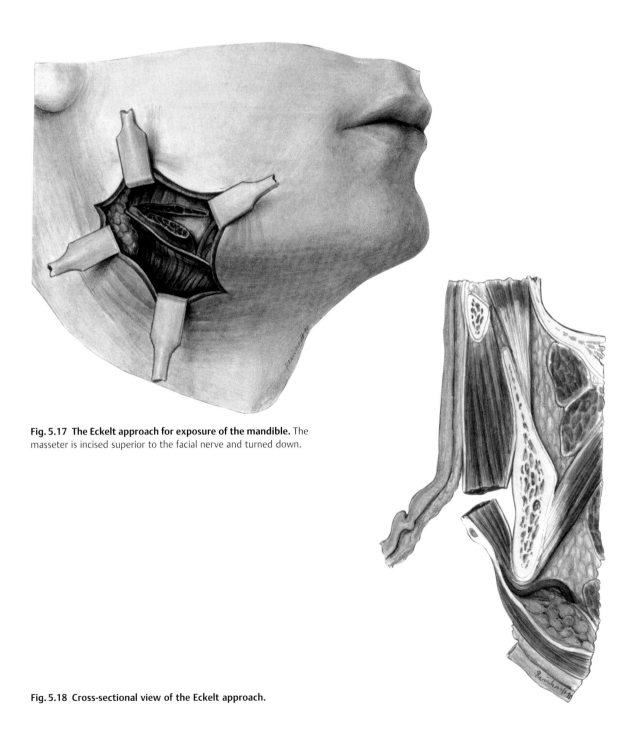

Fig. 5.17 The Eckelt approach for exposure of the mandible. The masseter is incised superior to the facial nerve and turned down.

Fig. 5.18 Cross-sectional view of the Eckelt approach.

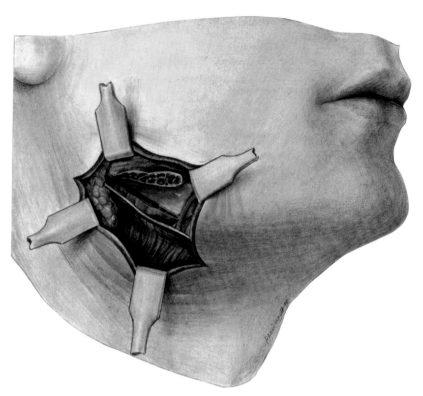

Fig. 5.19 The Wilk approach for exposure of the mandible. The masseter is incised superior to the facial nerve and turned upward.

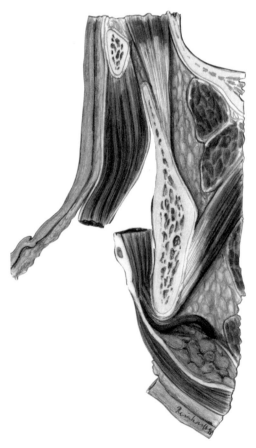

Fig. 5.20 Cross-sectional view of the Wilk approach.

Mid and Upper Face

Maxilla Intraoral Vestibular and Marginal Rim Approach

As already described for the mandible, exposure of the maxilla can be achieved by either a vestibular or marginal rim incision. In this way the lower half of the midface, including the infraorbital rim, can be exposed. A common complication of the vestibular incision is wound dehiscence. Such a dehiscence can be avoided with a marginal rim incision, which also offers enhanced healing due to the immunological defense mechanism of the periodontium (Schroeder and Page, 1977).

Lower Eyelid Approach

The lower orbital rim and orbital floor can be exposed transcutaneously through subciliary, lower eyelid, or infraorbital incisions. In the transconjunctival approach the incision is limited by the fornix. For more extensive exposure a lateral canthotomy and cantholysis are necessary. According to Bär et al. (1992), the lower eyelid incision showed the best results with a lower complication rate compared with other approaches. The lower eyelid inci-

sion is placed parallel to the ciliary margin at a level just caudal to the tarsus. The orbicularis muscle is exposed and, with blunt dissection in the direction of the muscle fibers, the orbital septum is exposed down to the infraorbital rim. After the orbital rim has been identified, an incision is made from the facial side of the rim, above the infraorbital nerve, through the periosteum. By subperiosteal dissection the orbital floor and the infraorbital rim will be exposed above the infraorbital nerve (**Fig. 5.21**). After osteosynthesis the periosteum is approximated and the skin is sutured without subcutaneous sutures.

Upper Lid Blepharoplasty Approach

The upper lid blepharoplasty approach provides excellent access to the frontozygomatic suture with good aesthetic results. This technique has been popularized by Kellmann and Marenette (1995) and Kung and Kaban (1996). The incision is placed in an upper lid skin crease extending from the mid pupil level to the lateral orbital rim. As usual in the orbital region, hemostasis is obtained with bipolar cautery and not monopolar cautery, which can damage the underlying sclera due to thermal conduction. The incision is continued on the level of the orbital septum and then directed to the frontozygomatic suture. The periosteum is incised and the fracture exposed (**Fig. 5.22**). After osteo-

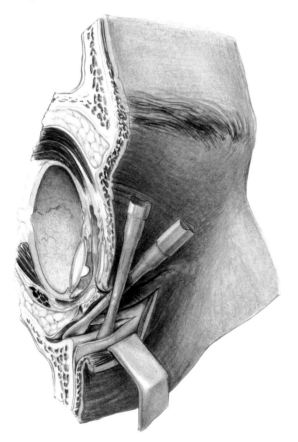

Fig. 5.21 Lower eyelid approach.

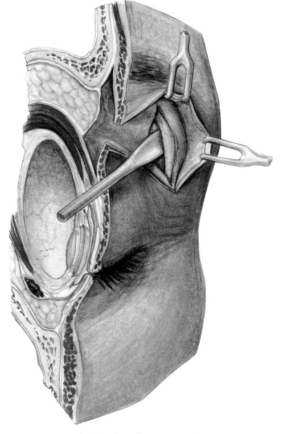

Fig. 5.22 Upper lid blepharoplasty approach.

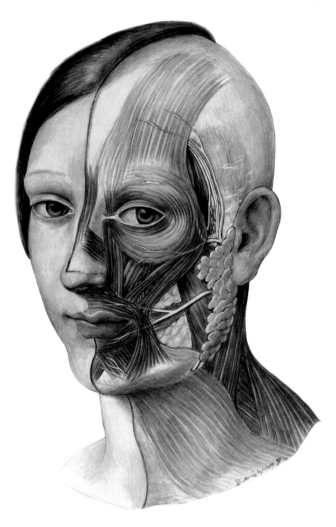

Fig. 5.23 Cross-sectional anatomy of the temporal branch of the facial nerve. Fusion of the temporal lines and position of the temporal branch of the facial nerve which passes over the zygomatic arch (Giovanni Antonio Boltraffio, *Portrait of a lady as St. Lucy*, ca. 1500, Foundation Museum Thyssen Bornemisza, Madrid).

synthesis the periosteum is approximated and the skin incision is closed using a running subcuticular or mattress suture. No subcutaneous closure is required.

Brow Approach

The brow incision for exposure of the frontozygomatic suture is the most common technique, with an extremely low complication rate. An incision is made through the skin, parallel to the hair follicles at the superior border of the lateral brow overlying the frontozygomatic suture. The muscle fibers are divided by blunt dissection down to the periosteum. The periosteum is divided by sharp dissection. After osteosynthesis the periosteum is ap-

proximated, and subcutaneous and skin sutures are performed. After surgery scars are sometimes visible and localized hair loss can occur.

Coronal Approach

The coronal approach provides excellent exposure of the cranium and upper craniofacial skeleton. Widening of the scar on the top of the head, paresthesias posterior to the incision, and weakness of the temporal branch of the facial nerve are common complications (**Fig. 5.23**). Shaving the head is not necessary if dural exposure is not required. The incision is made through the scalp, the subcutaneous tissue, and the galea until the loose layer of the scalp, between the galea and pericranium, is reached. Hemostasis can be obtained with cautery, scalp clips, or running silk locking sutures. The dissection in the layer over the pericranium down to the supraorbital rim is relatively bloodless. Care must be taken below the fusion of the temporal lines because of the temporal branch of the facial nerve which passes over the zygomatic arch. The pericranium is incised 2 cm superior to the supraorbital rim, and the dissection is continued over the bone to the supraorbital rim. When the neurovascular bundle of the frontal nerve is enclosed in a foramen, the bone bridge is excised (**Fig. 5.24**). To preserve the temporal branch of the facial nerve, the fusion of the temporal line and of the superficial and deep layers of the deep temporal fascia have to be identified (**Fig. 5.25**). If the dissection continues superficial to the fascia, the frontal branch of the facial nerve will be transected. A fat pad is seen inferior to this line of fusion. An incision in the superficial layer of the deep temporal fascia exposes the fat. The dissection continues through the fat pad and leads to the zygomatic arch.

After incision a subperiosteal detachment on the superior border of the zygomatic arch is performed. The temporal branch of the facial nerve is now retracted laterally with the periosteum of the arch and the superficial layer of the deep temporal fascia (**Fig. 5.26**). To prevent facial nerve injuries, never use sharp instruments since these may penetrate the nerve. Once the nerve has been protected the dissection can proceed in the subperiosteal layer to the lateral orbital rim. If the medial wall must be exposed, the anterior and the posterior limbus of the medial canthal ligaments and the lacrimal sac are identified. To avoid orbital hematoma, the anterior ethmoid artery should be dissected carefully, clipped, and divided.

Excessive traction over the eyes by the developed coronal flap can adversely affect the cardiac rhythm and may even cause a cardiac arrest.

If the canthal ligaments require reattachment they should be secured. Also the temporal fascia should be sutured to ensure proper soft-tissue configuration. Wound closing can be obtained with staples or suture.

Fig. 5.24 Coronal approach.

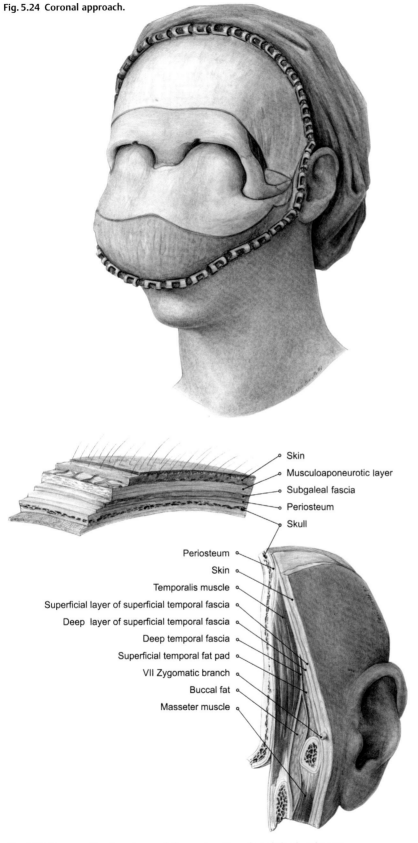

Fig. 5.26 After incision on the superior border of the zygomatic arch. The temporal branch of the facial nerve is retracted laterally with the periosteum of the arch and the superficial layer of the deep temporal fascia.

Skin
Musculoaponeurotic layer
Subgaleal fascia
Periosteum
Skull

Periosteum
Skin
Temporalis muscle
Superficial layer of superficial temporal fascia
Deep layer of superficial temporal fascia
Deep temporal fascia
Superficial temporal fat pad
VII Zygomatic branch
Buccal fat
Masseter muscle

Fig. 5.25 Cross-sectional anatomy of the zygomatic arch and the facial nerve.

6 Materials and Instrumentation

Leen M. de Zeeuw and Oliver Scheunemann

Introduction

The predominant aim of a manufacturer of osteosynthesis systems is to satisfy the aspirations of clinicians. The clinical challenges that physicians face nowadays in traumatology and reconstructive surgery require solutions that can only be achieved by innovation, extensive experience, and cutting-edge vision. Continuous dialogue and intensive collaboration between scientists and clinicians on the one hand, and the use of highly advanced manufacturing technology on the other, have always been necessary. Commercially available osteosynthesis systems exist in a variety of designs, materials, and mechanical properties (KLS Martin, Lorenz, Medartis, Medicon, Osteomed, Stryker Leibinger, Synthes, etc.)—it is the surgeon's choice which to use. Here, the different osteosynthesis systems manufactured by KLS Martin are discussed as general examples.

The Miniplate Osteosynthesis System was developed and modified by Champy and his coworkers (1975; 1976; 1977; 1978; Champy, 1983; 1986; Champy and Blez, 1992). The system based on miniplates (1 mm thickness, 2–9 mm length, **Fig. 6.1**) and miniscrews (2.0 mm diameter, 5–19 mm length, **Fig. 6.2**) was the point of origin for all today's miniplate systems. This system is made to satisfy the philosophy and aims of Champy and his colleagues, which means that the materials and instruments are manufactured to the highest standards.

Materials

Titanium and stainless steel are used in the manufacture of plates and screws of implant quality. To maintain consistently high levels of quality, all plates, screws, and instruments are subject to certificated international standards of control, with regard to both raw materials and laboratory standards. Quality is further assured by highly automated production methods. These processes guarantee the metallurgical standards for the composition, microstructure, and mechanical properties of the articles produced.

Osteosynthesis systems are basically available in two materials: titanium (pure titanium and titanium alloys) and stainless steel, both of implant standard (relevant standards are ASTM F 139/DIN 17443, ASTM F 67/ DIN 17850, and ASTM F 136/DIN 17851). Traditionally, stainless steel has been used widely as an implant material, but in maxillofacial surgery since the 1980s it has been substituted by titanium, owing to the latter's greater biocompatibility and corrosion resistance.

Osteosynthesis Technique and Equipment

The Champy Miniplate System was followed by several other osteosynthesis sets, mainly differing from each other in their screw diameter, depending on the bone pattern of application and the correspondingly necessary load-bearing abilities. Alongside the 1.0 mm and 1.5 mm micro and 2.0 mm mini systems, the 2.3 mm and 2.7 mm systems have been developed. While the micro osteosynthesis systems are mainly used in pediatric craniofacial surgery, neurosurgery, midfacial fracture management,

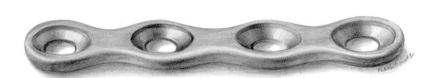

Fig. 6.1 Four-hole, 2-mm miniplate.

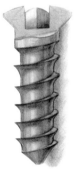

Fig. 6.2 Miniscrew, 2 mm in diameter.

orthognathic surgery as well as preprosthetic surgery, the 2.0 mm and 2.3 mm osteosynthesis systems mainly find application in all types of mandibular fracture treatment, such as primary mandibular reconstruction cases. The 2.7 mm system is suitable for primary and secondary reconstruction of the mandible.

The myriad of osteosynthesis systems available requires new storage concepts. Modularity for individual set creation and methodical color coding of sets and instrumentation to allow easy handling and assignment are as important as the development of multipurpose tools covering different functions for many osteosynthesis modules (**Fig. 6.3**). Thus it has been possible to reduce the amount of instruments required in the operating room to a reasonable and manageable number, which however is still sufficient for all-in-one osteosynthesis solutions.

The KLS Martin "Level One Fixation" modular concept (**Fig. 6.4**) has been developed to meet the requirements of osteosynthesis techniques for the craniomaxillofacial skeleton, by incorporating all the above-mentioned plate and screw systems into one integrated hardware. This system functionally addresses the following osteosynthesis indications:

- craniomaxillofacial trauma
- orthognathic surgery
- craniofacial surgery
- neurosurgery
- reconstructive surgery
- skull base surgery
- oculoplastic surgery
- guided tissue regeneration
- implantology
- preprosthetic reconstructive surgery

Screws

Screw Head Designs

Various types of screw head are available for different systems (**Fig. 6.5**). The first screw heads were based on simple cruciform or single-slot designs. To facilitate the osteosynthesis technique, self-retaining screw types like the Centre Drive and the Cross Drive have been developed by KLS Martin. The screw head is square in shape, whereas the screwdriver is slightly conical. This combination assures a secure connection between screw and screwdriver, with improved intraoperative visibility, especially when using angled screwdrivers in difficult-to-access intraoral regions. Additional self-retaining screw heads, like the star-shaped design, are also available.

Screw Thread Designs

In general, smaller screws are monocortical and self-tapping, for which careful and accurate drilling is essential. They are available in various lengths and their thread pitch may vary, depending on the outer thread diameter

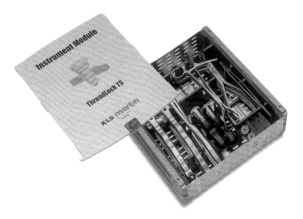

Fig. 6.3 Preconfigured, multipurpose instrument set.

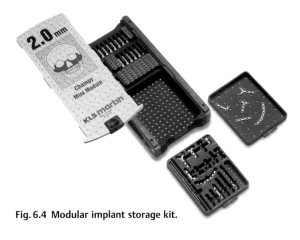

Fig. 6.4 Modular implant storage kit.

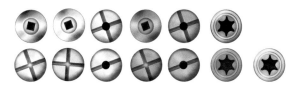

Fig. 6.5 Different screw head designs.

(**Fig. 6.6**). All these screw types require the drilling of a pilot hole, which generally corresponds to the core diameter of the screw's thread. In a further development, self-drilling screws with a different screw-tip design have been introduced (see Chapter 28) that do not require pilot holes to be drilled.

Plates

A wide selection of preshaped plates is available according to their range of application, to suit individual requirements (**Fig. 6.7**). They differ from each other in thickness, hole-to-hole distance, hole diameter, and design. Miniplates, for example, are excessively rigid in non load-

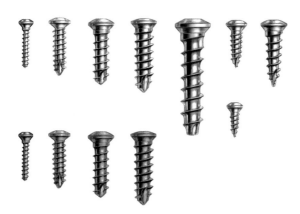

Fig. 6.6 Variety of screw types.

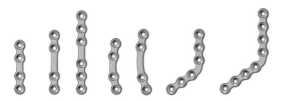

Fig. 6.7 Selection of preshaped plates.

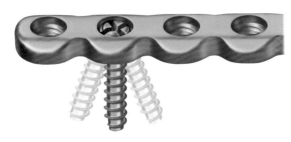

Fig. 6.8 Multidirectional locking plate system.

bearing areas with thin bones, and can be palpable through the skin where there is little interposing soft tissue. This is where micro osteosynthesis systems are applied following the aim of basic principles of general orthopedics—always to reduce the volume and quantity of any implanted material. For bridging large mandibular defects after tumor resection on the other hand, thicker and stronger reconstruction plates are used to withstand the high forces. To facilitate plate adaptation, templates are usually available for bending the plates in advance.

Locking Systems

Conventional bone plating systems achieve their stability when the head of the screw compresses the fixation plate to the bone as the screw is tightened. If plates are not precisely contoured, tight contact with the bone may lead to resorption and instability, which may be avoided by using locking plate systems. These systems achieve stability through an implant design that locks the screw to the plate while the screw shaft secures the bone. In the case of the KLS Martin ThreadLock TS System, the screw design uses the same thread and pitch throughout the entire screw. This taper screw (TS) design allows the screw to engage the bone prior to locking into the plate with the final turns (**Fig. 6.8**). In addition, the ThreadLock screws are designed to be inserted at an angle of ± 20° to the plate surface.

Currently, the locking system can be considered an inherent part of all modular osteosynthesis concepts.

7 Mandibular Fractures Including Atrophied Mandible

Hans-Dieter Pape, Klaus Louis Gerlach, and Maxime Champy

Introduction

The experimental and clinical investigations of Champy et al. (1976a, b, 1977) established the biomechanical preconditions and the surgical basis for successful miniplate osteosynthesis. The most important result of Champy's investigations was the determination of an ideal osteosynthesis line in the biomechanically favorable region at the base of the alveolar process. The strength of the plate and the diameter of the monocortical screws were adapted to the biomechanical demands of the mandible. Using these results, many companies developed osteosynthesis systems. The use of miniplate osteosynthesis in fractures of the horizontal mandible has become a generally accepted procedure. Nevertheless, the mechanical characteristics of the miniplate systems produced by different firms can vary widely.

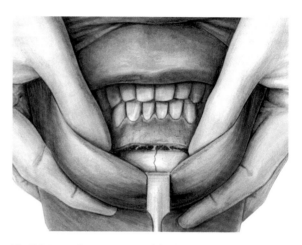

Fig. 7.1 Manual repositioning of the fracture parts.

Technique

The technical procedure is the same for all fractures of the mandible; the following points should be observed.

Time of Treatment

The treatment of all mandibular fractures should take place, if at all possible, during the first 12 hours after the accident (Champy and Lodde, 1976). There are various reasons for this recommendation, in particular the relationship between delayed treatment and increase in the rate of infection (Gerlach and Pape, 1988).

Anesthesia

Most mandibular fractures require intubation anesthesia. Our own experience showed that miniplate osteosynthesis under local anesthesia with premedication is also possible and saves staff time. The main indication for the use of local anesthesia is a simple or double fracture in the front part of the mandible or in the area of the wisdom teeth. Local anesthesia may also be favored in patients who have a poor general medical condition that is prejudicial to intubation anesthesia. Approximately 40 % of patients can be operated on using local anesthesia (Walz et al., 1996).

Re-establishment of Occlusion

The feasibility of manually repositioning dislocated mandible fragments should be checked. If correct occlusion to the upper jaw can be achieved without difficulty, intermaxillary fixation is not required. However, where problems arise, for instance in multiple fractures, preoperative splinting and intermaxillary fixation are necessary. With the help of a capable assistant, the experienced surgeon should be able to reposition many simple fractures manually (**Fig. 7.1**). An inexperienced surgeon, however, should certainly start with splinting of the upper and lower jaw by the eyelet method of intermaxillary fixation (Ivy, 1922; Obwegeser, 1952; Stout, 1942). Remember that each fractured fragment should be fixed individually to the upper jaw. A splint bridging the fracture makes correct occlusal reduction impossible.

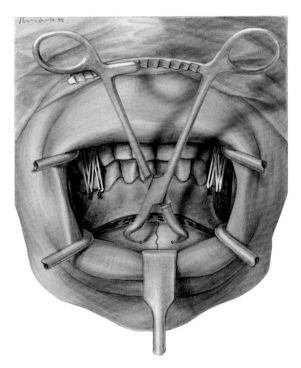

Fig. 7.2 Fractured jaw. Fixation with a bone clamp and intermaxillary fixation (for details of treatment, see **Figs. 7.15, 7.16**).

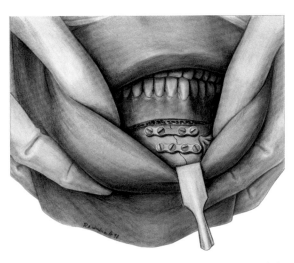

Fig. 7.3 Fractured jaw. Reposition and fixation by two four-hole plates.

Gingiva Incision

To avoid dehiscences, the rules for incisions, as described in Chapter 5 on Surgical Approaches, must be observed. The incision line should be 5 mm below the level of the attached gingiva (Champy and Lodde, 1976). Occasionally, a marginal rim incision is indicated. The length of the incision must allow free access to the fracture line and the surrounding area. If two plates are to be applied in the front area, an extension of the incision is necessary.

Miniplate Choice

The normal four-hole plate with screws of 5–7 mm diameter is preferred in most cases. Alternatively, four-hole plates with bar or six-hole plates with or without bar may be indicated for anatomical reasons (e.g., where there is involvement of the foramen mentale, danger of injury to root tips, or there are comminuted fractures).

Miniplate Osteosynthesis

After exposing the fracture line, the fragments are reduced manually. In difficult cases, a bone hook may be applied to the proximal fragment and countertraction applied simultaneously to the anterior fragment to facilitate reduction and interdigitation of the fracture ends. The use of bone clamps for the temporary immobilization of fragments simplifies the adaptation and fixation of a miniplate (**Fig. 7.2**). Following reduction, the occlusion is checked and secured by hand adaptation or through simple intermaxillary wiring. With modeling pliers and modeling lever, the osteosynthesis plate has to be precisely adapted to the outer cortical surface at the level of the osteosynthesis line. After drilling a hole, the screw is inserted and only then is the next hole drilled. After the plate has been fixed with two screws on one side of the fracture, care has to be taken before drilling the first hole in the other fragment, so that an optimal adaptation of the fragments can be achieved. Every plate must be fixed with at least two screws in each fragment. After inserting one or more screws, no attempts should be made to improve the adaptation of the plate, since this would result in the loosening of screws already inserted. Instead, the plate should be removed and adapted correctly. If a screw fails to gain a secure grip close to the fracture line, the position of the plate should be altered; alternatively, a plate with bar can be used (**Fig. 7.3**). In comminuted fractures or where there are detached triangular pieces of bone, longer plates with six or more screws should be used (see **Fig. 7.20**). The drill should, if possible, be held perpendicular to the bony surface (**Fig. 7.4**). An angulation up to 30° is allowed (Champy and Lodde, 1976), but it must be strictly monoaxial. Any change in the drilling angle during the drilling procedure results in a conical drill hole that fails to guarantee a firm grip on the screws (**Fig. 7.5**). The normal thickness of the cortical layer is 3 mm, and since the screw threads lie approximately 1 mm apart, screw fixation depends on three screw threads. A conical drill hole might reduce the grip of the screw to one or two threads. Excessive tightening of the screw produces microfractures within the drill hole (**Fig. 7.6**). When the osteosynthesis has been completed, stability and occlusion should be checked with the lower jaw in motion. After replacing the loosened soft tissue, the mucosa should be sutured, together with the periosteum.

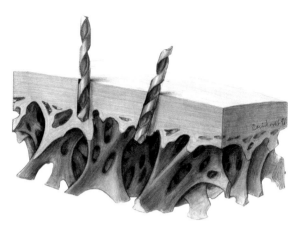

Fig. 7.4 Drill position.

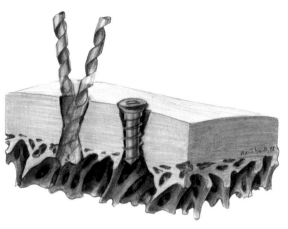

Fig. 7.5 Excentric drill.

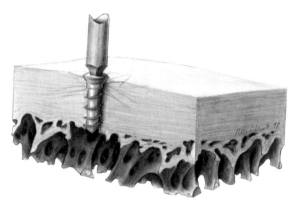

Fig. 7.6 Excessive tightening of a screw.

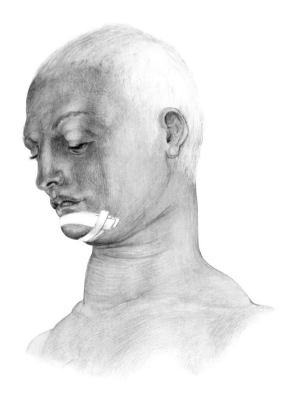

Fig. 7.7 Extraoral plaster dressing (after Albrecht Dürer, *St. Apollonia*, 1521. Kupferstichkabinett, Berlin).

To avoid a hematoma, the soft tissue of the chin should be stabilized against the chin bone with an extraoral tape dressing (**Fig. 7.7**). For the same reason, a Redon vacuum drainage or a simple piece of tubing should be used for drainage in the premolar and molar regions. Postoperative intermaxillary fixation is not required. If intraoperative splinting has been performed, this fixation can remain in place for some days. It may be helpful where the patient has difficulty in finding the correct occlusion. Immobilization also encourages soft-tissue wound-healing (Khoury and Champy, 1987).

Different Areas Require Special Measures

The Interforaminal Area

To neutralize torsion forces in the symphysis region between the mental foramina, two parallel plates should be used (Sustrac and Villebrun, 1976). The gap between them should be 4–10 mm. It is recommended that the lower plate be fixed first, then the subapical plate. Insertion of the screws should always follow the same sequence: first hole, first screw, then second hole, second screw, on one fragment (**Fig. 7.8**).

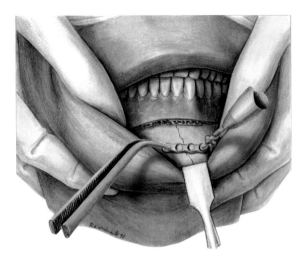

Fig. 7.8 Fracture in the symphysis region. Fixation of the lower plate first.

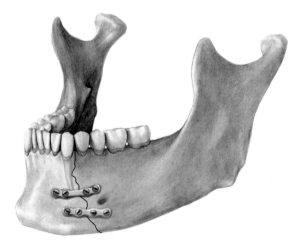

Fig. 7.9 Four-hole plate with bar for preservation of the apex of the canine.

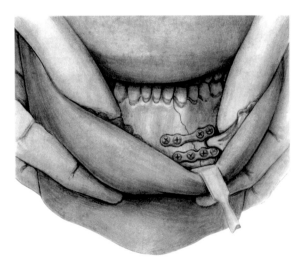

Fig. 7.10 Plate fixation above the foramen mentale. Surgical approach by means of marginal rim incision.

The Canine and Premolar Area

Fractures behind the mental foramen can be sufficiently stabilized by only one plate. In this area there are two anatomical danger points. The apex of the canine is normally long and may lie close to the osteosynthesis line. Therefore, it is necessary to make sure that the drill holes are placed beside the apex and do not damage them. If this is not possible with a simple four-hole plate, a four-hole plate with bar should be used (**Fig. 7.9**). In most cases this allows the correct positioning of the drill holes. The nervus mentalis lies below the osteosynthesis line. It emerges from the mandible between the apices of the two premolars through the foramen mentale. If care is not taken, the mental nerve may be damaged by the application of the plate. It is therefore advantageous to place the concave section of the plate between the screw holes exactly over the exit point of the nerve (**Fig. 7.10**), or to bend the plate in an edgewise direction over the exit point. With a fracture situated at the mental foramen, a second plate below the nervus mentalis can be necessary if some torsional instability is detected on checking the osteosynthesis.

The Molar Area and the Angle of the Mandible

If the mouth is small and the intraoral application of a drill and screwdriver becomes too difficult, either an angled screwdriver or the transbuccal approach can be used. After puncturing the soft tissue of the cheek, transbuccal instruments will facilitate the use of the drill and avoid injury to the cheek (**Fig. 7.11**).

In a fracture at the angle of the mandible, the plate should be located on the proximal fragment medial to the oblique line, so that it is bent over the surface and the proximal screws are placed in a nearly sagittal direction. The two screws in the distal fragment can then be fixed in a more horizontal direction (**Figs. 7.12, 7.13**). In certain cases—with simultaneous fractures of the alveolar process or when an impacted wisdom tooth is present—the plate may be fixed to the outer surface of the mandible, corresponding in position to the course of the tension line (**Fig. 7.14**).

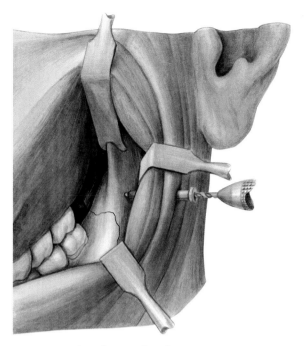

Fig. 7.11 Transbuccal approach with instruments.

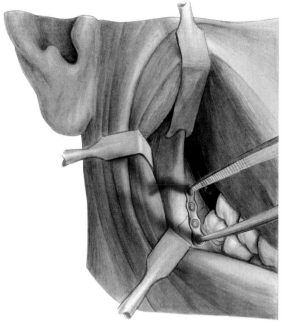

Fig. 7.12 Plate fixation at the angle of the mandible. Control of the position.

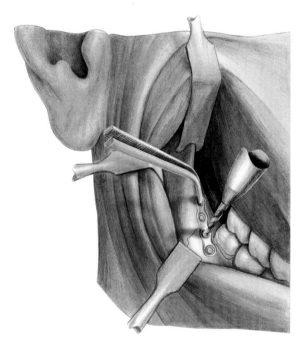

Fig. 7.13 Plate fixation at the angle of the mandible. Drilling of the first hole.

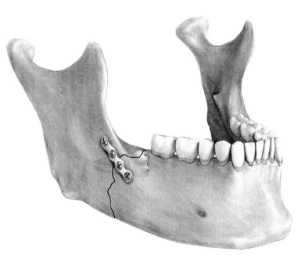

Fig. 7.14 Plate fixation at the outer surface of the mandible.

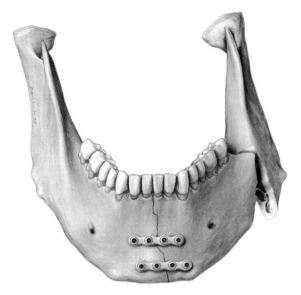

Fig. 7.15 Double fracture—first step. Fixation of the midline fracture.

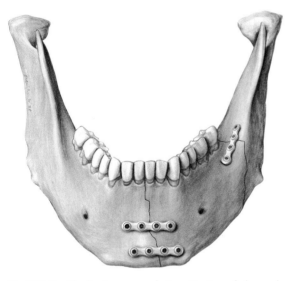

Fig. 7.16 Double fracture—second step. Fixation of the angle fracture.

The Ramus

Intraoral miniplate osteosynthesis can be recommended for use in fractures of the lower section of the ramus ascendens. For fractures below the incisura mandibula, adequate visual control of the intraorally applied plates and the correct insertion of the drill and screwdriver are possible.

In cases of fractures of the condylar neck of the mandible, lag screw or lag screw plate osteosynthesis with extraoral approach, or extraoral and intraoral miniplate

osteosynthesis as described in Chapters 11–18, should be considered.

Multiple Fractures

When there are two or more fractures of the mandibular body, the fracture lines are exposed first. Thereafter the fragments are reduced and held firmly in occlusion with intermaxillary wiring during the operation. The osteosynthesis is performed first in the tooth-bearing section of the jaw (Champy and Lodde, 1976). For example, in cases of fractures at both the midline and angle of the jaw, the midline fracture would be treated first. In this way it is easier to avoid malocclusion (**Figs. 7.15**, **7.16**).

Medicinal Therapy

A preoperative antibiotic medication is recommended on the day of the operation, either as one-shot medication 1 hour before surgery or three doses distributed over the operation day. Anti-edematous drugs are usually not prescribed. If the soft tissue is severely traumatized, intraoperative medication with 250 mg cortisone may be given and, to minimize hemorrhage, local anesthesia with adrenaline is recommended.

Postoperative Care

The patient is given soft food for approximately 7 days, following which the improving muscle activity allows a slow increase of chewing pressure. An oral hygiene regime must be observed. The sutures can be removed after 7–10 days. The miniplates should be removed under local anesthesia, usually after 2–4 months.

Special Fracture Situations

The particular anatomical conditions of a child's jaw, of the edentulous atrophied mandible of elderly patients, and of patients with comminuted jaw fractures or bone defects all call for changes in the normal miniplate treatment.

Mandible Fractures in Children

Fractures in children up to 6 years of age normally receive conservative treatment. An indication for osteosynthesis may be a simple or multiple fracture with displacement, especially when the possibilities of conservative fixation

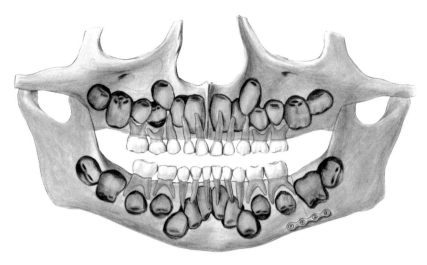

Fig. 7.17 Child up to 6 years of age. Jaw fracture in the molar region, stabilized by a microplate.

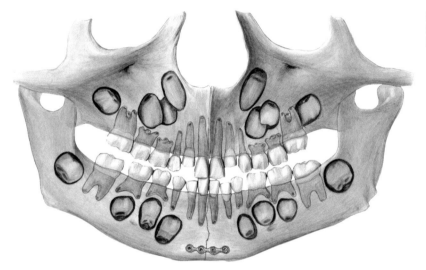

Fig. 7.18 Child 6–12 years of age. Jaw fracture in the front region, stabilized by one microplate.

are limited. In such cases two changes from the usual procedure should be made: a single microplate (1.5 mm system) is normally sufficient for the stabilization of a fracture, and because of the position of the teeth germs, the microplate should always be placed at the lower border of the buccal side (**Fig. 7.17**). Fractures of the jaw in children from 6 to 13 years of age also require that attention should be paid to the position of the teeth germs, particularly in the lateral side of the mandible. If the indication for osteosynthesis is given by dislocation or instability, a normal miniplate should be used. It should, however, as with younger children, also be placed at the lower border. The reduced chewing force in children and the much quicker healing of the bones make this shift from the tension line to the lower border possible, as pointed out by Champy and Lodde (1976) (**Fig. 7.18**). Young people between the ages of 12 and 18 years can be treated in the same way as adults—the plates are applied to the osteosynthesis line.

The Edentulous Atrophied Mandible

If the bone form is normal, fractures of the edentulous mandible are treated according to the same principles as mandibles with teeth. However, if an advanced atrophy of the mandible (< 10 mm) is evident, the tension zone shifts down toward the lower border, and the miniplate must be placed accordingly. Thus in cases of advanced atrophy the screws may endanger the nervus alveolaris inferior, particularly in the premolar region. Since the cortical bone on the occlusal side is normally thin, the miniplate may have to be fixated very close to the lower border (**Fig. 7.19**). With these patients bone is brittle and does not provide a solid grip for the screws. The use of a six-hole plate and fixation with three screws on each fragment can be recommended. As the chewing forces are reduced in edentulous atrophied jaws, there is no danger to the stability of the osteosynthesis. In cases of extreme atrophy the soft tissue is removed without the periosteum and the miniplate is fixed extraperiosteally. In this way a further re-

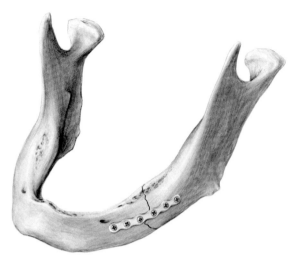

Fig. 7.19 Fracture of an edentulous mandible with advanced atrophy. Plate fixation.

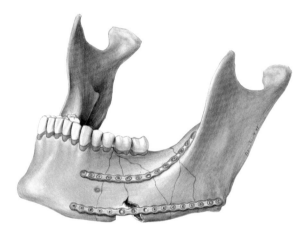

Fig. 7.20 Defect fracture with two plates in position.

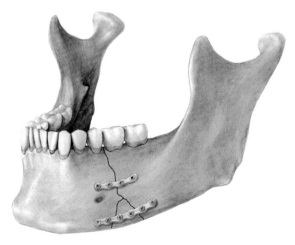

Fig. 7.21 Comminuted fractures with two plates in position.

duction of blood supply to the bone can be avoided. In cases of severe atrophy the miniplate is the most suitable osteosynthesis material; wire does not provide sufficient stability and fixation, and larger plates can lead to an even greater atrophy.

Defect and Comminuted Fractures

Where a bone fragment at the lower border is missing, the self-stabilization of the compression zone cannot function. It is therefore necessary to use two plates. One is placed in the tension zone above the missing fragment; the second plate is placed lower to bridge the defect and to stabilize the bone (**Fig. 7.20**).

Two miniplates also need to be used in comminuted fractures because multiple fragments cannot be stabilized with one plate (**Fig. 7.21**).

Teeth in the Fracture Line

The indications for extracting teeth along the fracture line, as well as the prognosis for such teeth as are retained, have been the subject of many papers. Removal of teeth along the fracture line is recommended when there is apical or marked periodontal bone loss, or when there is any sign of infection, or when teeth have been badly damaged by caries or trauma. It is also recommended that impacted wisdom teeth be removed from the fracture line, unless they can be utilized for the fixation of small-plate osteosynthesis, or their removal would cause a loss of bone from the fracture margins. In the former circumstances, the wisdom tooth should be removed together with the osteosynthesis material in a second procedure under local anesthetic 3 months after fracture reduction.

Applying these criteria, 18 (23%) of 78 line teeth were extracted as a primary measure in the cases reported on by Berg and Pape (1992). Only one of the teeth retained subsequently required extraction, so that 98% of these retained teeth were successfully salvaged. This result is comparable to that of Günther, Gundlach, and Schwipper (1983), but it is in contrast to those of Ewers, Reuter, and Stoll (1976), who subsequently extracted 14% of retained fracture line teeth, and Stoll, Niederdellmann, and Sauter (1983), who later extracted 20% of retained teeth.

Berg and Pape's findings (1992) showed that a higher proportion, 22%, of fracture line teeth became nonvital. Similar findings have been published by other researchers.

The periodontal condition of teeth retained in the fracture line is another consideration. There is no obvious reason why such teeth should show an increase in gingival pocket depth after postoperative healing is complete. Berg and Pape (1992) observed in their sample that 88% of the patients had no increase in pocket depth around such teeth when compared with the corresponding contra-lateral tooth. Hoffmeister (1985), Günther, Gundlach, and Schwipper (1983), and also other authors found no significant differences in similar studies.

Moreover, Hoffmeister (1985) reported that the horizontal mobility of retained fracture line teeth, once healing is complete, does not appear to differ from the normal physiological range for healthy teeth. Schmitz, Höltje, and Cordes (1973), and Krenkel and Grunert (1987) published

similar results. No periapical osteitis was reported by Berg and Pape (1992), Günther, Gundlach, and Schwipper (1983) or Schönberger (1956). However, Schmitz, Höltje, and Cordes (1973) and Fuhr and Setz (1963) reported periapical osteitis in 11 % and 11.7 %, respectively, of the teeth in their studies.

In conclusion, the good prognosis for retained teeth makes clear that fracture-line teeth should only be extracted when a definite indication exists.

8 Hooks for Intermaxillary Immobilization

Hendrik Terheyden

Introduction

Intermaxillary fixation is usually accomplished utilizing either interdental wiring or arch bars. This technique, however, is not possible in those patients who are either edentulous or have severe hypodontia.

Immobilization by Wiring

Immobilization can also be obtained utilizing circumzygomatic or piriform aperture suspension wires in combination with circumferential mandibular wiring to immobilize a mandibular fracture. Usually this method requires general anesthesia (Krüger, 1964).

Immobilization Using Hooks

Dal Pont (1965) described a less invasive method of achieving intermaxillary fixation with hooks that engaged the inferior mandibular border and the piriform aperture. The disadvantage of hooks is their tendency to dislocate.

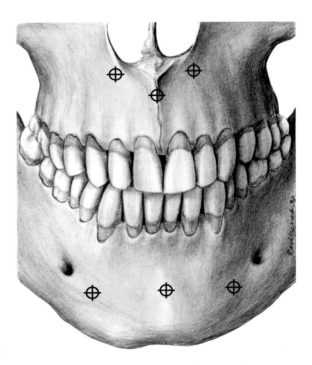

Fig. 8.1 Preferred sites for placement of miniscrew hooks.

Miniscrew Hooks

An elegant alternative is the insertion of miniscrew hooks. They are inserted subapically and bicortically into the anterior mandible, and into the anterior maxilla below the nasal spine. The procedure, originally described by Otten (1981), can be performed under local anesthesia. The regions can be exposed by small vertical incisions in the median labial frenulum. If more fixation is required, additional miniscrew hooks can be used laterally as well. With a 12-mm long miniscrew, hand-bent hooks of 1 mm steel wire can be secured (Car et al., 1986; Shetty and Niederdellmann, 1987; Ito et al., 1988; Toth-Bagi, Ujpal, and Gyenes, 1994). A second intervention under local anesthesia is required to remove the devices (**Fig. 8.1**).

Miniscrew hooks can be applied in children, after eruption of the central incisors, and in atrophic jaws in aged patients. Miniscrew hooks can be utilized in the edentulous patient and in the dentate patient as well. The insertion of an acrylic splint helps to stabilize the dentition and prevent unwanted tooth migration. In the edentulous patient dentures should be worn to maintain the vertical dimension (**Fig. 8.2**). If no dentures or splints are available, then long transmucosal miniplates can be placed in the midline (Reuter and Koper, 1985; Wolfe, Lovaas, and McCafferty, 1989) or bilaterally (Hori et al., 1992) from the nasal aperture to the anterior mandible to achieve intermaxillary immobilization (**Fig. 8.3**).

Ligatures

Transmucosal osteosynthesis screws also provide abutments for intermaxillary ligatures or elastic bands. Screws of different diameters have been recommended: 2 mm miniscrews (Arthur and Berardo, 1989; Onishi and Maruyama, 1996; Jensen, 1997); 2.7 mm screws (Busch and

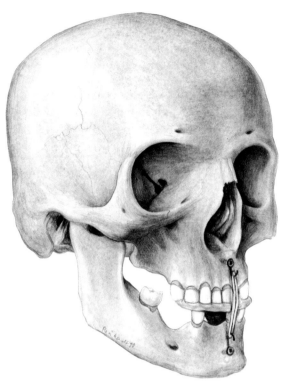

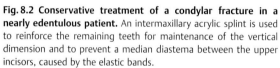

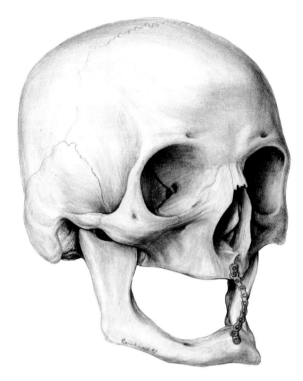

Fig. 8.2 Conservative treatment of a condylar fracture in a nearly edentulous patient. An intermaxillary acrylic splint is used to reinforce the remaining teeth for maintenance of the vertical dimension and to prevent a median diastema between the upper incisors, caused by the elastic bands.

Fig. 8.3 Intermaxillary immobilization of an edentulous mandible by a transmucosal miniplate.

Prunes, 1991; Busch, 1994; Isaacs and Sykes, 1995); and 3.5 mm screws (Win et al., 1991). A special transalveolar 2-mm screw with a capstan head was reported by Jones (1997).

9 Principles of Application of Lag Screws

Franz Haerle

Introduction

Lag screw osteosynthesis is a form of osteosynthesis in which absolute interfragmentary stability is generated by screws that transfix the fracture gap. The screw is under tension. The screw holes are prepared in such a way that when a screw is tightened, it engages the bone only in the distal fragment—not in the fragment adjacent to the screw head. With a minimum of hardware the lag screw produces interfragmentary stability directly in the center of the fracture line (**Fig. 9.1**). In contrast, plates apply stability indirectly from the external cortex by tension bending (see **Fig. 4.2**). The function of a lag screw provides mechanical rest and stability. Therefore, lag screws facilitate direct bone healing (Müller et al., 1991).

Toulouse Mini Lag Screw

The Toulouse mini lag screw is a further development within the Champy Titanium Mini Osteosynthesis System (Boutault et al., 1987, 1989). The same instruments and drills may be used for insertion (**Fig. 9.2**).

Cortical Lag Screw

To understand the concept of a lag screw it is necessary to understand the basic design of the cortical screw, which is the predominant type of screw used in the maxillofacial region (**Fig. 9.3**). Each cortical screw consists of a head and a shank; the entire length of the shank has threads and defines the screw length. Screw heads come in a variety of configurations; the popular ones have either a straight, cruciform, hexagonal, or square slot (**Fig. 9.4**). The shank has an internal diameter, also known as the core diameter, and an external diameter or thread diameter. The cortical screw can act as a lag screw only when the hole in the fragment adjacent to the screw head is over-enlarged. This is called the gliding hole. The diameter of the gliding hole is equal to or greater than the thread diameter of the screw. The diameter of the screw hole in the distal fragment is smaller than the gliding hole and corresponds to the core diameter of the screw. The hole in the distal fragment is called the traction hole (**Fig. 9.5**).

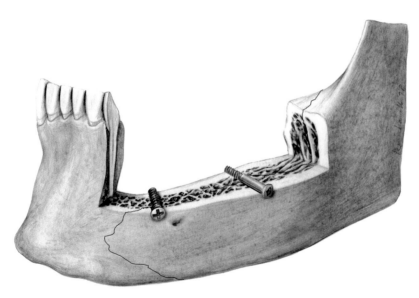

Fig. 9.1 Lag screw osteosynthesis produces interfragmentary rest and stability by interfragmentary friction due to the serration of the fragments with a minimum of hardware. Left: a cortical screw as lag screw; right: a typical lag screw.

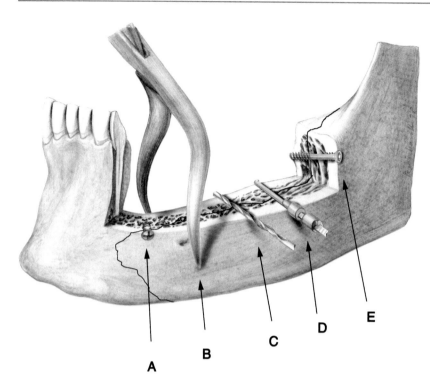

Fig. 9.2 Preparation for a Toulouse mini lag screw in mandibular fracture. (A) Toulouse mini lag screw applied to a lamellar fracture of the outer cortex. (B) Modified towel clip holds the bone fragments in reduction. (C) Bicortical drilling at the internal or core diameter of the screw. (D) Depth gauging. (E) Insertion of a screw resulting in compression of the fracture by bicortical application.

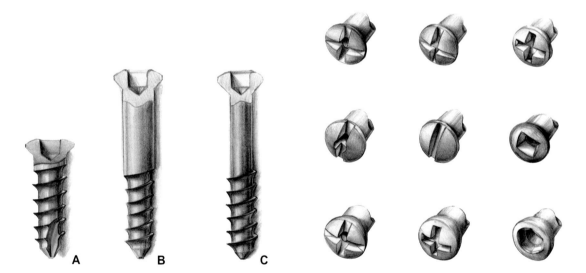

Fig. 9.3 Configuration of screws. (A) A cortical screw with a head and a shank. The entire length of the shank has threads and defines the screw length. The shank has an internal diameter, known as the core diameter, and an external or thread diameter. (B) A lag screw. Only the distal part of the screw has threads of the same diameter as the shank in the central part of the screw. (C) A special lag screw (Toulouse mini lag screw). Only the distal part of the screw has threads. The diameter of the shank in all parts of the screw is the same.

Fig. 9.4 Screw heads with a variety of configurations from different systems and companies. Top: cruciate and Phillips screw heads. Center: slotted and center drive screw heads. Bottom: special screw heads with cruciate, Phillips, and hexagonal socket heads.

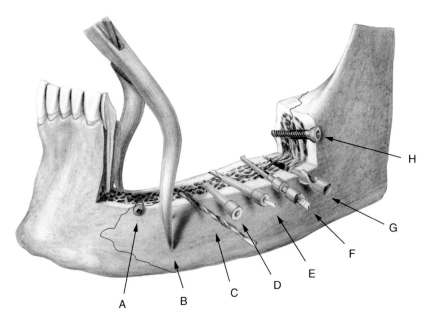

Fig. 9.5 Preparation for lag screws in mandibular fracture. (A) Lag screw applied to a lamellar fracture of the outer cortex. (B) Modified towel-clip type of bone holding forceps may be used to hold the bone fragments in reduction. (C) Drilling of a gliding hole in the outer cortex. (D) Insertion of a centering guide in the gliding hole. (E) Use of a centering guide to drill the traction hole coaxially. (F) Depth gauging. (G) Inlet countersinking in the outer cortex. With non self-tapping lag screws, tapping of the traction hole is necessary. (H) Insertion of a screw resulting in compression of the fracture by bicortical application.

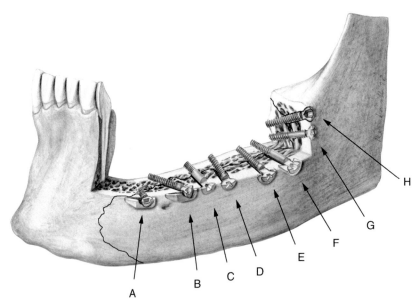

Fig. 9.6 Configuration of different types of lag screws and washers. (A) Monocortical lag screw with self-adapting spherical washer. (B) Bicortical lag screw with self-adapting spherical washer. (C) Bicortical lag screw with threads only in the distal part of the screw. (D) Bicortical lag screw with threads in the entire length. (E) Bicortical lag screw with a washer and threads in the entire length. (F) Bicortical lag screw with a biconcave washer. (G) Bicortical lag screw with a conical head. (H) Bicortical lag screw with a spherical head.

True Lag Screw

In contrast, a true lag screw has threads only at its terminal end. When used, the threads engage the distant cortex and the head sits against the proximal cortex, resulting in compression and mechanical rest (**Fig. 9.6**).

A depression or countersink corresponding to the screw head is created at the opening of the gliding hole. Screws with a spherical head provide an area of extensive surface contact of the screw head with the bone, thus avoiding stress concentration and micro fractures. Conical heads or screws with a washer used without countersinking produce a random, circular bone contact. Circular bone

contact by concave screws or spherical screws with biconcave washers (Krenkel, 1994) can produce stress concentration and local overload. This can result in a fracture of the cortical bone when tightening the lag screw and in complete failure of the osteosynthesis. All lag screws that are conical, conical with washers, spherical, spherical with biconcave countersink washers, or of concave head design can crack the thin cortex of craniofacial bones. Problems of transfer of load between the screw head and the bone are even more severe when the screw is inserted at an angle (**Fig. 9.7**). To prevent any fragmentation of bone by lag screw application, a technique has been developed that includes a self-adapting spherical washer (Terheyden, 1998). The spherical washer has a spherical hole on top,

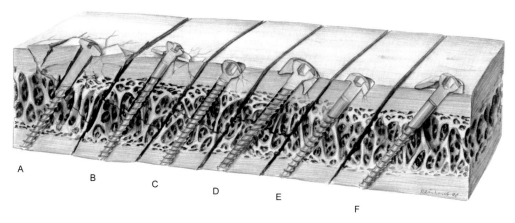

A B C D E F

Fig. 9.7 Stress concentration and microfractures produced by application of different screw heads in lag screw osteosynthesis. (A) Conical head produces maximum stress on the bone surface. (B) Conical head with a washer distributes the stress to the bone. (C) Spherical screw head with countersink puts less stress on the bone. (D) Spherical screw with biconcave washer puts even less stress on the bone. (E) Concave-shaped screw head shows a similar stress distribution effect. (F) Distribution of stress by application of spherical screw with a self-adapting spherical washer.

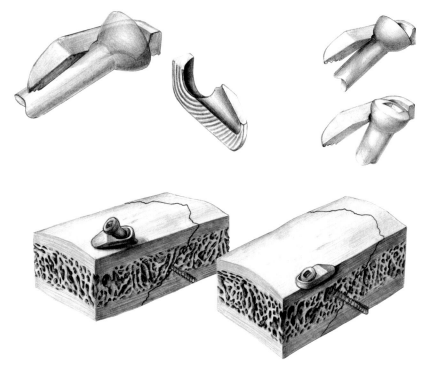

Fig. 9.8 Self-adapting spherical washer.

which corresponds to the spherical shape of the screw head. At the bottom it has an excentric slot, so that the washer automatically aligns its position with the cortical surface at any angle of the screw. In combination the screw and washer act like a spherical articulation. Countersinking of the bone is not necessary, thereby avoiding weakening it (**Fig. 9.8**).

The screws for maxillofacial applications must be remarkably strong and provide stability for early postoperative mobilization. Rotational forces on the fragments can be neutralized by the use of two or more lag screws. However, under compression there is a high interfragmentary friction because of the serrated surfaces of the fragments. In anatomical reduction, this may allow the use of a single lag screw in certain indications.

To avoid shearing forces on the fragments in mandibular fractures, the holes for lag screws should be drilled perpendicular to the fracture plane. It must be emphasized that the use of lag screws demands technical precision; however, limited exposure of the operative field

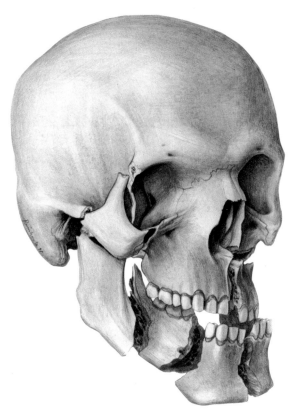

Fig. 9.9 Maxillofacial fractures.

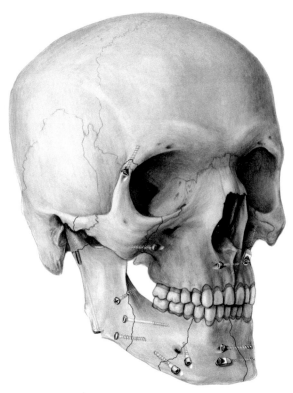

Fig. 9.10 Application of lag screws at maxillofacial fractures.

often makes it difficult to evaluate their placement. In some situations it may be necessary to perform a transcutaneous stab incision.

Position Screw

A lag screw effect can be achieved only if the screw can pass freely through the gliding hole and engage the cortex in the opposite fragment. If the diameter of the gliding hole is smaller than the screw thread diameter, the screw will engage bone in the gliding hole. In this situation, similar to that of two nuts on the same bolt, the fracture gap will remain open without any interfragmentary compression. There are certain clinical situations where this transfixation effect is desired. In such cases the screw is referred to as a "position screw." The position screw, using threaded holes in both cortices, finds application in orthognathic procedures, such as sagittal split-ramus osteotomies, where it helps to maintain spatial relationships and the position of the condyles (see **Fig. 24.7**).

Indications for Lag Screw Osteosynthesis

Lag screws have numerous applications in the mandible, but they have limited use in the midface region. With the exception of oblique fractures in the periorbital or subnasal regions, which can be reduced by lag screws, the bone elsewhere in the midface is too thin to permit placement of screws (**Figs. 9.9, 9.10**).

Simple fixation with lag screws is ideal for wide sagittal fractures, or for lamellar fractures that have a large area of interfragmentary contact and sufficient friction between the lamellae. If two, or even three, lag screws are used, shearing and bending forces can be neutralized and optimal interfragmentary contact and mechanical rest can be achieved (Niederdellmann and Shetty, 1987). A median fracture of the mandible in combination with a bilateral condylar neck fracture presents a problem of miniplate application because of the diastasis of the lingual cortical surface (**Fig. 9.11**). The fracture can be perfectly stabilized with lag screws (**Fig. 9.12**).

Short sagittal fractures may need additional stabilization by a miniplate. In comminuted fractures lag screws are used primarily to simplify the fracture situation. Several fragments can be transformed into a simple fracture

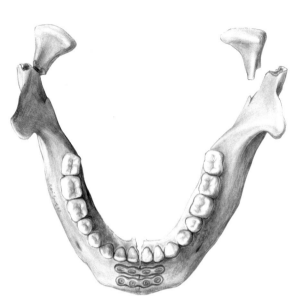

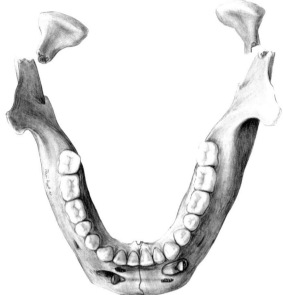

Fig. 9.11 Median fracture of the mandible in combination with bilateral condylar neck fracture treated with two miniplates in the fracture line. This has produced a diastasis of the lingual cortical surface.

Fig. 9.12 Median fracture of the mandible with bilateral condylar neck fracture perfectly stabilized by lag screws. On the inferior border it was necessary to drill a deep hole into the bone to countersink the screw head. Use of a self-adapting spherical washer on the superior border has kept the bone surface intact.

with the aid of lag screws, and additional stabilization is achieved by a plate.

Screws placed in lag fashion are also used to reduce condylar fractures, first described by Petzel (1982) and Kitayama (1989), and utilized by Eckelt (**Fig. 9.13**; see also Chapter 12) and Krenkel (**Fig. 9.14**). Lag screws are useful for fixation of inlay and onlay bone grafts. Stable fixation is obtained in various orthognathic procedures, such as genioplasties, subapical osteotomies, and sagittal split-ramus osteotomies, as well as in alveolar ridge augmentation procedures. For lamellar fractures, bone graft fixation, and small fragment fixation a lag screw can suffice.

When combined with a miniplate osteosynthesis system, the lag screw should have spherical screw heads that coincide with spherical holes in the miniplate (**Fig. 9.15**). Finally, we need a 2-mm drill for the gliding hole preparation, an inlet countersinker and a self-centering sleeve drill guide (see **Fig. 9.5**).

Lag screws can be applied in an increased range of situations by utilizing a self-adapting washer with spherical hole and eccentric slot. In a median mandibular fracture the screw load is greater. In such a situation a larger, 2.7-mm screw, with a core diameter of 2 mm, is necessary. This screw should be combined with the self-adapting spherical washer to prevent bone overload (see **Fig. 9.12**).

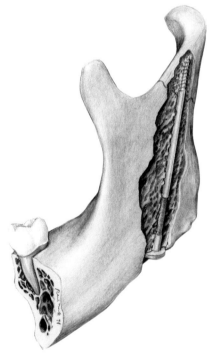

Fig. 9.13 The Eckelt technique for treatment of condylar neck fractures. (See Chapter 12 for further information.)

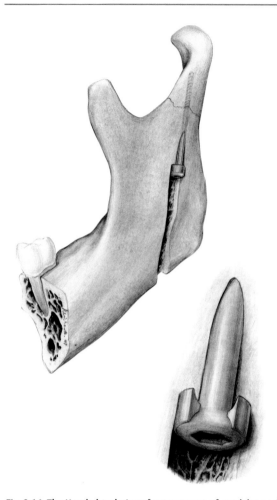

Conclusion

Any screw traversing a fracture should be inserted as a lag screw (Schwimmer, 1993).

Lag screw osteosynthesis is a very sensitive technique; any deviation from the standard lag screw procedure will affect the stability of the result.

To summarize, the advantages of the lag screw technique are:

- minimal hardware requirements
- the need for few special instruments
- possibility of application in combination with the miniplate system
- the direct central application of reduction forces
- an even distribution of forces on the fragment interface
- rotational stabilization by close interdigitation of the fracture serration
- interfragmentary mechanical rest and stability
- the best conditions for primary bone healing
- simple removal of screws

Fig. 9.14 The Krenkel technique for treatment of condylar neck fractures. (See also **Fig. 12.1**.)

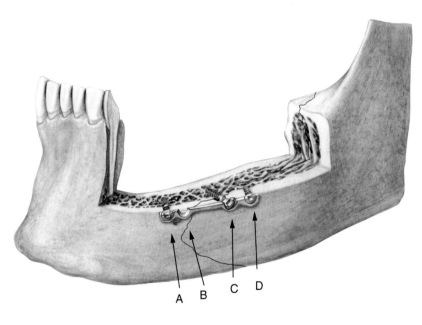

Fig. 9.15 Miniplate system with spherical screw holes and spherical plate holes. (A, D) Miniscrew positioned perpendicular to the bone surface. (B) Spherical hole in the miniplate. (C) Angulated lag screw traversing perpendicular to the fracture line.

10 Guided Lag Screw Technique in Mandibular Fractures

Gregory C. Chotkowski

Introduction

Under certain conditions the application of a lag screw can be difficult in mandibular fractures, and the direction and position of screws are not always predictable by the conventional lag screw technique. The drill guide developed for extremity traumatology (Müller, Allgöwer, and Willenegger, 1969; Müller et al., 1991) is not practicable in mandibular fractures (**Fig. 10.1**). For this reason special instruments for guidance of lag screws have been developed, to enable fractures of the mandible to be accessed and fixed through a transoral approach, by the guided lag screw technique (Chotkowski, 1997). The exceptions to a transoral approach are:

- severely atrophied mandibles
- severely comminuted fractures
- fractures of the condyle and high condylar neck

The guided lag screw technique utilizes precision instrumentation together with a specialized screw for the fixation of mandibular fractures (**Fig. 10.2**). It provides a predictable method of rigid internal fixation with minimal hardware through the use of conservative surgical access in a short operative time (Ellis and Ghali, 1991).

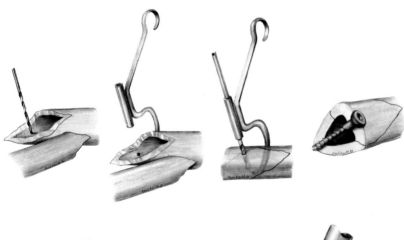

Fig. 10.1 Drill guide for lag screw technique in extremities. Application for tibia fracture.

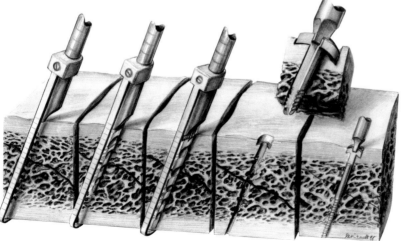

Fig. 10.2 Application of the screw and use of the drill guide. The undersurface of the head of the screw has a biconcave bevel. When the screw is tightened, it directs the compressive forces to the smooth surface of the shaft of the screw. This increases the overall frictional forces of the screw with the bone which, in turn, increase the total compressive forces across the fracture (see also **Fig. 9.7**, E).

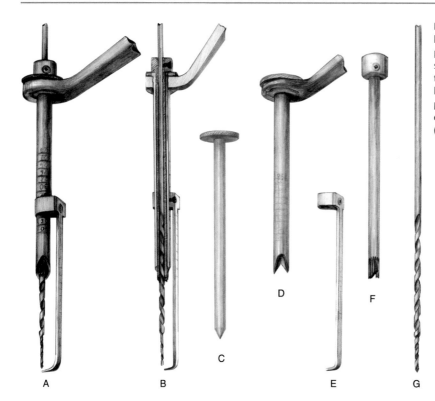

Fig. 10.3 Equipment for the guided lag screw technique. Drill guide, pointer, adjustable countersink and stepped drill bit (A), cross-section (B), trocar (C), calibrated drill guide with beveled end (D), adjustable calibrated pointer (E), adjustable biconcave beveled countersink (F), stepped drill bit (G).

The biomechanics of the mandible give the best preconditions for lag screw application (Rudderman and Mullen, 1992).

The guided lag screw technique differs from conventional lag screw techniques in that it eliminates uncertainties and reduces the number of operative steps (**Fig. 10.3**). The drill guide enables the surgeon to adjust the drill bit so that its point of exit can be predicted accurately. This ensures that anatomical structures, roots of teeth and their associated neurovascular bundles will be avoided when drilling. The pointer, which functions as an external depth gauge, runs parallel to the direction of the drill bit and measures the length so that the proper guided lag screw can be selected. Surgical time is also decreased with the use of the stepped drill bit and adjustable countersink. The stepped drill bit tapers from 2.3 mm to 1.7 mm. The countersink, gliding, and pilot holes can be prepared in one pass. This reduces the risk of misalignment of the holes, which can occur when multiple drill bits are passed.

The Surgical Technique

Stabilization of the Occlusion

The most important aspect of fracture management is to reproduce the occlusion that existed before the injury. The occlusion may be secured by using intermaxillary arch bars, Ernst ligatures, Ivy loops, or temporary intermaxillary fixation screws with interarch wires.

Surgical Approach

The recommended surgical approach is transoral. Local anesthesia, with a vasoconstrictor for hemostasis, is administered first. The incision is made in the mucobuccal fold, extending through mucosa, muscle, and periosteum, or as a marginal rim incision. The dissection is continued down to, and around, the inferior border of the mandible. Important anatomical structures are identified and protected throughout the procedure.

Reduction

The fracture is manually reduced after the fracture site has been cleaned of all debris (i.e., fractured roots, blood clots, and granulation tissue), which may interfere with the absolute reduction of the fracture. Intermaxillary fixation, applied while reducing angle fractures, may assist in maintaining this reduction. Fixation of the fracture should not be attempted until absolute reduction has been achieved. Reduction clamps may be applied to aid in reduction of the fracture (see **Fig. 7.2**).

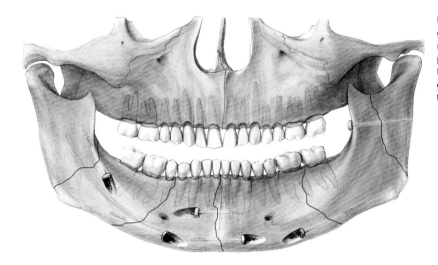

Fig. 10.4 Mandibular fractures and guided lag screw placement. Placement is shown for symphysis and parasymphysis fractures, anterior body fractures, posterior body fractures, angle fractures, and condylar neck fractures.

General Fixation Technique

Survey of the fracture. The tip of the pointer is extended 15 mm beyond the fracture and maintains contact with bone. The beveled end of the drill guide contacts the near cortex. The appropriate angle for screw placement is determined. The pointer is locked into this position (**Fig. 10.2**).

Adjustment of the drill bit. The stepped drill bit is advanced through the adjustable countersink until it is 2 mm beyond the pointer tip. The countersink is locked into this position (see **Fig. 10.3**).

Drilling. The drill guide and pointer are reapplied to the mandible. The tip and undersurface of the pointer must maintain contact with bone. The pilot hole, gliding hole, and countersink are prepared (see **Fig. 10.2**). The standard countersink is used to redefine the countersink hole.

Screw placement. The depth gauge is used to measure the guided lag screw hole preparation. The appropriate-sized screw is tightened (**Fig. 10.2**).

Wound closure. After copious irrigation the vestibular incision or the marginal rim incision is closed with a continuous resorbable suture or interdental nylon sutures.

Removal of intermaxillary fixation. The intermaxillary fixation is removed at the end of the procedure.

Specific Applications of the Guided Lag Screw Fixation Technique

Fixation of mandibular fractures using the guided lag screw technique is best explained for the area of the mandible in which the fracture has occurred (**Fig. 10.4**).

Symphysis and Parasymphysis Fractures

The guided lag screw technique is performed between the two mandibular canine teeth and the appropriate length screw is placed (**Fig. 10.5**). An additional screw—especially in sagittal fractures—is placed in the same or opposite direction, to prevent rotation about a single screw. Use of an additional screw is particularly critical with sagittal fractures (**Fig. 10.4**).

Body Fractures

Some differences in technique are required when the fractures occur around the mental foramen.

For anterior body fractures that occur around, or anterior to, the mental foramen, surgery is executed from an anterior approach (**Fig. 10.6**). No additional fixation hardware is needed, due to the angle at which the screw crosses the fracture (**Fig. 10.4**). In cases where rotation may occur around a single screw, a second screw or a four-hole monocortical 2-mm plate should be applied.

With posterior body fractures that occur anterior to the mandibular angle region, the lag screw technique is performed at the inferior border, from an anterior approach (**Fig. 10.7**). An additional four-hole monocortical 2-mm plate may be applied, but is not absolutely essential (**Fig. 10.4**).

Angle Fractures

Third molars must be removed if fractured, mobile, partially erupted, or when interfering with either fracture reduction or screw placement. The guided lag screw technique is performed superior to the neurovascular bundle (see **Fig. 10.8**). Niederdellmann et al. (1976), Shetty et al. (1995), and Weber (1997) pointed out that a solitary screw is sufficient fixation for angle fractures.

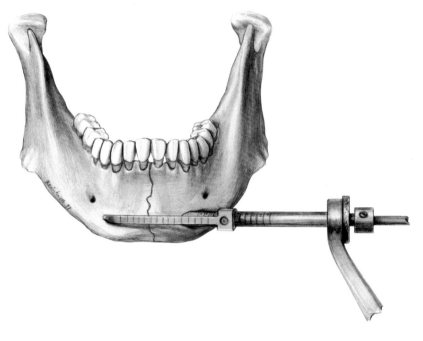

Fig. 10.5 Symphysis and para-symphysis fractures: proper placement of the drill guide and pointer. The tip of the pointer extends 15 mm beyond the fracture and is in contact with the lateral surface of the mandible. The undersurface of the pointer must maintain contact with bone during the drilling process.

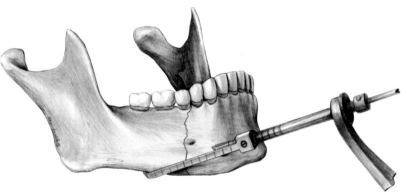

Fig. 10.6 Anterior body fractures: proper placement of the drill guide and pointer. The tip of the pointer extends 15 mm beyond the fracture and is in contact with the inferior border or lingual surface of the mandible. The pointer is angled to allow the drill to pass below the neurovascular bundle. The undersurface of the pointer must maintain contact with the lateral surface of bone during the drilling process.

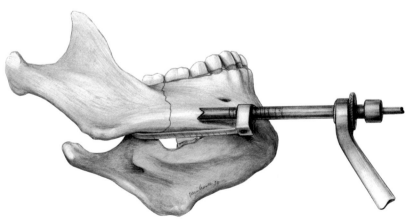

Fig. 10.7 Posterior body fractures: proper placement of the drill guide and pointer. The tip of the pointer extends 15 mm beyond the fracture and is in contact with the lingual surface of the mandible. The beveled end of the drill guide is in contact with the lateral surface or near cortex. The undersurface of the pointer maintains equal contact with the inferior border of the mandible during the drilling process. This ensures that the drill bit passes below, and avoids injury to, the neurovascular bundle (this should not be attempted in cases where there is a low-lying nerve).

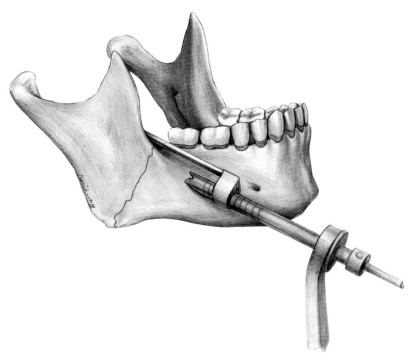

Fig. 10.8 Angle fractures. From an inferior anterior approach, the tip of the pointer extends 15 mm beyond the fracture and is in contact with the lingual surface of the ramus, anterior to the lingula. The pointer is angled on an axis that runs parallel to the course of the neurovascular bundle. This axis also runs parallel to the external oblique ridge and ascending ramus. The beveled end of the drill guide is in contact with the widest segment of the external oblique ridge, a minimum distance of 1 cm from the fracture. The undersurface of the pointer maintains equal contact with the superior border and ascending ramus. This ensures that the drill bit passes above, and avoids injury to, the neurovascular bundle (this should not be attempted in cases where there is a high-lying nerve).

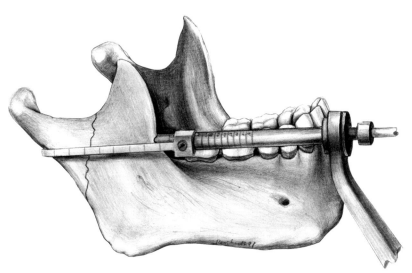

Fig. 10.9 Condylar neck fractures. From an anterior approach, the tip of the pointer contacts the posterior lateral surface of the condylar segment. The distance of the tip from the fracture is recorded using the calibration on the pointer. The stepped drill is adjusted and the hole is prepared. For optimal results, the fracture must be reduced and intermaxillary fixation applied prior to fixating.

Condylar Neck Fractures

Condylar neck fractures can be approached transorally and fixated using a lag screw if they occur low into the ramus and are not sagittal. An anterior approach is used (**Figs. 10.9**, **10.4**).

Complications

The guided lag screw technique accurately and predictably places screws, avoiding injury to important anatomical structures. However, the system has no emergency screws. In situations where the screw has lost retention, another screw or fixation device may be applied around it. Once the fracture has been secured, the loose screw is removed. In situations of unstable fractures, a period of intermaxillary fixation may be required for healing.

11 Condylar Base and Neck Fractures: What is to be Done?

Franz Haerle, Uwe Eckelt, Klaus Louis Gerlach, Guenter Lauer, Tateyuki Iizuka, Andreas Neff, Michael Rasse, Christian Krenkel, Juergen Reuther, and Christophe Meyer

As with the treatment of mandibular body fractures, the surgeon has two options for the treatment of condylar base (Loukota et al., 2005) and neck fractures: the closed and open treatments.

Conservative treatment is based on a centuries-old tradition, the first scientific publications having appeared more than 200 years ago (Desault, 1798; Malgaigne, 1847), whereas the open reduction has a relatively short history of just over than 80 years. The first report about an open reduction was published by Perthes in 1924; since then a continous development of open reduction procedures has taken place, whereas the modalities of closed treatment were largely exhausted in the mid-1930s by the introduction of functional treatment (Reichenbach, 1938). The introduction of functional treatmant affects the surgical approaches to the joint as well the techniques of reposition and osteosynthesis.

Up until the 1950s the osteosynthesis techniques were dominated by wire suturing, which is an unstable osteosynthesis technique. Subsequently, more and more reports about more rigid osteosynthesis techniques were published, for example wire suturing combined with an extraoral pin fixation (Thoma, 1954) or with an intramedullary nail (Cadenat and Cadenat, 1956). However, these treatment methods did not enable an immediate mobilization of the mandible after surgery. That was only possible after the introduction of function-stable osteosynthesis procedures for different indications, including the condylar neck, for example, by miniplate (Robinson and Yoon, 1960; Snell and Dott, 1969; Pape et al., 1980) and by lag screw (Petzel, 1980; Eckelt, 1981; Krenkel, 1992). Function-stable osteosynthesis enabled, for the first time, both basic demands of condylar neck fracture treatment to be met simultaneously, that is, the exact anatomical repositioning of the fragments and the immediate mobilization of the joint in order to restore functionality. Advancement in X-ray imaging methods like computed tomography enabled an improved preoperative evaluation of the position of the fragments, which led to a more accurate indication. Nowadays, computed tomography in addition to orthopantomography are required in diagnosis of possible temporomandibular joint fractures—even, for example, diacapitular fractures.

Indications for closed or open treatment of condylar base and neck fractures are controversial at present. There are many publications expressing quite different opinions about the issue.

For a long time, the only comparative studies were retrospective studies, with all their attendant disadvantages. However, Worsaae and Thorn (1994) in a prospective study were able to find better results for patients who had been treated with open reduction; the group receiving closed treatment particularly showed malocclusion, asymmetry of the mandible and an impaired mastication function, as well as impaired healing of the fragments, discus luxation, ankylosis, and pain.

In another prospective nonrandomized study Haug and Assael (2001) did not observe any statistical preference for either one of the two treatment techniques. However, they found out that the group who received closed treatment suffered from chronic pain to a larger extent. In a comparative study Ellis and Throckmorton (2001) detected no difference in mastication force between the two treatment techniques, but there was more malocclusion for the closed treatment (Ellis et al., 2000); they also considered open reduction to offer advantages.

In the first prospective randomized study of seven treatment centers Eckelt et al. (2006) found that the functional results, as well as the patient's subjective feelings, were significantly better after performance of the open reduction. This was based on parameters like the mouth opening, the lateral pathway and the range of protrusion as well as malocclusion. It was particularly notable that even the patient's subjective evaluation regarding pain and impairment during everyday life (assessed by Mandibular Function Impairment Questionnaire [MFIQ]; Stegenga et al., 1993) showed the advantages of open reduction.

At present, the surgeon is able to use safe operative approaches such as the oral periangular, retromandibular, preauricular, and retroauricular approaches for fracture localization of the condylar base and condylar neck, as well as for diacapitular fractures (Rasse, 1993; Neff, 2004). This enables the application of stable osteosynthesis methods like miniplate osteosynthesis, the trapezoid or delta plate, as well as the lag screw or position screw osteosynthesis, which will be described in the following chapters. Finally, the decision for open or closed treatment of dislocated and displaced fractures is one that concerns both the surgeon and the patient. Due to the availability of prospective and partly randomized studies, the patient can be informed in a preoperative consultation about the possible risks, such as facial nerve impairment after open reduction, or the disadvantage of an extraoral or intraoral scar. Moreover, surgery has to be performed under general anesthesia. Referring to closed treatment, the patient has to be informed that a longer lasting therapy including elastic immobilization will be necessary. Furthermore, the patient needs to be informed about a possibly higher risk for chronic pain and less favorable functional results in the future. In principle, it is a comparable situation to that of mandibular body fractures, having the option of closed treatment in small or undislocated fractures.

The circumstances are different for infant fractures. By today's standards, the decision to perform closed treatment is predominantly favored because of the well-known remodeling process. Closed treatment is generally the first choice for children up to 12 years of age. The indication for an open reduction is restricted to exceptional cases (Rasse et al., 1991), for example, severe dislocations, where a fragment dislocation makes it impossible to move the mandible. However, future developments also need to be monitored; possibly the decision for an open reduction in these cases may be taken more often than at present.

As a matter of principle, indications for open reduction in adults are dislocated and displaced fractures with a bending of the small fragment of more than 10° (Eckelt et al., 2006). That is particularly the case for bilateral fractures. The individual experience of the surgeon should always count when deciding on the kind of treatment to be carried out. Such osteosynthesis techniques should only be applied by skilled surgeons, who are able to perform a minimum of two surgical approaches, one for high condylar neck fractures and one for condylar base fractures.

It would even be preferable were the surgeon able to perform an intraoral approach. If these preconditions are not available at a treatment center, it should be the surgeon's free choice as to whether the patient is referred to a specialized treatment center, or whether a closed treatment is performed.

To avoid the complications of open reductions, the following preconditions should be met:
- There must be sufficient access to, and visibility of, the fracture site.
- There must be functionally stable fixation.
- Bilateral condylar fractures should be operated upon early.

12 Condylar Neck Fractures: Lag Screws

Uwe Eckelt

Introduction

The primary aim of the treatment of condylar neck fractures is the restoration of an undisturbed functionality to the temporomandibular joint. One method is lag screw osteosynthesis (see Chapter 9), which is used for achieving a stable fixation of the fragments, primary bone healing, and early mobilization to restore the functions of the joint.

Wackerbauer (1962) and Petzel (1980) first described a method of performing lag screw osteosynthesis of condylar neck fractures via a submandibular approach, using long lag screws. An intraoral lag screw method was described by Kitayama in 1989. Krenkel (Krenkel and Lixl, 1988; Krenkel, 1992) developed a method of lag screw osteosynthesis of condylar neck fractures by a submandibular approach, using a lag screw with a biconcave anchor washer to prevent microfractures (**Fig. 12.1**). Kuttner (1989) has demonstrated that lag screws with biconcave washers (anchor washers) can be turned twice as tightly as screws without washers before cracks occur in the bone. Eckelt (Eckelt and Gerber 1981; Eckelt, 1984) developed a special nut and screw for lag screw osteosynthesis of condylar neck fractures via a special surgical periangular approach (**Fig. 12.2**). This method has been especially developed to remove the osteosynthesis materials without reopening the joint region, which poses a further risk of facial nerve lesions.

Indication

Use of this technique is indicated in condylar base and neck fractures:
- with dislocation
- with significant displacement of more than 10° or contraction of the fragments by more than 2 mm or lack of bone contact in the fragments

Instruments

Special surgical instruments have been developed for secure execution of lag screw osteosynthesis. These include lag screws with diameters of 2 mm and 2.3 mm. The latter is used as an emergency screw only (**Fig. 12.3**).

The lag screws are 45–70 mm in length, in increments of 5 mm. The screws have a cortical thread of 10 mm at one end and a metric machine thread at the other. At this end is a square head which fits a special square spanner for insertion of the screws (**Fig. 12.4**). Interfragment pressure is caused by screwing a nut onto the lag screw at the mandibular base. The nut has a sleeve 6 mm long, projecting into the gliding channel, and is fitted against the base of the mandible (**Fig. 12.5**).

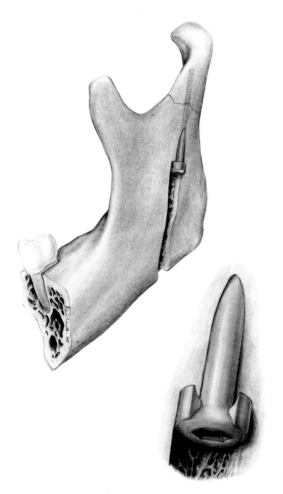

Fig. 12.1 Principle of lag screw osteosynthesis according to Krenkel, at the condylar neck of the mandible.

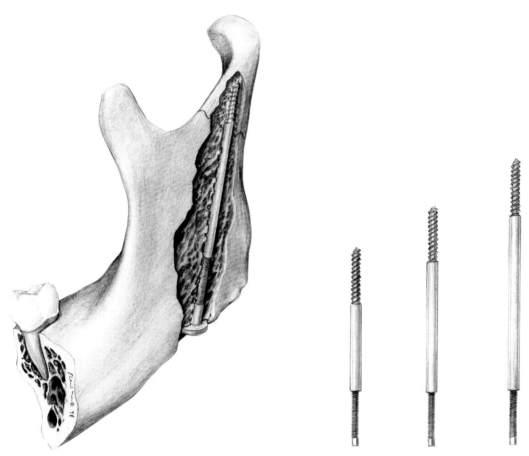

Fig. 12.2 Principle of lag screw osteosynthesis according to Eckelt, at the condylar neck of the mandible.

Fig. 12.3 Range of lag screws.

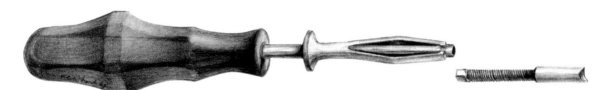

Fig. 12.4 Square spanner suitable for the lag screw.

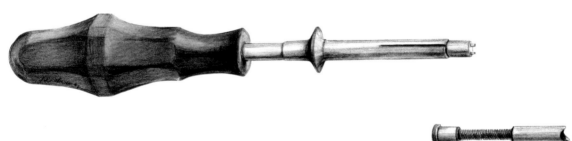

Fig. 12.5 Nut and special spanner.

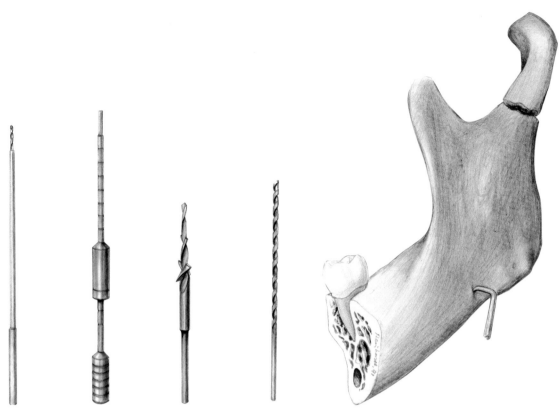

Fig. 12.6 Condylar drill, depth gauge, countersink, and twist drill.

Fig. 12.7 The mandible is pulled down with a single-forked hook to facilitate reduction of the condylar fragment.

In addition, a countersink has been developed to create a level surface at the base of the mandible, and a depth gauge for determining what length of lag screw is required.

For drilling into the condylar process, a special drill with a cutting length of only 10 mm has been developed; this ensures that drilling beyond the process does not occur. The gliding channel is created by a Lindemann drill with a length of 35 mm. To extend the gliding channel, especially at the upper part where the Lindemann drill ends in a point, twist drills of 2 mm and 2.3 mm diameter are available (**Fig. 12.6**).

Surgical Technique

For the surgical approach to the joint, a skin incision of 4 cm is made at the mandibular angle. When positioning the patient, a roll has to be placed under the shoulders so that the head is slightly inclined. This is the only way to direct the drills into the mandibular ramus without being impeded by the patients thorax.

After the skin incision on the first skin fold of the neck (1 cm below the mandibular edge), the platysma is ex-

posed to approximately 1 cm above the border of the mandible. Here, the fasciae of the masseter muscle are bluntly dissected carefully and the marginal ramus of the facial nerve is identified using a nerve stimulator. The masseter muscle is cut above the marginal ramus nerve, which is now displaced caudally to avoid its being traumatized by the retractor that will be used later to ensure good vision of the operating field (see **Figs. 5.17, 5.18**). This procedure has proved advantageous; no permanent damage of the facial nerve has been seen (Eckelt and Hlawitschka, 1999).

First step: After dividing the masseter muscle the lower part of the muscle is turned down and the edge of the mandible is exposed (the lower part of the masseter muscle is connected to the medial pterygoid muscle). A hole is drilled into the mandibular body and the ramus pulled caudally with a bone hook (**Fig. 12.7**). This makes surveying the joint area and preparing the fracture site easier.

Second step: Repositioning the condylar process is often only possible by gliding a periosteal elevator medially alongside the ramus, which relocates the condyle in the articular cavity.

With severely dislocated fractures this is often not sufficient. A repositioning forceps has been developed

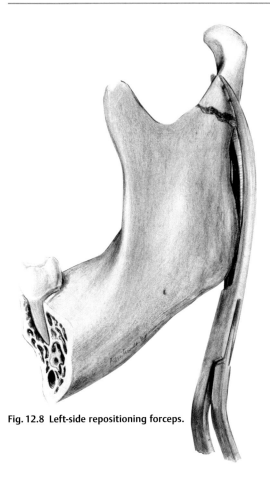

Fig. 12.8 Left-side repositioning forceps.

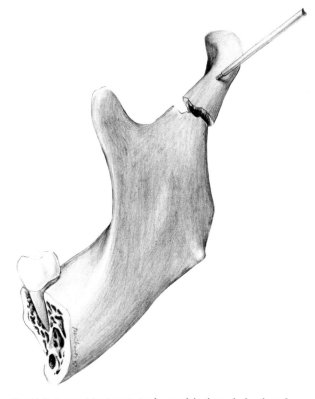

Fig. 12.9 A repositioning pin in the condyle through the skin of the cheek, placed using a trocar.

especially for the right and left side of the mandibular ramus, which allows the condylar neck to be seized and repositioned in its former situation (**Fig. 12.8**).

A third way of repositioning is to fasten a special repositioning pin in the condyle through the skin of the cheek by means of a trocar. In this way the condyle can be moved and repositioned in its former situation (**Fig. 12.9**).

Repositioning the condyle is very difficult, requiring all the skill and experience of an experienced surgeon.

Third step: After repositioning, a groove of 10–15 mm is created in the outer cortex, extending caudally from the fracture. This groove indicates the direction of the later gliding channel (**Fig. 12.10**). This "window" in the outer cortex permits a good view of the tip of the drill. It can be directly observed when drilling into the condylar head, whether the drill tends to glide medially or laterally at the fracture surface. This is especially important for oblique fractures.

Fourth step: After creating this window in the outer cortex, the direction of the gliding channel from the base of the mandible is determined by setting a mark with a round burr at the corresponding place on the mandibular base (**Fig. 12.11**).

Starting from this point, the gliding channel is made in the mandibular ramus with the Lindemann bone drill (**Fig. 12.12**). If the ramus is sufficiently wide, the Linde-

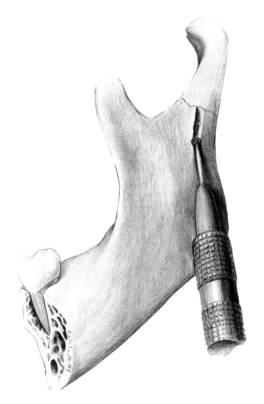

Fig. 12.10 A 10–15 mm long groove in the outer cortex, extending caudally from the fracture line, is created using a round burr.

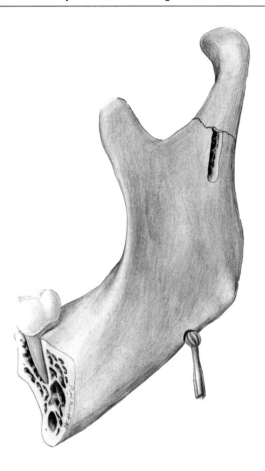

Fig. 12.11 The bone surface at the mandibular base is flattened using a round burr.

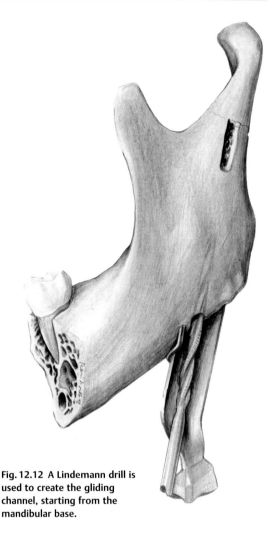

Fig. 12.12 A Lindemann drill is used to create the gliding channel, starting from the mandibular base.

mann drill glides upward, between the outer and inner cortex, and the window in the outer cortex is reached. If the ramus is extremely thin, the gliding channel may be open in some parts. Normally this does not impair stability of the osteosynthesis. If it is not stable enough the screw can be stabilized by a microplate or a miniplate osteosynthesis. Whether a lag screw is indicated or not can be estimated preoperatively by examining the preoperative CT scan (Schneider et al., 2005). Necessary adjustments to the direction of the gliding channel can be made using the Lindemann bone drill. Special retractors have been developed to protect soft tissues at the base of the mandible while drilling the gliding channel.

Execution of lag screw osteosynthesis is especially difficult where the ramus is narrow and in oblique fractures. In these cases the groove from the outer cortex into the small fragment is extended so that there is sufficient

thickness of bone in the upper part of the condyle to give a good position for drilling into the condyle (**Fig. 12.13**).

Fifth step: After the gliding channel is finished, a level base for the nut has to be created at the base of the mandible (**Fig. 12.14**).

Sixth step: Next, the 10-mm drill is bored into the condyle (**Fig. 12.15**). The "window" in the outer compact bone allows an excellent view of the fracture surface. Slippage of the drill can be immediately observed and corrected. The length of the lag screw needed is determined (**Fig. 12.16**) and the screw is then screwed into the condyle (**Fig. 12.17**). When the nut at the base of the mandible is tightened, the osteosynthesis is functionally stable (**Fig. 12.18**). The patient can move the mandible directly after surgery.

A functional treatment is indicated in all cases.

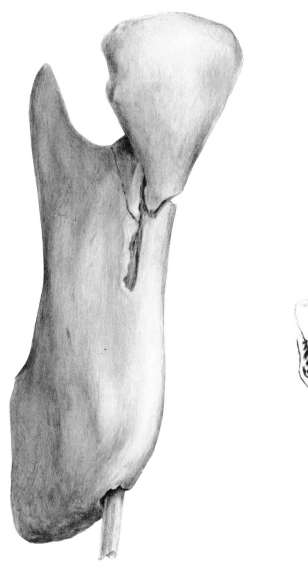

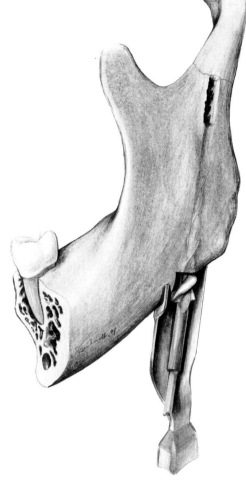

Fig. 12.13 Extension of the groove in the outer cortex of the small fragment.

Fig. 12.14 A countersink is used to create a level surface for the nut.

Removal of Osteosynthesis Material

The lag screw is removed under local anesthesia after 4–6 months by a stab incision in the old scar without exposing the joint. After the nut has been removed, the screw is extracted. Ease of removal of osteosynthesis material and less dissection of the displaced or dislocated fragment are the most important advantages of this technique over other functionally stable methods.

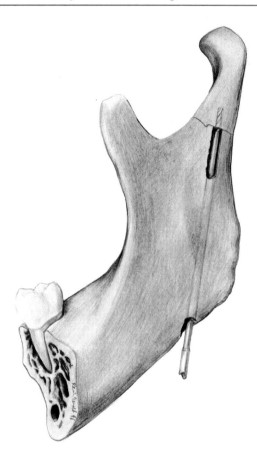

Fig. 12.15 The condyle is bored using a 10 mm drill.

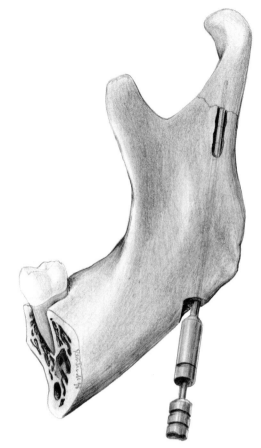

Fig. 12.16 Measuring the length of the lag screw.

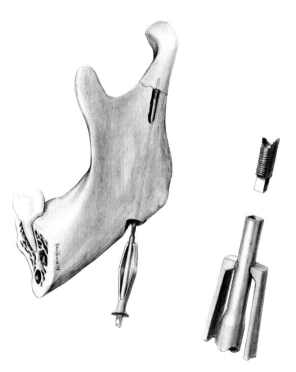

Fig. 12.17 Screwing the lag screw into the condyle.

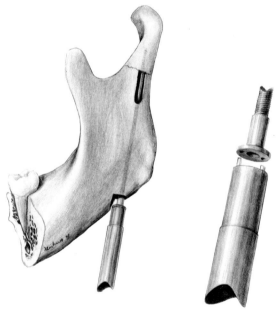

Fig. 12.18 Interfragmentary compression is created by tightening the nut at the mandibular base.

13 Condylar Neck Fracture Miniplates: Extraoral Approach

Tateyuki Iizuka and Christian Lindqvist

Introduction

Early mobilization and functional rehabilitation are considered important in the treatment of condylar neck fractures (Zide and Kent, 1983; Upton, 1991). Although indications for various treatment methods remain controversial, open reduction and internal fixation are generally required for fractures with severe displacement or dislocation (Zide, 2001). Anatomically correct repositioning and functional stabilization of such a severely displaced fracture require sufficient exposure of the fracture site, with good access and visibility through an extraoral approach. The miniplate is one of the most commonly used devices for fracture fixation.

Indication

Simple radiographic measurements (panoramic, radiograph, and Towne's view) are used to identify difficult condylar fractures. Silvennoinen et al. (1994) found that fractures with marked reduction in ramus height, irrespective of presence or absence of condylar displacement, frequently resulted in occlusal and functional disturbances (**Figs. 13.1–13.3**). Condylar displacement from the fossa is not the only deciding factor. Where the condyle is still in the fossa, reduction of more than 8 mm in ramus height is frequently associated with a therapy-resistant occlusal change. In cases in which the condyle is dislocated from the glenoid fossa, overriding is also evident. Because of condylar displacement, marked reduction of ramus height is also observed (mean 10.3 mm). Thus we consider traumatic reduction of more than 8 mm in ramus height to be an indication for surgery. In an extensive epidemiological study on different patterns of condylar fractures, Silvennoinen et al. (1992) pointed out that 15 %

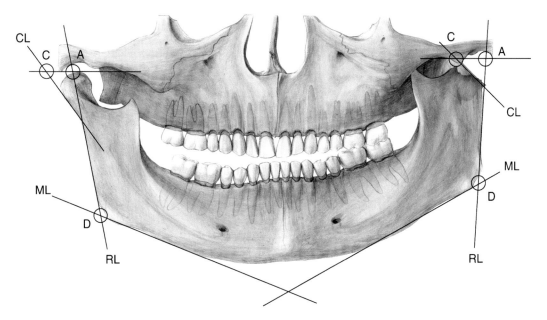

Fig. 13.1 The method of radiological measurement. Ramal height is the distance between the mandibular line (ML) and a tangent to the superior point of the condyle (CA) measured along the ramus line (RL) on the fractured and nonfractured sides (from point A to point D). Reduction of ramus height is represented by the difference in length between the fractured and nonfractured sides. The mandibular line is the tangent to the lower border of the mandible.

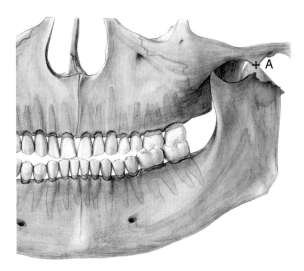

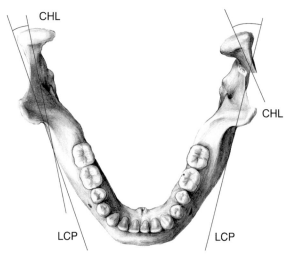

Fig. 13.2 Dislocation. The fracture is considered to be dislocated when the condyle is located in front of the lowest point of the articular eminence, or when the angulation in an oblique frontal projection (Townes view) is more than 50°.

Fig. 13.3 Measurement of fracture angle. Angulation of the fractured and nonfractured condylar processes is measured in the oblique frontal projection as the difference between a midcondylar line (CHL) and a line along the lateral cortical plate (LCP) of the mandibular ramus. Angulation of the fractured side is represented by the difference, in degrees, between the fractured and nonfractured sides.

of patients were retrospectively considered to have had an indication for open reduction.

Surgical Approaches

Two main approaches are preferred: the preauricular approach and the retromandibular approach, with the rhytidectomy (face-lift) approach as a modification (**Fig. 13.4**). The level of the fracture and the degree of displacement are the most important factors in selecting the approach. Preauricular incision is the most direct approach to high subcondylar and neck fractures. It is especially useful for fracture displacements where medial exploration is desired, with the potential for surgical manipulation of soft tissues within the joint (Chuong and Piper, 1988). On the other hand, access to the ramus fragment is often too limited to allow enough space for a miniplate. A retromandibular approach provides good access in cases of low subcondylar fractures, and more space for placing the plate and screws. Subcondylar fractures and fractures extending into the upper ramus region are best addressed using the retromandibular approach. However, reduction of the medially dislocated condyle is often difficult due to the limited access. In severe anteromedial fracture dislocations an additional vertical ramus osteotomy, followed by removal of the osteotomized segment, may be necessary (Boyne, 1989; Ellis, Reynolds and Park, 1989; Mikkonen et al., 1989). Occasionally a combination of approaches is needed, particularly in fracture dislocations

in which a preauricular approach may be necessary to retrieve the condylar segment, while fixation is performed through a retromandibular approach (Takenoshita, Ishibashi, and Oka, 1990).

Surgical Technique

The preauricular approach (Al-Kayat and Bramley, 1979) is recommended.

The Preauricular Approach

The skin incision is carried through the skin and superficial fascia to the level of the temporal fascia. This layer is dissected downward, along and posterior to the temporal vessels, until the lower end of the skin incision is reached. Then the posterior end of the zygomatic arch can be palpated easily. At a point roughly 2 cm above the zygomatic arch, the temporal fascia splits into the lateral and medial layers. The pocket formed by the division of the temporal fascia contains fatty tissue, which is visible through the thin lateral layer (**Fig. 13.5**). Starting at the root of the zygomatic arch, an incision running at 45°–60° upward and forward is made through the superficial layer of the temporal fascia. From inside this pocket, the periosteum of the zygomatic arch can be safely incised and reflected forward as one flap with the outer layer of the temporal fascia. The flap can be raised anteriorly, as far as

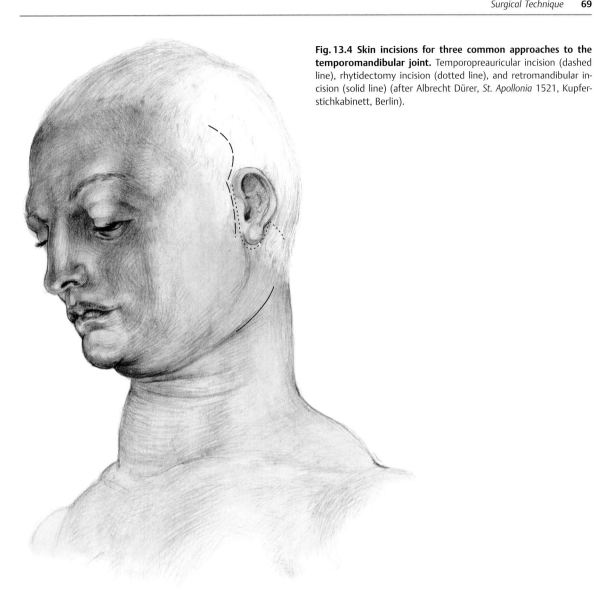

Fig. 13.4 Skin incisions for three common approaches to the temporomandibular joint. Temporopreauricular incision (dashed line), rhytidectomy incision (dotted line), and retromandibular incision (solid line) (after Albrecht Dürer, *St. Apollonia* 1521, Kupferstichkabinett, Berlin).

the posterior border of the frontal process of the zygomatic bone, and caudally, closely following the cartilaginous external auditory canal beneath the superficial temporal vessels and the glenoid lobe of the parotid gland (**Fig. 13.6**). As the temporal vessels cross under the branches of the facial nerve, the nerves are safely embedded in the flap. Until the flap is elevated, the temporal vessels are left intact as an important landmark. Proceeding downward from the lower border of the zygomatic arch and articular fossa, the tissues lateral to the joint capsule are dissected and retracted until the neck of the condyle is exposed.

The Retromandibular Approach

The retromandibular approach was first described by Ellis, Reynolds, and Park (1989).

The skin incision begins 0.5 cm below the lobe of the ear and continues inferiorly for 3–3.5 cm. It is placed just behind the posterior border of the mandible and usually does not extend inferiorly below the level of the mandibular angle. The dissection is performed through the skin, subcutaneous fat, and the platysma muscle to the parotid gland. After the parotid capsule has been entered, blunt dissection begins in an anteromedial direction toward the posterior border of the mandible. The marginal mandibular and cervical branches of the facial nerve will frequently be encountered during this dissection. The cervical nerve is of no consequence, because it usually runs

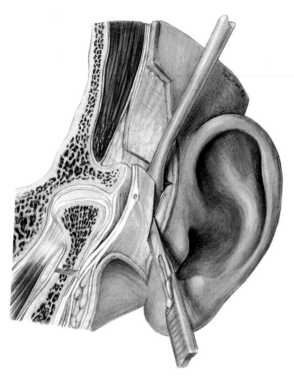

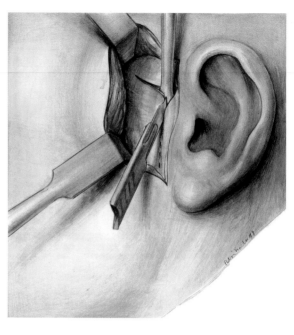

Fig. 13.5 Coronal section showing the layer of dissection. The position of the temporal branch of the facial nerve is shown during exposure of the temporomandibular joint by preauricular approach.

Fig. 13.6 Preauricular approach to the temporomandibular joint.

vertically out of the operation field. The mandibular branch must be retracted either superiorly or inferiorly, depending on its location. Once the nerve is retracted, the pterygomasseteric sling can be readily exposed at the posterior border of the mandible. The retromandibular vein runs vertically in the same plane of dissection, and is commonly exposed along its entire course. This vein rarely requires ligation. The periosteum along the posterior border of the mandible and partially around the mandibular angle is incised, from as far superiorly as is reachable, to as far inferiorly around the gonial angle as is possible (**Fig. 13.7**). The periosteum and the masseter muscle are then stripped from the ramus.

Rhytidectomy, Face-lift Approach

The incision for the rhytidectomy, face-lift approach differs from that of the retromandibular approach. It employs the more hidden cutaneous incision that was originally used for face-lifts (Zide and Kent, 1983) and was recently described by Anastassov et al. (1997) for exposing posterior mandibular fractures. The incision begins approximately 1.5–2 cm superior to the zygomatic arch, just posterior to the anterior extent of the hairline. From this point the incision curves posteriorly and inferiorly,

bending into a preauricular incision in the neutral crease anterior to the pinna. The incision continues under the lobe of the ear and posteriorly in the lobular fold, and then curves superiorly. The incision extends roughly 3 mm onto the posterior surface of the auricle. This modification prevents a noticeable scar, which occurs during contraction of the flap, from being visible in the mastoid region. Instead, the scar ends up in the crease between the auricle and the mastoid skin. When the incision is at a point where it is well hidden by the ear, it curves posteriorly toward the hairline. It then runs along the hairline—or just inside it—for a few centimeters. A skin flap is elevated with sharp and blunt dissection. The flap must be widely undermined so that a subcutaneous pocket is created that extends below the mandibular angle and a few centimeters anteriorly to the posterior border of the mandible. If one stays in the subcutaneous tissue, there are virtually no anatomical structures of any clinical significance. Once the skin has been retracted anteriorly and inferiorly, the soft tissues overlying the posterior half of the mandibular ramus will be seen (**Fig. 13.8**). From this point the dissection proceeds exactly as described for the retromandibular approach.

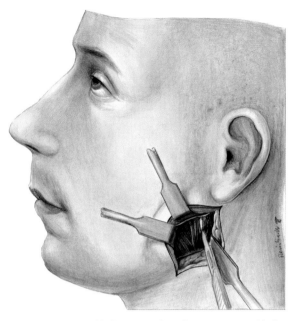

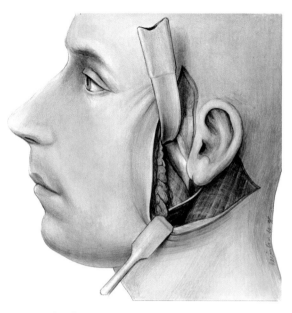

Fig. 13.7 Retromandibular approach to the temporomandibular joint (after Franco-Flamish Master, *Portrait of Wencelas of Luxembourg, Duke of Brabant*, ca. 1405–1415).

Fig. 13.8 Rhytidectomy approach to the temporomandibular joint (after Franco-Flamish Master, *Portrait of Wencelas of Luxembourg, Duke of Brabant*, ca. 1405–1415).

Osteosynthesis Technique

When the preauricular approach is used, the condylar neck is first exposed, and the condyle is localized. In case of medial displacement, the fossa is empty, and usually only the distal border of the condylar fragment, which is at an angle to the ascending ramus, is visible. Repositioning of the condyle in the fossa takes place by careful lateral traction using hooks, periosteum elevators, or both (**Fig. 13.9**). After the condyle has been repositioned, the distal end of the fragment is adapted to the stump of the ascending ramus and is maintained by rigid intermaxillary fixation (**Fig. 13.10**). Based on the results of recent biomechanical (Choi et al., 1999; Wagner et al., 2002; Asprino et al., 2006; Lauer et al., 2007) and clinical (Choi et al., 2001, 2003) studies, the fracture should ideally be stabilized using two miniplates (double miniplate technique) to achieve sufficient functional stability (**Fig. 13.11**). However, a condylar neck fracture rarely allows the application of two plates in the proximal segment. Consequently, the fracture is fixed using a single miniplate on the lateral surface. In this case, for functionally stable fixation that avoids resilient movements of the condylar fragment, at least two screws should be used on each side of the fracture. Because access below the fracture is limited with the preauricular approach, plating may involve using a transcutaneous trocar to aid in placing the most inferior screws (**Fig. 13.12**). As another alternative,

an L-shaped plate can be used, with both screw holes at the same level below the fracture line (**Fig. 13.13**).

When the retromandibular approach is used, repositioning of the condylar fragment is undertaken using a hooked clamp or forceps. Osteosynthesis is performed using a straight four-hole miniplate. To achieve more rigid stability, screws of 2 mm diameter are recommended (Ellis and Dean, 1993). Bicortical screws may also be used. If the condyle is severely displaced in the medial direction, it is often difficult to locate the fractured fragment. To obtain better access to the condyle, one option is the use of the osteotomy–osteosynthesis technique (Boyne, 1989; Ellis, Reynolds and Park, 1989; Mikkonen et al., 1989), in which a vertical osteotomy is performed from the sigmoid notch to a point 1.5 cm above the posterior border of the mandible, and then posteriorly through the posterior border. After this segment of bone has been removed, there is unlimited access to the lateral pterygoid muscle and the displaced condyle. The condyle can then be distracted into position and a plate applied. The condylar head usually remains attached to the lateral pterygoid muscle. In some cases, it may be necessary to totally remove the condyle and perform osteosynthesis extracorporeally. Rigid fixation with plates is performed between the ramus segment and condylar head. The unit is returned as a free autogenous bone graft, and the osteotomy is plated. Based on previous orthopedic studies, it has been assumed that the replanted condylar fragment can better heal to the ramus if it is rigidly stabilized (Ellis and Throckmorton, 2005).

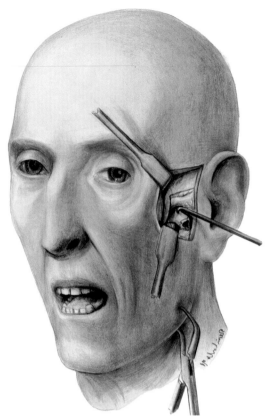

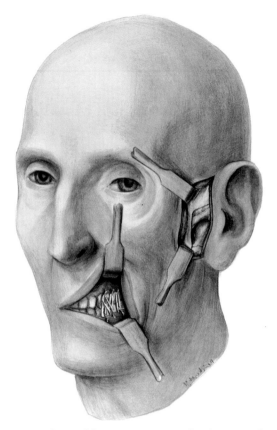

Fig. 13.9 Repositioning a medially luxated condyle through a preauricular approach. Inferior traction of the mandible is accomplished through a clamp placed percutaneously, which the assistant pulls downward (after Jacopo Tintoretto, *Portrait of a Senator*, ca. 1580, Foundation Museum Bornemisza, Madrid).

Fig. 13.10 The condyle is now repositioned and intermaxillary fixation is applied (after Jacopo Tintoretto, *Portrait of a Senator*, ca. 1580, Foundation Museum Bornemisza, Madrid).

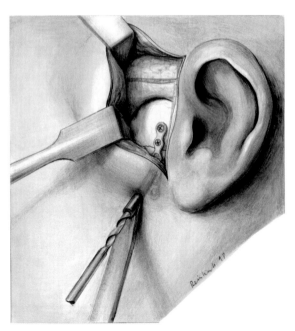

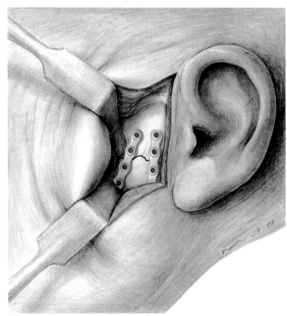

Fig. 13.11 Miniplate osteosynthesis with a six-hole plate. A transcutaneous trocar is used to facilitate the placing of the three inferior screws.

Fig. 13.12 Miniplate osteosynthesis with two miniplates.

Complications

Problems such as limited opening interfering with function, occlusal shifts, late arthritic changes, dysfunction, and deformities such as asymmetry and open bite have been previously noted. Such problems have also been noted with closed reductions (Jeter and Hackney, 1992). Hemorrhage and development of a hematoma are possible. Some patients have motor weakness of the lower lip at the immediately postoperative stage. This damage is temporary and is most likely caused by tension in the surrounding soft tissues during the surgical procedure. No damage to the facial nerve has been observed in any cases operated on via the preauricular approach. The risk of auriculotemporal syndrome in connection with a preauricular approach is low (Swanson, Laskin and Campbell, 1991). Postoperatively, partial resorption and positional changes of the condylar head are possible (Ellis, Simon, and Throckmorton, 2000; Sugiura et al., 2001). The most severe complication was described by Iizuka et al. (1991). One patient had persistent joint pain and limited mouth opening with a total condylar resorption and plate fracture after extraoral miniplate osteosynthesis, which made a subsequent arthroplasty with an autogenous costochondral graft necessary. Plate fracture is considered to be caused by an alteration of the condylar position, as a result of incorrect fracture reduction and unphysiological functional loading.

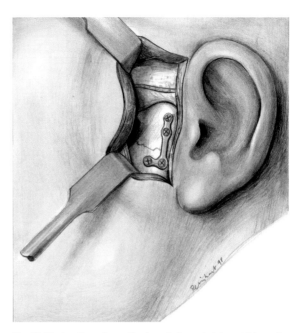

Fig. 13.13 Another alternative is an L-shaped plate, which can be applied without the use of a trocar.

14 Condylar Neck Fracture Miniplates: Intraoral Approach

Klaus Louis Gerlach and Steffen Mokros

Introduction

Surgical treatment of condylar neck fractures is indicated where the dislocated proximal fragment is in such an unusual position that purely conservative treatment does not guarantee any success.

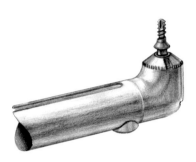

Fig. 14.1 Right-angled drilling and screwdriving instrument.

The risk of damaging the facial nerve, which exists in open reduction via an extraoral approach, is avoidable when using intraoral access. This approach was first described by Silverman (1925) and later recommended by Steinhäuser (1964). Pape, Hauenstein, and Gerlach (1980) were the first to present a larger series with miniplate osteosynthesis of condylar neck fractures after an intraoral approach. In a later follow-up, published by Horch, Gerlach, and Pape (1983), the poor results in some cases were explained by access difficulties; the approach was indicated only for low condylar fractures where the fracture line was running through the sigmoid notch. Later on, further recommendations for an intraoral approach were made by Jeter, van Sickels, and Nishioka (1988), Lachner, Clanton, and Waite (1991), Ellis and Dean (1993), Nehse and Maerker (1996), and Hochbahn et al. (1996). The difficulties previously described, involving access and control of the reduced condyle fragments, had been solved by using a right-angled drilling and screwdriving instrument (**Fig. 14.1**), and by the addition of endoscopic monitoring (Fritzemeier and Bechthold, 1993; Mokros and Erle, 1996; Gerlach, Mokros, and Erle, 1996).

Surgical Approach

The condylar neck is approached through an incision over the anterior border of the ascending ramus extending into the lower buccal sulcus. The temporalis muscle is stripped from the anterior border and the masseter is reflected laterally by subperiosteal dissection. Soft tissue reflection is enhanced by a special retractor placed at the dorsal border of the ramus. An additional notched retractor at the anterior border of the coronoid process allows good inspection of the sigmoid notch and the coronoid process (**Figs. 14.2, 14.3**). The periosteum of the proximal segment is then elevated cranially for approximately 1 cm, which is necessary to position the plate.

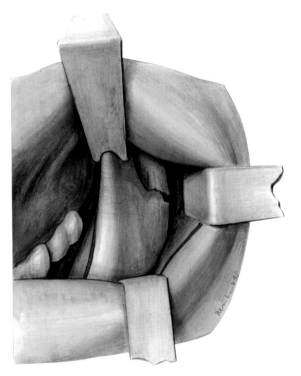

Fig. 14.2 Intraoral surgical approach to the condylar neck.

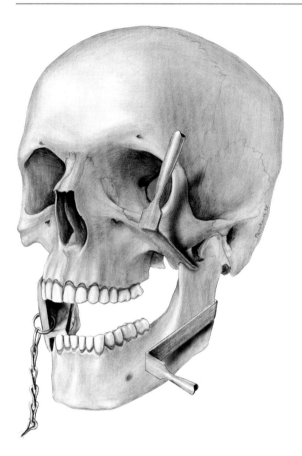

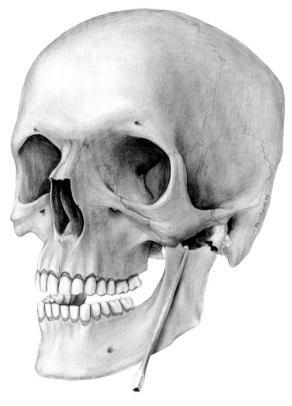

Fig. 14.3 Exposure of the condylar neck using a notched retractor at the anterior border of the coronoid process and a second retractor placed at the dorsal border of the ascending ramus.

Fig. 14.4 A sharp hook placed into the sigmoid notch allows the anterior fragment to be displaced caudally, so enabling the condyle to be repositioned.

Technique

The repositioning of the condyle fragment is aided by displacing the anterior fragment caudally using a sharp hook, which is placed either into the sigmoid notch (**Fig. 14.4**) or in a special bore hole made in the anterior aspect of the ascending ramus (**Fig. 14.5**).

A bent four-hole plate is then adapted so that it lies parallel to the dorsal border of the ascending ramus with two holes covering each fragment.

The plate is removed, the proximal fragment is moved laterally and a hole is prepared with a right-angled drilling instrument (**Fig. 14.6**).

A 5 mm screw, together with the plate, is attached to the right-angled screwdriver by the aid of a fixing clip and placed over the drill hole in the dislocated proximal fragment. For this purpose the use of center-drive screws is convenient (**Fig. 14.7**). After the first few turns of the screw, when it threads into the bone, the plate-securing fixing clip is pushed away and tightening is continued.

Following this, the second screw is inserted into the proximal fragment.

The condylar fragment is repositioned, occlusion is established by temporary intermaxillary wiring, and the reduction of the fragments checked with an endoscope. The remaining screw holes in the distal fragment are drilled, and the screws inserted and tightened (**Figs. 14.8–14.10**).

As an alternative to the use of a right-angled drilling and screwdriving system, insertion and tightening of the screws may be performed transcutaneously. For this, a trocar is inserted in the preauricular region for the instrumentation. Drilling is done via the trocar. The adapted osteosynthesis plate is transferred through a transoral incision and aligned over the drill holes; the screwdriver with the attached screws is inserted through the trocar, and the screws are tightened. It is recommended that the plate should be secured to the condyle fragment first, as previously described, and the reduction confirmed before the plate is secured to the ramus.

A perioperative antibiotic prophylactic and the use of suction drainage are also recommended.

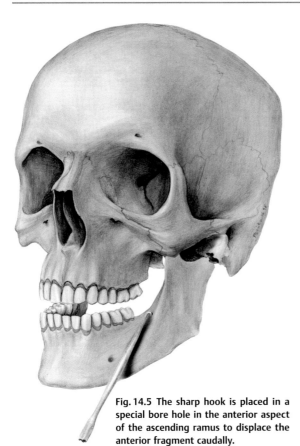

Fig. 14.5 The sharp hook is placed in a special bore hole in the anterior aspect of the ascending ramus to displace the anterior fragment caudally.

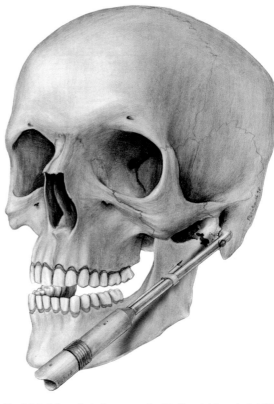

Fig. 14.6 A bore hole is prepared with the right-angled drill in the proximal fragment.

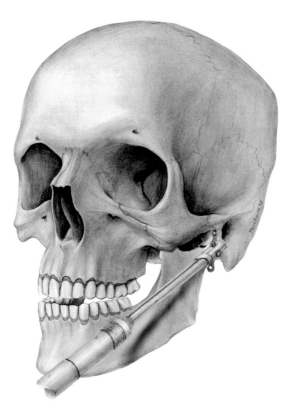

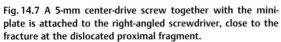

Fig. 14.7 A 5-mm center-drive screw together with the miniplate is attached to the right-angled screwdriver, close to the fracture at the dislocated proximal fragment.

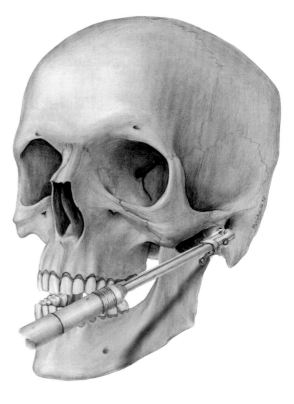

Fig. 14.8 The second screw is placed into the proximal fragment

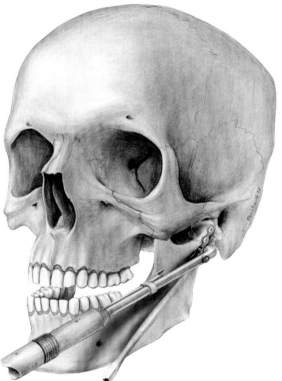

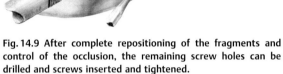

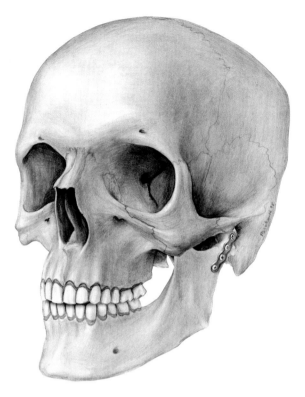

Fig. 14.9 After complete repositioning of the fragments and control of the occlusion, the remaining screw holes can be drilled and screws inserted and tightened.

Fig. 14.10 Situation after performed osteosynthesis.

Advantages of Technique

The operative repositioning and fixation of condylar fractures by miniplates via an intraoral approach is comparatively difficult because of limited access. Therefore this method is especially recommended for laterally and—with some restrictions—for medially dislocated subcondylar fractures. In the case of luxation of the condyles out of the fossa, an alternative extraoral approach is preferred.

Confirming the reduction by endoscopic examination avoids postoperative complications. Further advantages of this technique are the avoidance of visible scars and the minimized risk of damage to the facial nerve. A further advantage (Ellis and Dean, 1993) is the familiarity that surgeons have with this approach, which is used during transoral vertical ramus osteotomy.

15 Condylar Neck Fractures: Delta-Shaped Plate and Endoscopic Approach

Guenter Lauer

Introduction

Condylar fractures are frequent (Ellis et al., 1985, Silven-noinen et al., 1992), and there is growing evidence that their surgical treatment grants better results than conservative treatment (Worsaae and Thorn 1994, Eckelt et al., 2006). To minimize the risks of extraoral approaches—facial nerve damage, visible scars (Weinberg et al., 1995)—the endoscopically assisted intraoral approach has gained increasing attention.

Endoscopically assisted condyle fracture reduction and osteosynthesis was introduced into the German literature by Fritzemeier and Bechthold (1993), then Mokros and Erle (1996). In the more international, English literature Lee's group from San Francisco (Jacobovicz et al., 1998; Lee et al., 1998) were the first to describe this approach. Special devices to attach the endoscope and apply the osteosynthesis plates were developed by Lauer and Schmelzeisen (1999). Meanwhile the effectiveness of the technique has been demonstrated in several reports on a few cases as well as clinical follow-up studies (Chen et al., 1999; Kellman, 2004; Schön et al., 2005). Despite the progress in instrumentation technique and the increased popularity of this approach, open reduction with internal rigid fixation is still challenging, the reasons being:

- confined space at the condylar neck
- size and design of the osteosynthesis plate
- biomechanical stability requiring two four-hole plates and eight screws

To address and overcome these obstacles, the delta-shaped plate was designed with the gliding hole feature and four holes only. The biomechanical properties of the plate have been compared with other osteosynthesis systems in cadaver studies, and the clinical application of the plate has been tested in a recent follow-up study (Lauer et al., 2007a, b).

The endoscopically assisted surgery requires a special set of instruments. In addition, it is helpful if the surgeon has some experience in treating subcondylar fractures openly and is used to performing orthognathic surgery. Besides the delta-shaped plate and the endoscope, additional instruments have proved to be helpful for performing this type of fracture surgery (**Fig. 15.1**), namely, two different types of low-profile right-angled drill and screw-

driver, a drill guide, and a modified Schuchardt retractor with a suction and an endoscope attached.

Further, it is particularly important to gain familiarity with the technique of performing surgery while visualizing the surgical site on a TV monitor. The monitor should be positioned so that direct viewing of the surgical field and the endoscopic picture are possible without turning the head.

Particularly when starting the technique, simple fractures should be chosen. Low fractures with little displacement are ideal; for the more experienced surgeon all subcondylar and condylar neck fractures or fractures of the Spiessl and Schroll classification (Spiessl and Schroll, 1972) may be chosen. These authors differentiate six different types of fracture, of which Spiessl I–IV are approachable for repair with plates. Spiessl V and VI can be treated with screws and pins (see Chapters 17 and 18). Fresh fractures are best for surgery, when the initial swelling has settled. Delayed fracture repair makes what is already a technically demanding procedure, even more challenging.

Surgical Approach

At the start of surgery, Ivy or Ernst ligatures are applied for intermaxillary fixation in the premolar region. The condyle fracture is exposed via one major and two additional small incisions (**Fig. 15.2**), which are referred to as "ports" in minimal invasive surgery. Most of the surgery is performed via the major port, and the additional ports facilitate the instrumentation. After infiltration with local anesthetics containing a vasoconstrictor (1% lidocaine and epinephrine 1 : 400 000), an S-shaped intraoral incision 3.5 cm long is made along the anterior border of the ramus of the mandible. To create the optical cavity for the endoscope between the mandibular ramus and the masseter muscle, careful dissection and elevation of the periosteum proceeds, avoiding disruption of the muscle (**Fig. 15.3**). Thus, troublesome bleeding and collapse of shredded muscle fibers into the cavity are avoided.

Long periosteal elevators help with the wide subperiosteal undermining on the entire lateral surface of the mandible. A Langenbeck retractor is placed at the upper border pointing toward the sigmoid notch along the

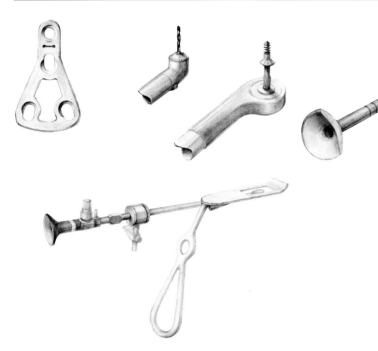

Fig. 15.1 Delta-shaped plate with gliding hole feature; two types of right-angled drilling and screwdriving tools (there is a difference in profile depth); a transbuccal drill-guide in the form of a concave, semicircular disc; and a specially modified Schuchardt retractor with a fenestration for transbuccal tool insertion and an attachment to take up a 4-mm endoscope.

upper border of the dissection cavity. A Schuchardt retractor taking the endoscope is placed with its tip around the posterior border, which helps to keep open the optical cavity. Periosteal elevation proceeds superiorly toward the fracture. Often the fracture is encountered, the end penetrating the masseter muscle or the angulated medial surface of the laterally displaced fragment. In the case of medial fragment displacement the superior edge of the distal fragment is reached without finding the proximal fragment.

This is a good time to place the transbuccal drill guide in the area of the fracture, to insert the pointy reduction forceps (pointy towel clamp) through the skin gripping the angle of the mandible, and to establish intermaxillary wiring (**Fig. 15.4**). The endoscope is placed to control fracture reduction.

Technique

To reduce the fracture or to develop the medially located proximal fragment laterally (**Fig. 15.4**), the angle of the mandible is pulled inferiorly, distracting the fracture while intermaxillary fixation is maintained via the Ivy ligatures at the premolar teeth bilaterally. This creates leeway for fragment manipulation. A muscle relaxant

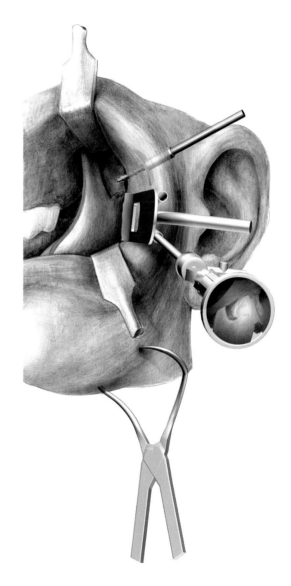

Fig. 15.2 **Intraoral surgical approach via an S-shaped incision as the major port, and meticulous subperiosteal dissection along the ramus to the condylar neck.** The endoscopically equipped Schuchardt retractor and a Langenbeck retractor are inserted. Inset: Endoscopic view of the fracture.

should be given to the patient. The bony lateral surface of the proximal fragment may then be further exposed to identify the anatomy and allow for proper reduction and fixation of the fracture.

Various techniques are used for fragment reduction. After approximate reduction by distracting the fracture and manipulating the proximal fragment, with either a freer, periosteal elevator or a scaler, holes are drilled in the proximal fragment starting with the one closest to the fracture line (**Fig. 15.5**). If the fracture is low, the low-profile angulated drill and screwdriver is used via the major port, otherwise instruments are inserted transbucally. The four-hole delta-shaped plate is placed via the intraoral port onto the lateral surface of the proximal fragment. Now the first screw closest to the fracture is inserted and driven home in the proximal fragment (**Fig. 15.6**). Then the second hole cranially is drilled and the screw inserted (**Fig. 15.7**). Once the plate is fixed to the fragment it can be used for fine-tuning of fracture reduction (**Figs. 15.8, 15.9**).

Therefore, the plate can be gripped and pulled downward by a special plate retractor (see **Fig. 15.8**). A reliable method also is to manipulate the proximal fragment via the screwdriver, which is inserted into the screw head (see **Fig. 15.8**). Thus, the proximal fragment with the plate attached can be moved in all dimensions to achieve ana-tomical alignment (see **Fig. 15.8**), while the distal fragment is manipulated via the towel clamp. Now, in particular, the alignment of the posterior border and of the lateral surface should be checked carefully via the endoscope. To enable manipulation and the control under endoscopic visualization, a special instrument was designed: a Schuchardt retractor modified by attaching the endoscope (see **Fig. 15.1**).

After achieving complete anatomical fracture reduction, the holes are drilled and screws inserted in the mandible fragment, usually with the low-profile angulated drill and screwdriver (**Fig. 15.10**).

Generally, the plates are fixed with 2.0 mm diameter screws of 5–6 mm in length. Once the screws have been placed into the bone, it might be advisable to loosen the screw a little so that the plate can be moved within the dimensions of the plate hole, for final corrections to the fragment position (**Fig. 15.11**).

The effectiveness of the delta-shaped osteosynthesis plate has been assessed in a clinical follow up study, where it showed good results. No displacements of the plate, fracture or proximal fragment occurred (Lauer et al., 2007a). Further, in cadaver studies comparing different plating systems for condylar neck fractures, the delta-shaped plate appeared to be nearly as effective as two miniplates (Lauer et al., 2007b).

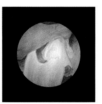

Fig. 15.3 The Langenbeck retractor along the lateral border of the ramus toward the sigmoid notch and the endoscopically modified Schuchardt retractor help to expose and visualize the condylar neck fracture and create the optical space. Inset: Endoscopic view of the fracture.

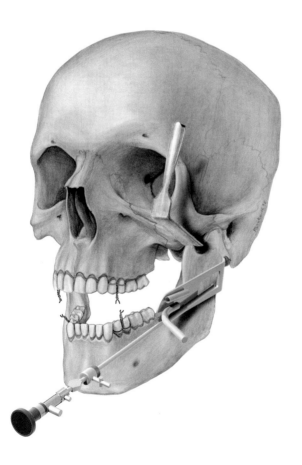

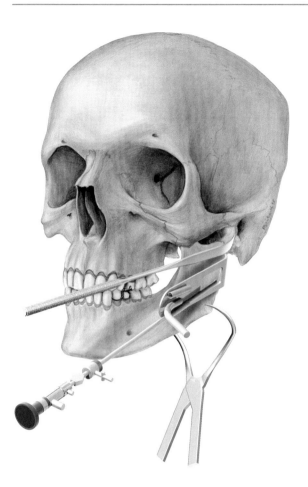

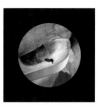

Fig. 15.4 Reduction of the fracture distracting the angle of the mandible caudally using a transcutaneously inserted towel clamp. The proximal fragment is manipulated applying a freer, scaler or a periosteal elevator. At the premolars, occlusion is fixed via Ivy ligatures or Ernst ligatures. Inset: Endoscopic control of the reduced fracture and the tip of the bent periosteal elevator.

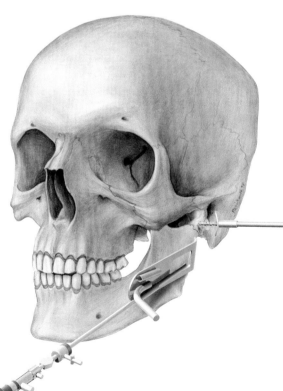

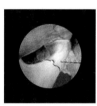

Fig. 15.5 The first hole is made in the proximal fragment close to the fracture line. For the high condylar neck fracture, drilling is via the transbuccal drill guide; otherwise the right-angled drill may be used. Inset: Endoscopically controlled transbuccal drilling.

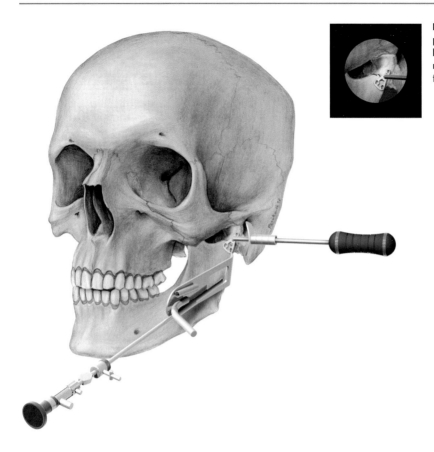

Fig. 15.6 The delta-shaped plate is placed via the transoral port at the lateral surface of the proximal fragment. Inset: Transbuccal insertion and fixation of the first screw.

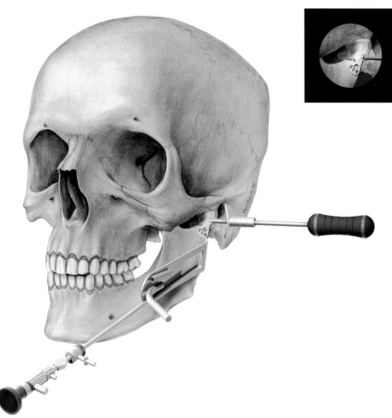

Fig. 15.7 The second hole is prepared cranially to the first screw in the proximal fragment, and the screw is inserted. Inset: Insertion of the second screw.

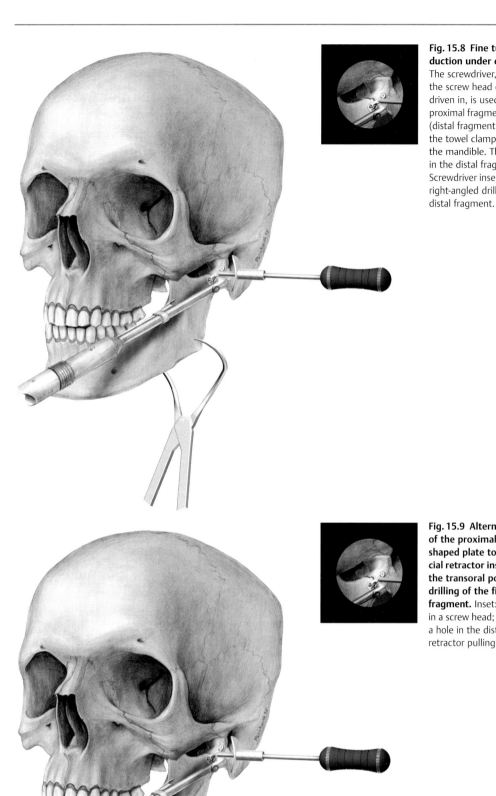

Fig. 15.8 Fine tuning of fracture reduction under endoscopic control. The screwdriver, which is pressed into the screw head of a screw already driven in, is used to manipulate the proximal fragment, while the mandible (distal fragment) is positioned using the towel clamp gripping the angle of the mandible. The first (anterior) hole in the distal fragment is drilled. Inset: Screwdriver inserted in the screw head, right-angled drilling of a hole in the distal fragment.

Fig. 15.9 Alternative manipulation of the proximal fragment and delta-shaped plate together, using a special retractor inserted in the plate via the transoral port, and right-angled drilling of the first hole in the distal fragment. Inset: Screwdriver inserted in a screw head; right-angled drilling of a hole in the distal fragment; special retractor pulling the plate.

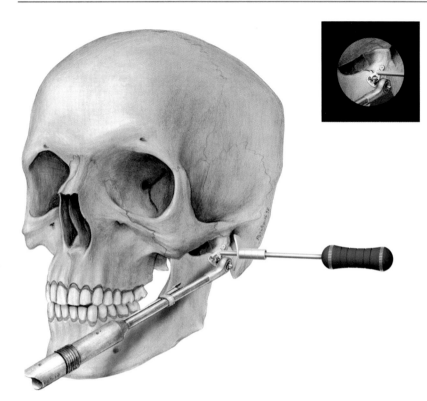

Fig. 15.10 Insertion of the first screw in the distal fragment with the low-profile, right-angled screwdriver. Drilling of the second screw hole and insertion of the screw. Inset: Low-profile screwdriver and screwdriver inserted in the proximal fragment screw head, still stabilizing the fracture.

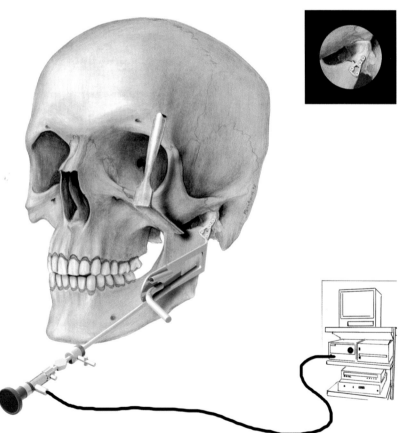

Fig. 15.11 Endoscopic control of fracture reduction and control of occlusion after performing osteosynthesis of a condyle neck fracture using the delta-shaped plate. Inset: Control of fracture alignment at the posterior border.

16   Condylar Neck Fractures: Lag Screw Plates

Juergen Reuther

Introduction

Reliable fixation and sufficient fragment stability cannot always be achieved with lag screws and plates (Petzel, 1982; Hidding, Wolf and Pingel, 1992; Krenkel, 1994; Ziccardi, Schneider, and Kummer, 1997), due to the aforementioned variations in bone thickness in the ascending ramus. To address this problem a combination of lag screws and miniplate rigid fixation using special instruments has been developed. The advantages of the technique are highlighted here.

The gliding hole in the lag screw plate allows the screw to be moved to ensure better interfragmentary compression. The plate is secured at a distance of 5–8 mm from the fracture line, at the posterior border of the ramus. The guide sleeve at the upper end of the lag screw plate has an angle of inclination of 10° to the bone surface. The lag screw is inserted through this guide sleeve into the small fragment, thus securing it to the larger fragment.

Technique

In slightly displaced condylar neck fractures the large fragment is exposed by an extraoral approach. It is slightly contoured from a buccal direction with a bone burr and then milled with a diamond-coated grooved cutter, with the groove pointing to the center of the small fragment and parallel to the posterior border of the ramus (**Fig. 16.1**). The plate is pre-fixed in the milled recess with a fixation screw in the middle portion of the gliding hole. The distance of the plate from the fracture gap is determined by the thickness of the condylar neck and by the 10° angle of inclination of the guide sleeve. As a rule, this distance is 5–8 mm, which presupposes a condylar neck thickness of approximately 5 mm in the area of the fracture. Then the condylar neck fracture is reduced. The medulla of the small fragment is pre-drilled with a twist drill through the guide sleeve in the plate (**Fig. 16.2**) and the lag screw is tightened. Often, the screw can be placed and tightened without pre-drilling. If the thread strips, a longer lag screw can be used. After the fragment has been

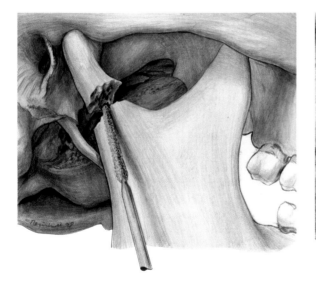

Fig. 16.1 The large fragment is slightly contoured from a buccal direction with a bone burr and then milled with a diamond-coated grooved cutter, with the groove pointing to the center of the small fragment and parallel to the posterior border of the ramus.

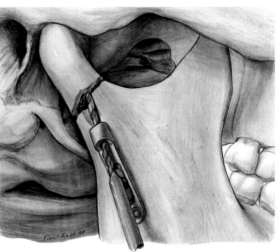

Fig. 16.2 The plate is pre-fixed in the milled recess with a fixation screw in the middle portion of the gliding hole. Then the condylar neck is reduced. The spongy space of the small fragment is slightly pre-drilled with a twist drill through the guide sleeve in the plate, and a screw inserted.

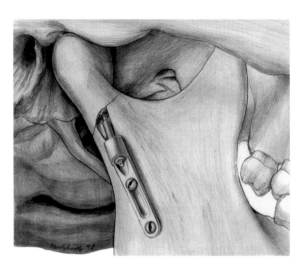

Fig. 16.3 Fixation is performed by tightening the bone screws in the gliding hole and in the fixation hole of the plate.

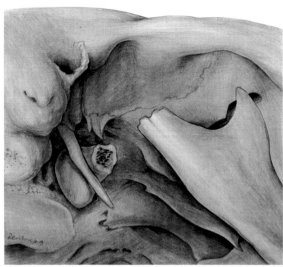

Fig. 16.4 In a severely displaced condylar neck fracture, the large fragment is exposed; it is centered, milled, and pre-drilled.

reduced satisfactorily, final fixation is performed by tightening the bone screws in the gliding hole and in the posterior fixation hole of the plate (**Fig. 16.3**). If the lag screw cannot be sufficiently secured in the small fragment, then the system can only be used for fragment positioning and immobilization has to be achieved with intermaxillary fixation.

In severely displaced condylar neck fractures the large fragment has to be exposed by an extraoral approach and it is centered, milled, and pre-drilled, as described before (**Fig. 16.4**). Then the lag screw is inserted into the center of the displaced fragment if possible (it is already connected with the plate through the guide sleeve) with a minimum of two turns (**Fig. 16.5**). Utilizing the lever action, the condylar neck is carefully pulled back into the mandibular fossa (**Fig. 16.6**). When the lag screw is placed in the recess

that has been milled in the bone, the small fragment should be in its correct anatomical position. The plate is then pre-fixed in the middle of the gliding hole with a bone screw and, by pulling the plate close, adaptation is achieved between the condyle and large fragment (**Fig. 16.7**). The plate is finally secured by tightening the first bone screw in the gliding hole and with a second bone screw in the posterior fixation hole (**Fig. 16.8**). Slightly varying the direction of the plate in the recess of the large fragment can, in some cases, ensure good adaptation. It must be kept in mind that the bony consistency of the small fragment varies and usually is not very strong. Therefore, care must be taken when tightening the lag screw to avoid producing high torque; surgeons should realize that there may be variance in the subsequent union between the large and small fragment.

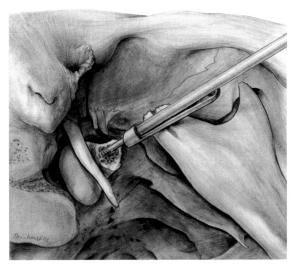

Fig. 16.5 The lag screw is inserted into the center of the displaced fragment (the lag screw is connected with the plate through the guide sleeve) with a minimum of two turns.

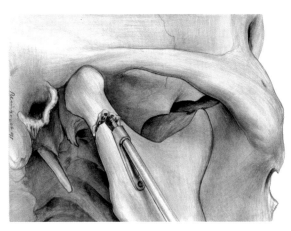

Fig. 16.6 The condylar neck is pulled back in the mandibular fossa.

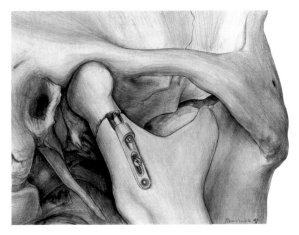

Fig. 16.7 The plate is pre-fixed in the middle of the gliding hole with a bone screw, and adaptation is achieved by pulling the plate close.

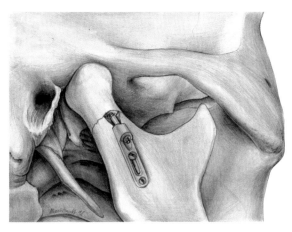

Fig. 16.8 The plate is fixed by tightening the first bone screw in the gliding hole and with a second bone screw in the posterior fixation hole.

17 Osteosynthesis of Condylar Head Fractures by Retroauricular Approach

Andreas Neff

The Retroauricular Approach

Due to its dorsolateral access to the temporomandibular joint, the retroauricular approach (Bockenheimer, 1920 and Axhausen, 1931) can be recommended, especially for condylar head traumatology, as it provides an excellent view of the typical fracture lines of the condylar head and high upper neck.

The skin incision runs 2–3 mm behind the dorsal conchal fold, reaching from the cranial dorsal fold of the concha until slightly above the earlobe (**Fig. 17.1**). Cranially, identification of the deep layer of the temporal fascia avoids lesions to the frontal branch of the facial nerve. This layer is bluntly dissected toward the zygomatic arch and

articular fossa. Caudally, starting from the mastoid fascia level, a blunt epiperichondral dissection in a strictly horizontal plane follows the chondral portions of the auditory canal, which is then transsected using, for example, a blade 20 scalpel. Cutting near the bony external acoustic meatus should be strictly avoided, to prevent postoperative cicatricial stenoses (**Fig. 17.2**).

The dissection can now proceed toward the articular fossa and articular eminence, following the deep layer of the temporal fascia; medial temporal vessels that cross the dissection path should be closed by ligatures. The zygomatic periosteum, however, should be left intact. Instead, a blunt dissection of the periarticular soft tissue strictly follows the lateral ligament plane using a pair of periostium elevators. As a rule, it is not necessary to expose the articular eminence in condylar head traumatology. As the joint space itself is entered directly over the fracture gap via a vertical incision into the posterior recess, the attachments of both lateral ligament and capsule can be left intact. The fracture gap can then be visualized by exposure of the upper parts of the condylar process, especially regarding the medio-caudal aspects (**Fig. 17.3**).

For wound closure of the external auditory canal, a multilayered suturing technique (including chondral layers), which is performed as long as the auricle is still folded anteriorly, will avoid postoperative stenoses. In addition, the posterior membranaceous part of the auditory canal should be kept open by two to three subcutaneous basal sutures.

Osteosynthesis of Condylar Head Fractures

Open reduction and internal fixation in condylar head traumatology has to secure not only an anatomically precise reduction of the small condylar fragment; equally important is the restoration of the physiological function of the disko-ligamental structures. Therefore, a functionally stable osteosynthesis, allowing the preservation of both disk and condylar mobility, is the basis for free postoperative functional movements and the prevention of degenerative long-term sequelae.

For reduction of the condylar head, distraction is performed near the fracture site using an ancillary screw

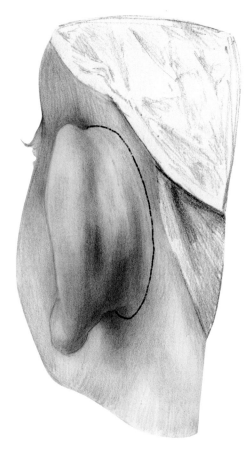

Fig. 17.1 Retroauricular skin incision line.

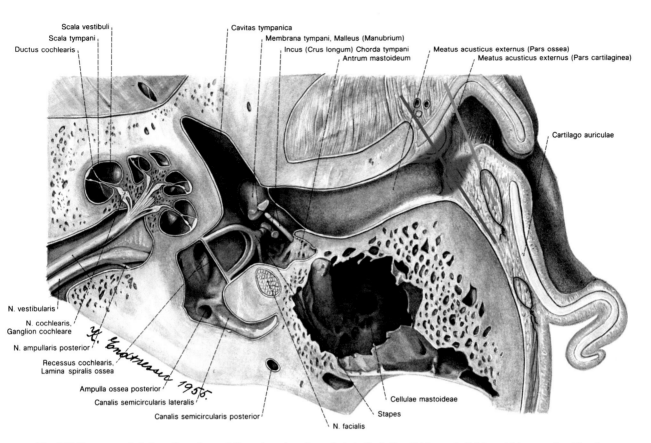

Scala vestibuli
Scala tympani
Ductus cochlearis
Cavitas tympanica
Membrana tympani, Malleus (Manubrium)
Incus (Crus longum) Chorda tympani
Antrum mastoideum
Meatus acusticus externus (Pars ossea)
Meatus acusticus externus (Pars cartilaginea)
Cartilago auriculae
N. vestibularis
N. cochlearis,
Ganglion cochleare
N. ampullaris posterior
Recessus cochlearis,
Lamina spiralis ossea
Ampulla ossea posterior
Canalis semicircularis lateralis
Canalis semicircularis posterior
Cellulae mastoideae
Stapes
N. facialis

Fig. 17.2 Recommended dissection plane of the external auditory canal (green line). Basal sutures (purple) keep the meatus open, whereas dissections near the bony external acoustic meatus (red line) lead to cicatricial stenosis (adapted from Pernkopf, E. Part 4, Kopf, Das Gehör- und Gleichgewichtsorgan. In: *Atlas der topografischen und angewandten Anatomie des Menschen*, Ferner H. (Ed.), Urban & Schwarzenberg, Munich–Vienna–Baltimore, 1979, Fig. 59).

8–9 mm long, placed in the upper condylar process, and a special retractor, which will avoid trauma to the auriculotemporal and facial nerves and allows a refined, three-dimensional guidance regarding the fracture gap (**Figs. 17.4, 17.5**).

The small fragment is reduced (**Fig. 17.6**) together with the disk under full muscular relaxation, as the lateral pterygoid muscle must never be detached from the small fragment. The correct, three-dimensional position can then be secured, for example, by a rectangular ancillary microplate, which may also be used for further positional optimization of the small fragment.

Next, internal fixation of the condylar head is performed, usually with at least two or three screws. Most common are self-cutting positional screws, which are predrilled over the lateral condylar pole, strictly below the lateral attachment of the capsule, or over the upper condylar neck (**Figs. 17.7, 17.8**). This procedure will secure an extra-articular position of the screwheads to minimize trauma to the periarticular soft tissues. During the whole drilling procedure the correct anatomical position of the condylar head can be secured, for example, by the ancillary microplate, which may be removed before wound closure if stability of the osteosynthesis allows this (**Fig. 17.9**).

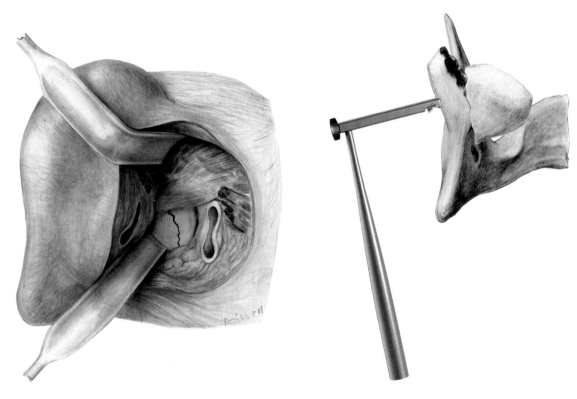

Fig. 17.3 Dorsolateral view of the condylar head with typical fracture line. The auricle is folded back after dissection of the external auditory canal.

Fig. 17.4 Ancillary screw and retractor for improved guidance of the condylar process.

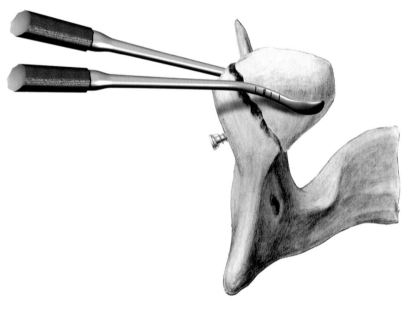

Fig. 17.5 Blunt reduction forceps with length markings for an atraumatic reduction of the small fragment.

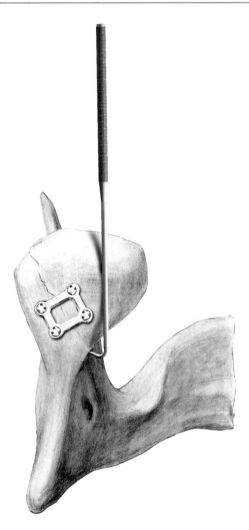

Fig. 17.6 For optimum reposition, the dorsomedicaudal fracture line can be adjusted by a fine hook. The position of the small fragment is secured by an ancillary rectangular microplate.

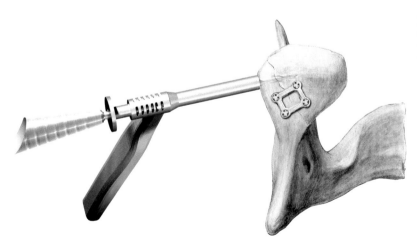

Fig. 17.7 Drilling guide for tissue protection and length adjustment for drilling in the direction of the transversal condylar axis.

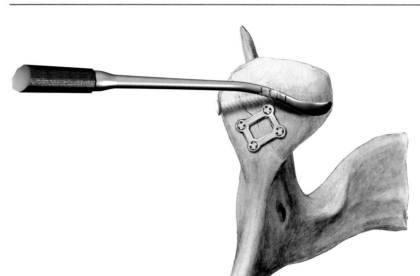

Fig. 17.8 The screw length and direction are given by the reduction forceps with length markings (at 11, 13, 15, and 17 mm). During the drilling and screwing procedure the ancillary microplate will secure the correct anatomical position of the small fragment.

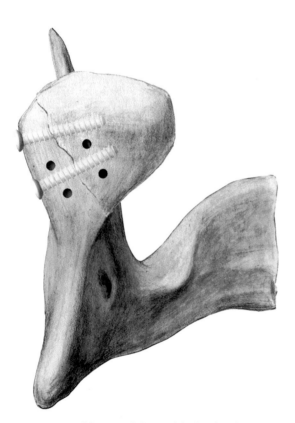

Fig. 17.9 Internal fixation of the condylar head with two positional screws. The ancillary microplate is removed.

18 Condylar Head Fractures: Screw and Pin Fixation

Michael Rasse

A close look at the clinical and functional outcomes of condylar head fractures stresses the need for a surgical approach in dislocated fractures of the condylar head, especially if more than two-thirds of the head is displaced. The favorable results of operated diacapitular fractures have been reported and also compared with the functional outcomes in conservatively treated cases (Rasse, 1993, 2000; Kermer, Undt, and Rasse, 1998; Neff, Kolk, and Horch, 2000; Neff at al. 2002, 2005; Hlawitschka, Loukota, and Eckelt, 2005). Safe procedures to guarantee the survival of the proximal fragment, good mobility (including disk mobility), and preservation of the facial nerve have been described by these authors.

Auricular Approach

An auricular approach (Rasse et al., 1993) to expose the fractured condylar head can use the almost invisible line along the tragus and helix, and may be extended to the temple (**Fig. 18.1**). Too limited an incision may necessitate undue traction for exposure, a possible cause for temporary weakness of the frontal and orbicular branch of the facial nerve. The dissection follows the ear cartilages as a safe plane. The temporoparietal muscle is cut to the depth of the superficial temporal fascia. The dissection proceeds anteriorly on the fascia and the zygomatic arch. The middle temporal vein, which emerges from under the superficial temporal fascia and crosses the zygomatic arch to the superficial temporal vein, is ligated and cut. From this point the superficial temporal fascia is cut cranially and anteriorly. Further dissection anteriorly is performed below the fascia and below the periosteum of the zygomatic arch. The facial nerve is thereby secured safely. In a plane parallel to the zygomatic arch the temporomandibular ligament is exposed downward until the superficial temporal vessels and the auriculotemporal nerve are identified. They are held laterally. Now the periosteum is incised horizontally under the lateral pole of the condyle, if the end of the distal fragment is not already visible. The periosteal incision turns perpendicular downward on the dorsolateral aspect of the condylar process, and the periosteum is lifted to gain access to the dorsal aspect of the condylar head. At this point the patient should be completely relaxed to make possible an extension of the

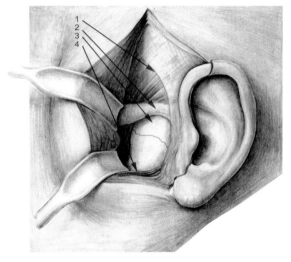

Fig. 18.1 Access to the condylar head.
Arrows:
1: Incision of superficial temporal fascia
2: Zygomatic arch
3: Temporomandibular ligament (joint)
4: Temporal vessels and auriculotemporal nerve

performed by means of a special clamp, which is placed transcutaneously on the mandibular angle area. This exposes the fracture site. The typical fracture area and lines were described by Rasse et al. (1993) and are shown in **Fig. 18.2.** A classification was given by Loukota et al. (2005). The proximal fragment is turned upright with two hooks and reduced by slow motions, overcoming the contraction of the lateral pterygoid muscle, which would have displaced the fragment anteriorly, medially, and caudally.

Osteosynthesis

After correct realignment (the dorso-caudal end of the fracture line giving a crucial hint), the proximal fragment can be fixed with a Kirschner wire of 1.2 mm diameter. This comes in a set with metal sleeves for the wire and applicators for the polydioxanon-pins that replace the wire later. The wire may be placed transcutaneously or through the access. The realignment should be checked

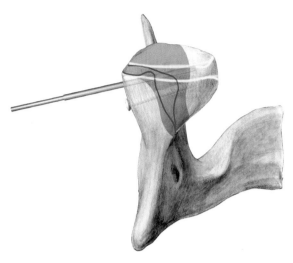

Fig. 18.2 Area of condylar head fractures and osteosynthesis.
Yellow lines: Confinement of capsular attachment
Dark area: Preferred area of diacapitular fractures (blue line: example with small extra fragment dorsally)
Screw and pin ostosynthesis of the condylar head

again. A screw of 2 mm diameter and a length of approximately 13–17 mm can now be placed more or less perpendicular to the fracture line (**Fig. 18.2**). A special transbuccal set is available to hold the soft tissue away from the drill (**Fig. 18.3**). Once the screw is positioned the wire can be replaced by a resorbable pin, which prevents rotation of the proximal fragment. If there is enough bone available, two screws can be placed instead of one screw and a pin. Small additional fragments may be fixed with additional pins, which is also possible on the articulating surface. If the diskocondylar ligament is torn, it can be sutured and the disk replaced in the same way. The wound is closed in layers. A drainage is applied. No intermaxillary fixation is necessary, neither during surgery nor afterward. A soft diet is recommended for 4 weeks (Rasse et al., 1993).

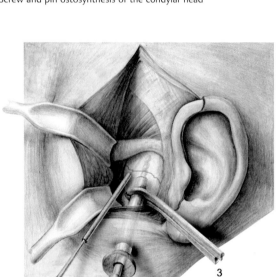

Fig. 18.3 Osteosynthesis of diacapitular fracture.
1: Pin
2: Drill for screw
3: Special clamp of the transbuccal sleeve

19 Midface Fractures

Klaus Louis Gerlach and Hans-Dieter Pape

Introduction

The aims of treatment of midface fractures are to re-establish midfacial height, width, depth, and projection together with the occlusion and the integrity of the nose and the orbit (Manson, 1986). These requirements can only be achieved by a stable osteosynthesis of the different fractured bones, using, for example, miniplates and microplates.

Technique

Access via intraoral, paraorbital, or bitemporal incisions allows the use of miniplates or microplates at all levels for the fixation of reduced maxillary fractures. Only some parts of the craniofacial skeleton constitute compact and solid bone: the cranium, especially at the level of the superior orbital rims, the zygomatic bone, the orbital margins, the nose and the supporting pillars of the maxillary skeleton including the zygomaticomaxillary buttresses, and the piriform aperture (Mariano, 1978). Evaluations of skulls showed that the bone thickness of these regions is strong enough for fixation of plates with screws 5–7 mm long (Ewers, 1977). Therefore, in these regions the application of standard miniplates is recommended. However, the role of miniplates in the midface has been superseded by different microplates developed during recent years. These are especially recommended for other anatomical structures whose lamellar structure has a thickness of only 1–1.5 mm. Generally, a microplate is used to span comminuted areas from solid bone to solid bone. First, the contoured plate has to be fixed at the solid bone parts, then the various comminuted fragments are repositioned and fixed against the plate with the aid of a small hook or an elevator. A hole is drilled through the plate into the fragment and a screw placed, thereby stabilizing the fragments to the plate. Examinations by computed tomography (CT) or magnetic resonance imaging (MRI) are often required preoperatively and postoperatively, especially in cases of combined injuries of the cranium and face. It is recommended, therefore, particularly in the midface, that osteosynthesis material made of titanium is used, to avoid distracting artifacts (Hoffmeister and Kreusch, 1991).

Fractures of the Zygoma

For the stable restitution of anatomical form, after repositioning fragments, the application of only one miniplate is recommended, preferably at the frontozygomatic process (**Fig. 19.1**). Alternatively, a plate at the zygomaticomaxillary buttress may be used. This "one point fixation" renders a solid stability to the cheek-bone, as demonstrated in large numbers of clinical follow-ups (e. g., Michelet, Deymes, and Dessus, 1973; Champy et al., 1977; Iatrou et al., 1991; Krause, Bremerich, and Kreidler, 1991; Zingg et al., 1991).

A further alternative, recommended by Pape (1997), is the use of one or two microplates at the zygomaticomaxillary buttress to stabilize the reduced zygoma.

The frontozygomatic process is approached either by an S-shaped incision below, or a straight one within the eyebrow. After exposure of the fracture line at the lateral orbital rim, the reduction is performed by a temporal or oral approach (Keen, 1909; Gillies, Kilner, and Stone, 1927). In German-speaking countries, reduction using a single-pronged bone hook is customary (Stromeyer, 1844). The hook is placed below the body of the zygoma after a stab skin incision; the displaced zygoma is then grasped from below, behind the zygomatic buttress, with the point of the hook and reduced by pulling on the hook until the bone is in place (**Figs. 19.2, 19.3**). While the bone fragment is maintained in the correct position with the aid of the hook, the plate is adapted at the bony surface and fixed to the bone. Normally, a four-hole plate with four screws of 5 mm or 7 mm in length is sufficient (see **Figs. 19.1–19.3**).

In those cases where stability is questionable, an additional plate may be placed at the zygomaticomaxillary buttress by an intraoral approach. Comminuted fractures of the infraorbital margin have to be reconstructed with a microplate. This is also recommended when a simultaneous orbital exploration is required, but from a mechanical point of view the infraorbital margin offers less additional stability.

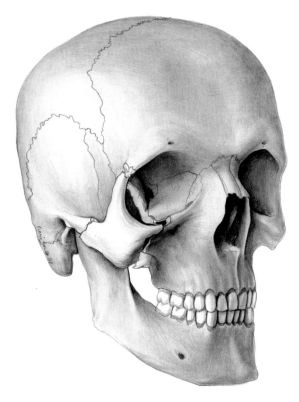

Fig. 19.1 Fractures of the zygoma with inferior displacement.

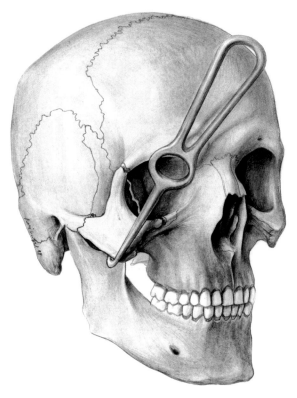

Fig. 19.2 Reduction of a fractured and displaced zygoma with a single-pronged bone hook.

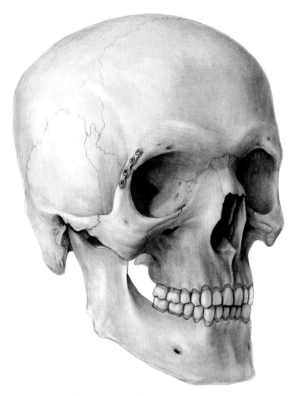

Fig. 19.3 Condition after stabilization of a repositioned cheek-bone with a four-hole miniplate osteosynthesis at the lateral orbital rim.

Le Fort I Fractures

Performing a plate osteosynthesis for a Le Fort I fracture requires prior intermaxillary fixation to establish the occlusion (**Fig. 19.4**). Locations for the plates are the zygomaticomaxillary buttress and the lateral margins of the piriform aperture. For this, the surgical approach to the lower portion of the maxilla is exposed through a maxillary degloving or marginal rim incision. Standard four-hole straight plates or L-shaped plates with 5 mm or 7 mm screws are usual. The use of microplates is recommended, especially when the fracture line is near to the root apices. Any additional associated midline separation has to be bridged with a plate at the lower margin of the piriform aperture. The osteosynthesis procedure starts from the stable parts of the midface bones to the unstable ones. The plates must be accurately adapted to the surface of the bone to avoid displacements of the fragments causing disturbances of the occlusion (**Fig. 19.5**).

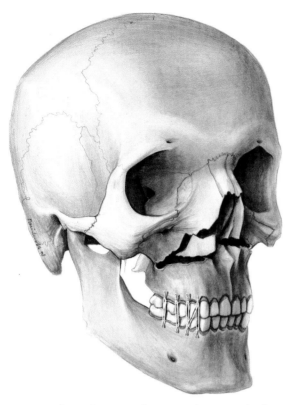

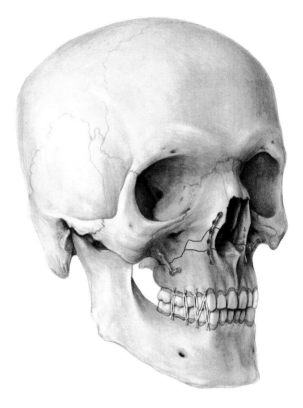

Fig. 19.4 Dislocated Le Fort I fracture with a triangular bone fragment on the right side after fixation of the occlusion by intermaxillary fixation.

Fig. 19.5 Reposition of a Le Fort I fracture by means of intermediate intermaxillary fixation and stabilization with a six-hole microplate on the right and a four-hole microplate on the left side at the zygomaticomaxillary buttress and the lateral margins of the piriform aperture.

Le Fort II Fractures

The treatment of central midface fractures starts with the application of arch bars and the re-establishment of the occlusion by means of intermaxillary fixation (**Fig. 19.6**). Surgical approaches are the intraorally degloving incision and, for instance, a subciliar or infraorbital incision to expose the lower infraorbital margin. If a proper reduction cannot be achieved by intermaxillary fixation, the maxilla will need to be mobilized with Rowe impaction forceps. A proper stabilization with plates has to be performed at the zygomaticomaxillary buttress using straight, four-hole, L- or Y-shaped miniplates or microplates. Additional microplates placed at the infraorbital margins allow a secure stabilization of the maxilla without the need for postoperative intermaxillary fixation. Persistent depression of the nose skeleton requires a stabilization of the nasal bones, in some cases. After a coronal incision, or a midline vertical incision from the frontal bone, the detached nasal pyramid fragments have to be reduced and a T-shaped or double Y-shaped microplate has to be adapted accurately to the bony surface. Two screws on the anterior aspect of the frontal bone and one or two screws at the nasal bones give a solid support to maintain the anterior projection of the nasal frame (**Fig. 19.7**).

Le Fort III Fractures

According to Champy, Lodde, and Wilk (1975), the application of a single miniplate at the frontozygomatic fracture lines after repositioning of the midface offers good stability for treatment of fractures of the Le Fort III type, especially in relatively nondisplaced ones (Champy, 1980). However, complete craniofacial disjunctions are very rare. More often, combinations of fractures of the zygomas with Le Fort I fractures are found. In those cases, after fixation of the zygomatic and nasal bones to the skull, any remaining Le Fort I and II fractures have to be stabilized (**Fig. 19.8**). Alternatively, it is sometimes useful to start with the reduction of the central part after re-establishment of the occlusion by intermaxillary fixation. In complex fractures a coronal incision is recommended. After proper reduction, the fragments have to be stabilized at the nasal root, the lateral orbital rims and the zygomatic arches; additional Le Fort I and II fractures are treated as described above (**Fig. 19.9**).

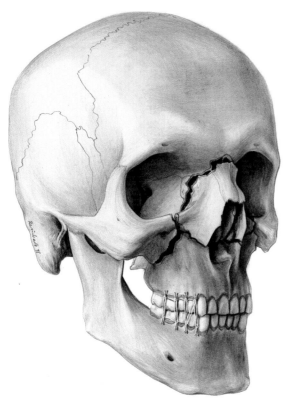

Fig. 19.6 Re-establishment of the occlusion by means of inter-maxillary fixation in a Le Fort II fracture.

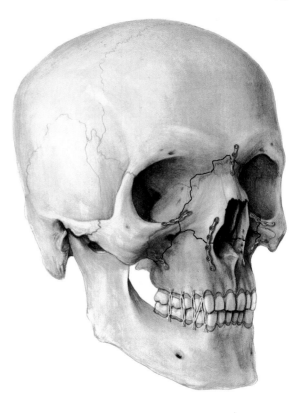

Fig. 19.7 Repositioning of a Le Fort II fracture with intermediate intermaxillary fixation and fragment stabilization by means of microplates in typical locations.

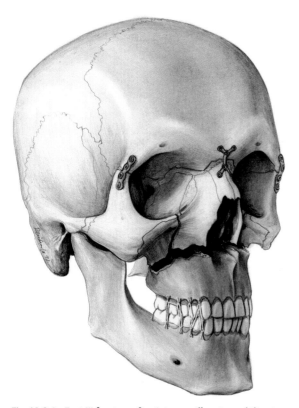

Fig. 19.8 Le Fort III fracture after intermaxillary immobilization and fixation of the zygomatic and nasal bones.

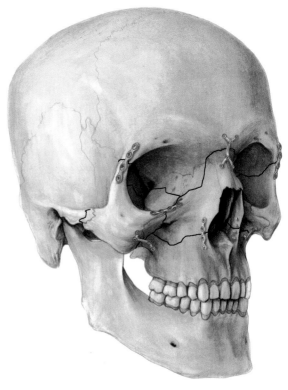

Fig. 19.9 Stabilization of midface Le Fort III fractures with mini-plates and microplates at typical locations, after reduction and intermediate intermaxillary fixation.

20 Naso-ethmoid Fractures

Peter Ward Booth

Introduction

Naso-ethmoid fractures represent a spectrum of injuries, from simple nasal fractures with undetectable ethmoid involvement through to grossly comminuted and compounded naso-ethmoid fractures involving the base of the skull and significant displacement.

Anatomical Considerations

The tentlike nasal bone is relatively thick, especially in the bridge area, but it is the triangular shape that provides the strength. Further strengthening is given by the "tent pole" of the vertical bony septum. Thus, there is considerable strength against fracture from a direct anterior blow. A blow laterally, however, meets little structural resistance; hence the relative frequency of simple fractured noses that have minimal effect on the ethmoids or the base of the skull. Once the nasal "tent" collapses, forces are dissipated into the air cells, which act like air bags. While this mechanically protects the base of the skull, collapse of the naso-ethmoid complex may occur relatively easily if these air cells are large and pneumatized. With minimal force the whole complex may collapse, frequently as one unit, into the frontal sinus. Thus a naso-ethmoid fracture may occur with relatively minimal injuries in some patients. Severe forces, however, may extend the fracture into the base of the skull, frequently seen as a cerebrospinal fluid leak, as the cribriform plate is ruptured.

The medial canthus has a small attachment point to the lacrimal crest. Loss of this attachment leaves an ugly, "blunt" medial canthus that is further damaged by the inevitable lateral drift. The resultant defect is very unsightly.

The lacrimal apparatus is more frequently damaged by lacerations and more rarely by secondary bony injury. On occasion, damage may be iatrogenic during osteosynthesis stabilization of the fractures.

Clinical Examination

Soft-tissue injuries are readily evaluated by clinical examination. Gross swelling may obliterate the canthal attachment but careful exploration normally overcomes this confusion. This exploration should be particularly directed at pulling the canthus to ensure that it is still attached to stable bone. If the bone attachment has itself been fractured, lateral displacement of the canthus should be evaluated.

When the lacrimal apparatus is damaged, it is most frequently by direct laceration. However, this is a rare complication. Lacerations in this area must be carefully explored. If doubt remains, radiological examination may be indicated.

However, even where swelling is pronounced, careful clinical examination will normally yield a clear understanding of the extent of the fractures. This is important

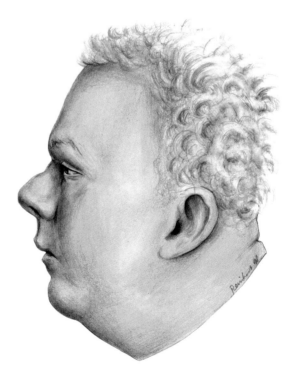

Fig. 20.1 A simple naso-ethmoid fracture illustrating the depression of the soft-tissue nasion. This tilts the nose back producing the "pig snout" appearance of the nares.

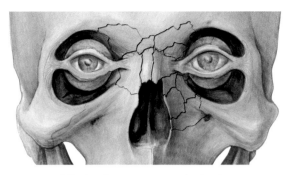

Fig. 20.2 Ayliffe classification type 0. Undisplaced.

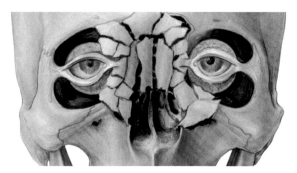

Fig. 20.3 Ayliffe classification type I. Comminuted but "platable."

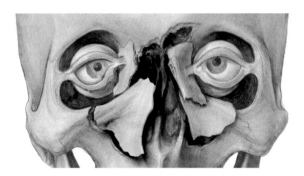

Fig. 20.4 Ayliffe classification type II. Requiring bone graft.

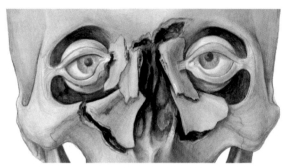

Fig. 20.5 Ayliffe classification type III. Canthal disruption, requiring canthoplexy.

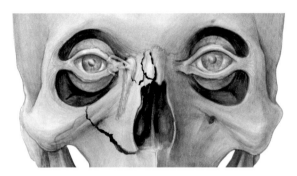

Fig. 20.6 Ayliffe classification type IV. Lacrimal reconstruction.

for requesting radiographic examinations that are well "targeted," so that maximum information is generated.

Clinically, the naso-ethmoid fractures may present with traumatic telecanthus and impaction of the bridge of the nose, producing a characteristic appearance. The nasal tip is elevated, the bridge depressed, and the nares projecting almost horizontally, to give the "pig snout" appearance (**Fig. 20.1**). The possibility of a cerebrospinal fluid leak should be eliminated.

Markowitz et al. (1991) have attempted to classify these bony fractures. This has not provided much useful correlation with outcome, but is frequently used. However, as with any fractures, it is important to determine their severity. Clearly, greater problems occur with compound, comminuted fractures with gross displacement than with simple fractures (Leipziger and Manson, 1992). In naso-ethmoid trauma, comminution and the actual detachment of the canthus from bone are severe findings and are a poor prognosis for satisfactory outcome.

Of all the classifications the least well know seems to offer the most useful data collection, identifying the "difficult" cases. This means outcomes can be meaningfully compared (**Figs. 20.2–20.6**). The diagrams illustrate the Ayliffe classification (P. Ayliffe, personal communication, 2006):

- type 0 (**Fig. 20.2**): undisplaced
- type I (**Fig. 20.3**): comminuted but "platable"
- type II (**Fig. 20.4**): requiring bone graft
- type III (**Fig. 20.5**): canthal disruption requiring cantoplexy
- type IV (**Fig. 20.6**): lacrimal reconstruction

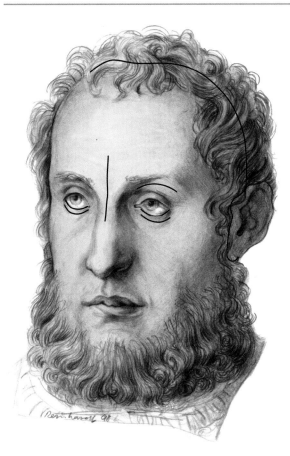

Fig. 20.7 Skin incisions for exposure of naso-ethmoid fractures (after Hans Burkmeir, *Portrait of a gentleman*, ca. 1505/1520, Amsterdam Rijksmuseum).

Radiological Examination

Occipital mental and lateral skull views (at 10° and 45°) are most helpful as an initial screening examination. Computerized tomographic (CT) scans are extremely valuable, perhaps even essential. Three-dimensional images are illustrative, but rarely add more information than a good, conventional CT scan.

Treatment

As with any soft tissue injury, treatment consists of:
- examination
- debridement
- closure

In the case of trauma to the naso-ethmoid area, care must be taken to diagnose any damage to the canthi and lacrimal system, as mentioned above. The canthi are rarely detached without damage to the underlying bone. Pure soft-tissue injuries to the lids may result in lacrimal system damage. Careful exploration and suturing is required. The vulnerable part is the short medial segment of the canaliculus before it enters the sac, lying between the medial canthi. Fine bore polyethylene or silicone tubes may be inserted into the canaliculus to prevent stenosis.

The principle of hard-tissue treatment is simple: reduce the fractures and stabilize (Champy et al., 1978b). In practice, there is significant difference between achieving this in a simple, noncomminuted, minimally displaced fracture, compared with a grossly comminuted compound, "bag of bones" fracture.

There is little doubt, however, that with any fracture, the best results are achieved using the following principles:
- good surgical exposure, either through existing lacerations, or via a coronal flap
- reduction and stabilization using low-profile, small osteosynthesis plates
- prompt treatment, as an aid to good reduction
- immediate bone grafting, if this is indicated

Surgical Exposure

The potential use of existing lacerations is obvious, but is not without its complications, mainly of infection, as these may be contaminated. Under such circumstances, surgery should be performed as soon as possible.

There are few skin incisions around the nose and forehead that are satisfactory (**Fig. 20.7**). This is in marked contrast to the excellent cosmetic results and superior access produced by the coronal flap (Shepherd, Ward Booth, and Moos, 1985). Even with this flap, care must be taken to place it well into the hair line to avoid exposure of the scar should balding occur (see **Fig. 5.22**). On rare occasions an incision over the nasion is possible (see **Fig. 20.7**). The coronal incision is combined with subciliary periorbital and upper buccal sulcus incisions as needed. The zygomatic arch is exposed through the coronal incision when necessary (Gruss, 1992).

Reduction and Stabilization

Microplates will stabilize very small fragments and provide a good three-dimensional stability (**Figs. 20.8, 20.9**). Particular care must be taken to stabilize any bone that has the canthi attached. In cases of gross comminution it may be helpful to place a plate over the bridge of the nose horizontally, to pull the fragments into a good sharp narrow arch (**Figs. 20.10, 20.11**).

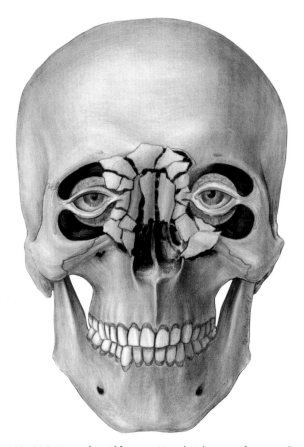

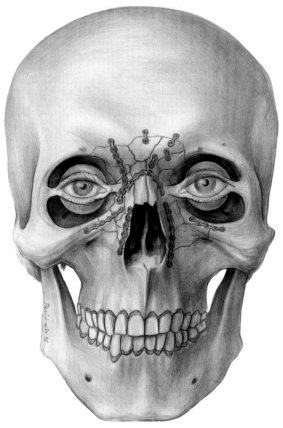

Fig. 20.8 Naso-ethmoid fracture. Note that the strong frontonasal buttress is detached superiorly and inferiorly, taking the medial canthal ligament with it.

Fig. 20.9 Microplates in the typical naso-ethmoid injury. The upper plates are placed across the upper portion of the fractures in the frontonasal region. The lower portions of the microplates are placed in such a way that they are adjacent to the canthal ligament, which is exactly repositioned.

Bone Grafting

This is rarely required, but in cases of gross comminution an immediate bone graft is indicated. If this is delayed, then the soft tissues contract, making later secondary grafting difficult, and possibly leading to erosion through the tight skin. Unfortunately, these grossly comminuted fractures are often compound, making a less-than-ideal environment for immediate grafting.

Detached Canthus

Often when the canthus is described as "detached," in reality it is attached to a small bone fragment. Under these circumstances, with modern microplates it is possible to "capture" the canthus and reduce it. In true detachment, it is difficult to hold the canthus. The canthus is first located by passing a needle through the canthal angle, easily

identified on the cutaneous surface (**Fig. 20.11**). Once it is located, a fine wire suture is passed through the deep surface of the canthal ligament. This wire is either passed transnasally (Hofmann, 1966; Tessier et al., 1967; Härle and Lange, 1975; Freihofer, 1980) to the opposing canthus, if this is attached, or through a bony point on the other side of the nose. The wire is placed so that it pulls medially and posteriorly.

While this technique is easily described, those experienced in the procedure recognize its shortcomings. The fine wire cuts through the fine canthus very easily, especially if edema puts any significant pressure on the reduction, or if the treatment is forced to be delayed. For this reason it may be helpful to support the canthal reattachment from the cutaneous surface. This can be performed using a preformed, clear acrylic button (**Fig. 20.12**). The risk of this procedure is skin necrosis, but with clear acrylic the status of the skin can be monitored.

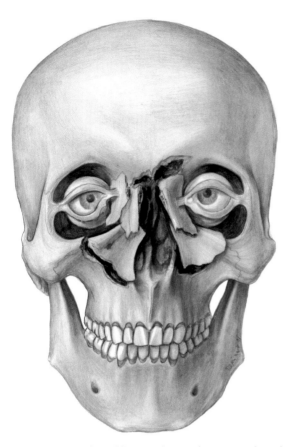

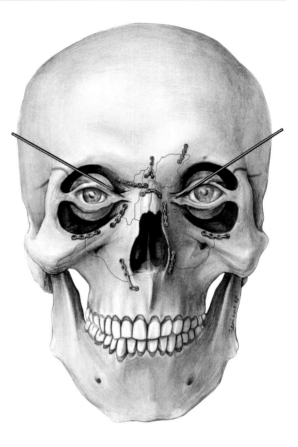

Fig. 20.10 Naso-ethmoid fracture showing bony naso-ethmoid–orbital injury in combination with orbital detachment and displacement.

Fig. 20.11 The plate is being inserted over the fragments to define the nasal form. Also note the needles being run through the medial canthus from the cutaneous side as identification of detached canthi from the periosteal side is very difficult.

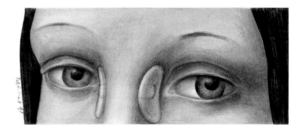

Fig. 20.12 Clear acrylic buttons can usefully support those rare cases of total canthal detachment. In late-treated cases, the transnasal wire used alone frequently cuts through the delicate canthal tendon if there is any tension (after Giovanni Antonio Boltraffio, *Portrait of a lady as St. Lucy*, ca. 1500, Foundation Museum Thyssen Bornemisza, Madrid).

21 Panfacial Fractures: Planning an Organized Treatment

Rudolf R. M. Bos

Introduction

In the treatment of panfacial fractures all treatment modalities for single fractures of the craniomaxillofacial area, described in other chapters, come together. A successful outcome of panfacial fracture treatment, however, demands a systematic approach by an experienced team of specialists, working in a trauma center that has all facilities for proper patient care. Developments during the last quarter of the 20th century (such as computed tomography [CT], wide-open reduction, internal fixation, immediate bone grafting, and soft-tissue handling) have revolutionized the potential for restoring the pre-injury appearance and function of panfacial fracture patients. The keys to successful treatment of panfacial trauma remain good exposure, careful reduction and fixation of the fractures.

The craniofacial skeleton consists of 22 different bones. These bones surround the different cavities that together form the head. These cavities are the cranium, the orbits, the sinuses, the nose and the mouth. In the craniofacial skeleton, thicker portions of bone are connected to thinner bony walls. These thicker bony structures are called "buttresses" and maintain the craniofacial proportions in height, width and anterior–posterior projection (**Fig. 21.1**; see also **Fig. 1.8**).

The buttresses form the key to the reconstruction of panfacial fractures and were originally described by Sicher and Tandler (1928), then Merville (1974) and later expanded by Gruss and Mackinnon (1986).

Wide exposure of fractures was also advanced by Merville (1974), using the principles of craniofacial surgery transferred to fracture repair. Exposure of the buttresses allows alignment and fixation of the fractures and so provides the potential for anatomical reduction of the bones. Internal fixation with combinations of different sizes of plates and screws provides three-dimensional stability and makes postoperative intermaxillary fixation almost superfluous. (A guide to the use of different plate–screw osteosynthesis systems in the craniofacial area is given in **Fig. 21.4**.)

Highly comminuted bones are replaced by bone grafts. Bone grafting is also used to supplement missing bone or bone volume. However, the need for primary bone grafting is largely reduced because of the stability provided by plate and screw fixation. It is still unclear how long plate–screw fixation provides stability when bridging an

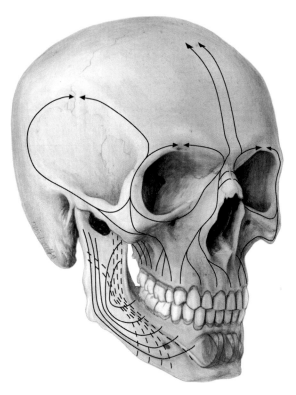

Fig. 21.1 The different buttresses, marked by arrows, that determine the width, height, and projection of the head. These buttresses form the key to the reconstruction of panfacial fractures (see **Fig. 1.8**). Biting forces produce tension forces (dashed lines) at the upper border and compressive forces (solid line) at the lower border of the mandible. Torsion forces are produced anterior to the canines of the mandible.

area of bone loss. In case of substantial bone loss or gross comminution, bone grafting may still be necessary to guarantee long-term stability (Klotch and Gilliland, 1987).

Diagnosis

In this specific sequence a careful history, physical examination, and radiographic evaluation are essential to get a proper understanding of a panfacial injury complex. Whenever possible, information should be gathered about the pre-injury appearance, occlusion, and function. Photographs and dental records can be very helpful.

Physical examination should consist of static and dynamic inspection and palpation from chin to crown, in order to identify injuries of the soft tissue, bone, and neurovascular bundles.

Special attention should be given to the naso-ethmoid region, the palate, the eye and the condylar process, where injuries are easily overlooked. All patients with severe craniofacial trauma deserve a complete ophthalmological evaluation.

CT scanning has replaced most conventional plain radiographs except for those that image the ascending ramus of the mandible, including the condylar process. For initial evaluation, plain radiographs like the Waters view in combination with a submentovertex view and a left and right half mandibular view, described by Eisler, provide valuable overall information. Detailed CT scanning in axial planes provides important information concerning the extent of craniomaxillofacial injuries. Two-dimensional coronal and sagittal reconstructions are most valuable for evaluation of fractures of the orbital walls, maxillary buttresses, and mandibular ascending ramus. The role of three-dimensional imaging is inconclusive. One has to be cautious in evaluating three-dimensional images in areas where the bone is thin or where there is minimal or no displacement. False positive as well as false negative findings are possible. As technology advances, three-dimensional imaging may become of more importance (**Fig. 21.2**).

Currently, magnetic resonance imaging (MRI) seems of little importance in the initial assessment of a panfacial trauma patient.

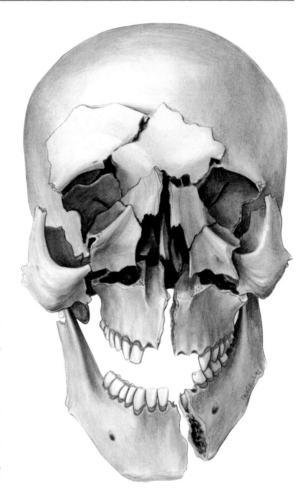

Fig. 21.2 Panfacial fracture.

Treatment Planning

Plate and screw fixation has significantly influenced the sequence of panfacial fracture treatment. It makes possible a full reconstruction of the mandible including subcondylar fractures, which is important to preserve vertical mandibular height. By complete mandibular internal fixation the craniomandibular relation is restored, so turning a panfacial fracture into an isolated midface fracture. However, this implies that one has to perform an open reduction and internal fixation of subcondylar fractures, which is not favored by many surgeons because of the anatomical hazards and the difficulty encountered during this operation. It is also a time-consuming procedure. On the other hand, one should realize that unilateral and, even more so, bilateral condylar neck fractures are looked upon more and more as an absolute indication for open reduction and fixation when part of a panfacial fracture. To prevent shortening of the vertical height of the face, due to telescoping of bone fragments and loss of antero-posterior dimension, fixation of the condylar fractures is essential. One also should think of the potential for further displacement of initially undisplaced or dislocated condylar fractures during the process of fracture reduction (Zide and Kent, 1983; Hayward and Scott, 1993).

Plate and screw fixation also creates a stable base in the midface. So, instead of starting with complete restoration of the mandible, internal fixation of the midface with plates and screws is performed to offer a stable and anatomically correct base for subsequent mandibular fracture treatment (Merville, 1974; Gruss and Mackinnon, 1986). The advantage of this sequence is that one can possibly omit open treatment of subcondylar fractures. A prerequisite of such a sequence is that there are enough bony landmarks available to allow anatomical reduction of the midface, including the maxilla. Gruss and Mackinnon (1986) advocated the need to always reconstruct first the so-called "outer facial frame" in panfacial fractures. This should start at the root of the zygomatic arch, advancing to the malar complex and the frontal bar, followed by "the inner facial frame" or naso-orbito-ethmoidal complex, when necessary using bone grafts to recon-

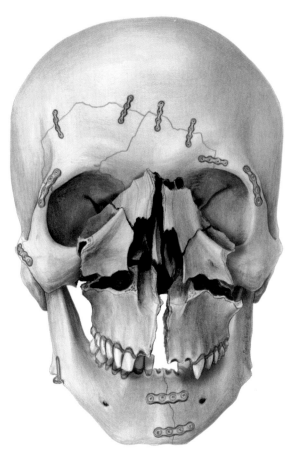

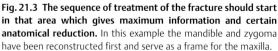

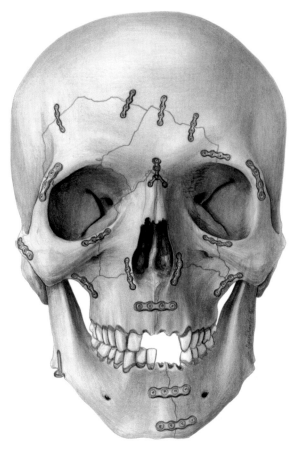

Fig. 21.3 The sequence of treatment of the fracture should start in that area which gives maximum information and certain anatomical reduction. In this example the mandible and zygoma have been reconstructed first and serve as a frame for the maxilla.

Fig. 21.4 Complete reduction and internal fixation of a panfacial fracture using different types of plates and screws. When mandible and zygoma are reconstructed, the maxilla can be set up like a key in a lock. Main frame for the use of different plate–screw osteosynthesis systems in the craniofacial area: cranial vault: microsystems; midface: microsystems; lateral orbital rim: from microsystems to minisystems; mandible: from minisystems to reconstruction systems.

struct orbital walls (**Fig. 21.3**). Then the maxilla is fixed by plate and screw fixation along the buttresses at the Le Fort I level, when necessary using bone grafts (Gruss and Mackinnon, 1986). Eventually, intermaxillary fixation is performed to place the mandible in its normal position, after which mandibular fractures are fixed by plates and screws. Fractures of the condylar process can be treated closed using this sequence (**Fig. 21.4**).

Kelly et al. (1990) and Manson et al. (1995) proposed complete reduction and fixation of the mandible, including fractures of the condylar process, as the base for proper intermaxillary fixation. If there is a sagittal fracture of the maxilla, this is reduced and fixed to re-establish the pre-injured maxillary arch that is necessary to establish the correct position for the mandible using intermaxillary fixation (**Figs. 21.5, 21.6**).

After reconstruction of the mandibulomaxillary block, the cranial vault is reconstructed including the forehead.

Then the naso-ethmoid complex is reduced and fixed to the forehead in the region of the glabela. Subsequently the outer facial frame is reconstructed starting at the dorsal root of the zygomatic arch and advancing to the lateral orbital and intra-orbital rims (see **Fig. 21.3**). Final correction at the Le Fort I level is performed with plates and screws over the buttresses (see **Figs. 21.4–21.6**), when necessary using bone grafts. Bone grafts are used for reconstruction of the orbital walls and the nose (**Fig. 21.7**).

There is no consensus as to which sequence in the management of panfacial fractures is the best. It becomes more and more obvious that factors like fracture displacement and amount of comminution are important for determining the choice. However, one thing is clear: the decision for one or another sequence should be based on a careful diagnosis.

Complete exposure of panfacial fractures is the essential first step in treatment by internal fixation. The need

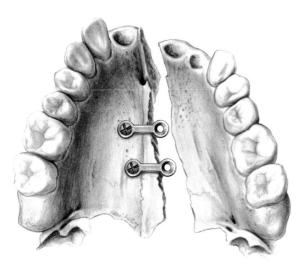

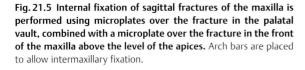

Fig. 21.5 Internal fixation of sagittal fractures of the maxilla is performed using microplates over the fracture in the palatal vault, combined with a microplate over the fracture in the front of the maxilla above the level of the apices. Arch bars are placed to allow intermaxillary fixation.

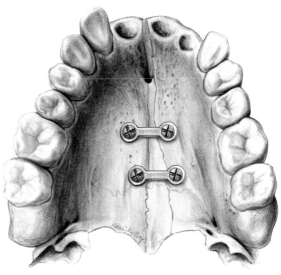

Fig. 21.6 Sagittal fracture of the maxilla is repositioned and fixed by microplates.

for different incisions is dependent on the treatment plan based on a careful diagnosis. The entire facial area can be exposed and reconstructed using a combination of coronal incision, one of the different lower eyelid incisions, the mandibular and maxillary gingivobuccal sulcus and a preauricular, retromandibular, or submandibular incision.

With the increased use of the coronal incision, other local facial incisions can be omitted. If a coronal incision is not used, different local periorbital incisions are required. Exposure of the zygomatic arch is then not possible. For reduction and plate and screw fixation of the outer facial frame and cranial vault, a coronal incision is a prerequisite. The coronal incision gives a wide exposure of the cranium and upper craniofacial skeleton. It gives the surgeon the optimal access for proper reduction and fixation of fractures and to a useful site for bone grafting, so avoiding another donor site. Simple fractures can be reduced and fixed through local incisions, while complex fractures demand wider exposure through a coronal incision. The use of traumatic lacerations may also be helpful.

The majority of patients with panfacial fractures have other injuries. Most of them are candidates for immediate surgery. There are only a few contraindications for immediate surgical intervention, such as cardiopulmonary instability, coagulopathy, and severe neurological trauma with high intracranial pressures. Delayed surgery causes scarring to develop, impeding anatomical reduction of the fractures. Therefore, immediate definitive repair within 48–72 hours is advocated.

If there are no contraindications for surgery, the multisystem injuries are normally treated first. However, it is important not to neglect control of bleeding, first from existing intraoral or extraoral lacerations, by cautery, suturing, or temporary tamponade. Before closing a laceration, it is important to determine whether reduction and fixation of an underlying fracture could be performed through that laceration.

Special attention should be given to the patients presurgical and post-surgical airway. In cases of panfacial fractures, a tracheotomy is preferred. It not only provides an adequate perioperative and postoperative airway, but also allows the surgeon optimal access to the craniomaxillofacial regions. However, if no indication for tracheotomy exists other than surgical convenience, the submental route for endotracheal intubation can be easily used (Altemir, 1986).

At the end of what is normally a long operation to reduce and fix panfacial fractures, proper handling of the soft-tissue incisions and lacerations deserves attention. To prevent "sag" of the facial soft tissues, careful management of the subcutaneous layers is necessary, closing periosteal incisions at specific points of the skeleton. The coronal incision is closed in at least two layers (galea and scalp). Closure of the periosteum over the zygomaticofrontal suture, at the lateral canthal ligament area and at the infraorbital rim, is necessary to reposition the soft tissue at its proper location on the underlying skeleton. A layered closure (muscle and mucosa) of the gingivobuccal sulcus incision is performed. Careful closure of the skin in layers provides less risk for visible scars, as it prevents widening of the scar.

Special attention should be given to difficult reattachment of the medial canthal ligament using microplates or

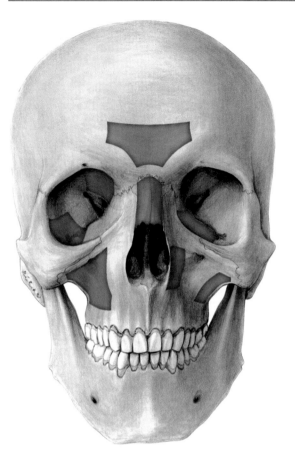

Fig. 21.7 Regions that more often demand reconstruction with bone grafts in panfacial fractures: frontal sinus wall, orbital walls, dorsum of the nose, malar complex, and maxillary sinus walls. The use of split calvarial bone is preferred.

transnasal wires (see **Figs. 20.4, 20.6, 20.7**) to prevent very unaesthetic traumatic telecanthus (Markowitz et al., 1991).

Conclusion

A planned sequence of surgery, based on a careful diagnosis, enables the surgeon to restore the appearance and function of patients in even the severest cases of panfacial fractures. The surgeon must choose the sequence of treatment for each individual case, based on detailed clinical and radiographical diagnosis in which fracture displacement and amount of comminution are especially important factors.

To ensure a precise anatomical reduction, reconstruction should be started in the area that gives maximum information. Fixation of fractures with different plates and screws is nowadays state of the art, providing excellent three-dimensional stability and quick recovery to normal function.

Wide exposure, using the buttresses, and the immediate use of bone grafts when necessary, are important ingredients for a successful outcome. Careful management of lacerations and incisions is necessary for an aesthetic and functional result. Immediate definitive repair within 48–72 hours is advocated to prevent scarring, which impedes anatomical reduction of the fractures. Information on the exact surgical techniques for treatment of different types of fracture is given in the relevant chapters.

22 Osteotomies of the Mandible

Paul J. W. Stoelinga

Sagittal Split Osteotomy

Introduction

The sagittal split osteotomy described by Obwegeser (Trauner and Obwegeser, 1957) is probably the most frequently used osteotomy to correct mandibular anomalies including hypoplasia, hyperplasia, and asymmetries. Miniplates can be used to stabilize these osteotomies, allowing for early release of, or even no, intermaxillary fixation. Studies have proven that the stability achieved, in advancement as well as setback cases, is adequate and highly predictable (Borstlap et al., 2004, 2005). The advantages of using plates as compared with positional or lag screws can be summarized as follows:

* Plates can be bent to adapt to the anatomical situation caused by the positional changes of the fragments; excessive, unwanted torquing, particularly of the proximal fragments, can thus be avoided.
* Extraoral stab incisions are not necessary when using miniplate fixation.
* Damage to the inferior alveolar nerve can be minimized because the nerve cannot be injured by the screws; since the fragments are not pulled together by screws, the nerve cannot be damaged by compression either.
* If, after the patient is awake and sitting up in a natural position, the occlusion is found to be inadequate because of a changed position of the distal fragment, the plates may be adjusted without a further general anesthetic. The procedure can be done under local anesthesia, several days after the first operation, when the swelling has subsided. Adjustment usually only includes repositioning of the screws in the distal fragment, after fine adjustment of the occlusion with temporary intermaxillary fixation.

Disadvantages include the following:

* The bone cuts have to be brought relatively further forward to allow for easy application of the plates; this may increase the risk of buccal plate fractures (bad splits).
* Ischemic necrosis of parts of the buccal plate around the screws is sometimes seen. This gives rise to an inflammatory reaction but does not usually interfere with overall bone-healing.

Technique

The sagittal split osteotomy (Trauner and Obwegeser, 1957) is performed using the modifications of Dal-Pont (1961), Hunsuck (1968) and Epker (1977). The anterior vertical cut is situated approximately between the first and the second molar. Following placement of an acrylic splint and intermaxillary fixation, the proximal fragment has to be positioned with a gauze-packing instrument. In cases of setback of the distal fragment, the appropriate amount of bone to be cut from the proximal segment can now be calculated (**Fig. 22.1**). An appropriate miniplate is selected, long enough to include two holes in the proximal and distal segment. The plate is bent to lie passively against the bone fragments. A straight Kocher clamp is then applied to the proximal segment and the segment is rotated anteriorly and superiorly. A hole in the proximal segment is drilled and the plate screwed in position using a 5-mm or 7-mm screw (**Fig. 22.2**). Plate position may now be checked and adjustments can be made. Following this, a second hole is made while the proximal fragment is

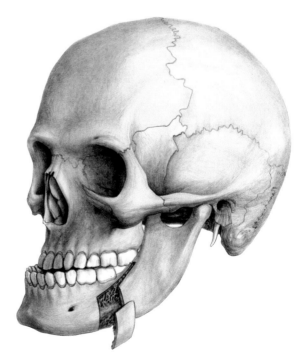

Fig. 22.1 Buccal cortical fragment to be removed to allow the mandible to be set back.

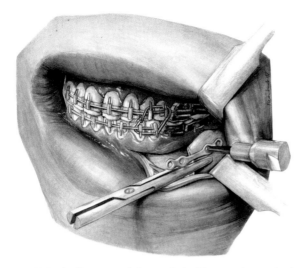

Fig. 22.2 The first screw is inserted. At this stage the proximal fragment may be placed in its proper position, to check plate alignment.

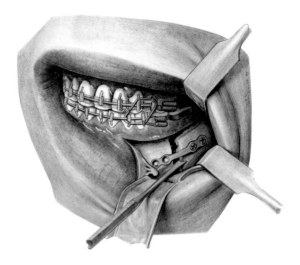

Fig. 22.3 A gauze-packing instrument is used to hold the proximal fragment in position while screws are inserted in the distal fragment.

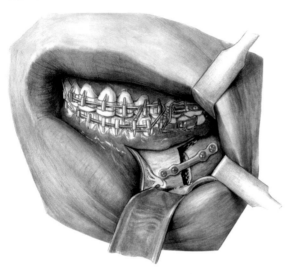

Fig. 22.4 The screws have been inserted in the proximal fragment and the distal fragment is in place.

again pulled forward and slightly rotated upward. The second screw is then placed and tightened. Next, the gauze-packing instrument is used to push the proximal fragment into its proper position, taking care to correctly align the lower margin in relation to the distal segment (**Fig. 22.3**). Holes are drilled in the distal segment and screws placed and tightened (**Fig. 22.4**). A similar procedure is performed on the other side, after which the intermaxillary fixation is released. The occlusion can now be checked by manually manipulating the chin with the condyles seated in their fossae. If an error is noted, intermaxillary fixation can be reapplied and the plates readjusted, which involves repositioning the distal screws only.

In Angle class II cases the osteotomy is performed using the same technique as in Angle class III patients. After osteotomy the mandible is positioned forward and the cortical bone gap is bridged with a four-hole or six-hole miniplate (**Figs. 22.5, 22.6**).

If the buccal plate is inadvertently fractured while splitting the mandible (bad split), the loose fragment can be fixed to the proximal fragment using a miniplate. In these circumstances it is best to complete the splitting first. The proximal fragment can then be mobilized and pulled forward to allow the miniplate to be fixed (**Fig. 22.7**). The fixed fragment can thus be used for fixation of the osteotomy site, but clearly this type of fixation cannot be described as rigid. A period of intermaxillary fixation of at least 4 weeks is recommended for such patients.

Vertical Ramus Osteotomy

Introduction

The vertical ramus osteotomy has frequently been used in the past for the correction of mandibular hyperplasia (Robinson, 1956). The application of an intraoral vertical ramus osteotomy, however, almost precludes the use of rigid fixation, including miniplates, because of lack of access and the risk of damage to the inferior alveolar nerve.

This osteotomy, however, is still the best option if vertical movements of the ascending ramus are needed, or in cases where extreme rotations of the distal fragments are anticipated. This may occur in patients with facial asymmetries. Lengthening or shortening of the ascending ramus, using the vertical ramus osteotomy, can

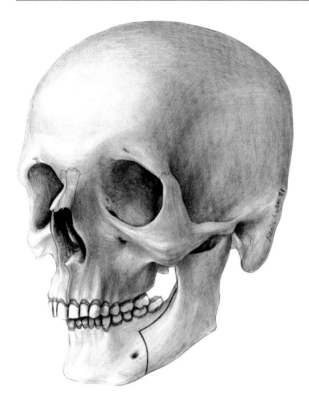

Fig. 22.5 Osteotomy design for advancement of the mandible.

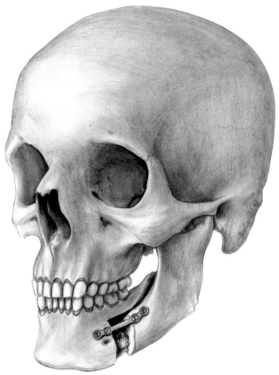

Fig. 22.6 A six-hole plate or a four-hole plate with a bridge is used to fix the fragments.

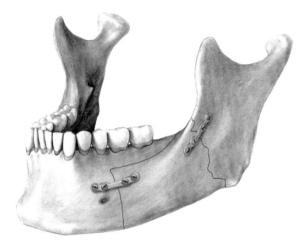

Fig. 22.7 A four-hole plate, used to fix an inadvertently fractured buccal fragment.

only be done through an extraoral route (extraoral vertical ramus osteotomy). Proper access to the fragments enables the surgeon to reduce the amount of bone needed (**Fig. 22.8**), or to position the proximal fragment with the condyle properly seated in the fossa. It also allows for the application of miniplates under controlled conditions.

Technique

Access is gained through a submandibular incision. Careful dissection, to avoid damage to the mandibular branch of the facial nerve, should expose the lateral aspect of the ascending ramus, up to the sigmoid notch. A vertical bone cut is made from the sigmoid notch to the angle of the mandible, its design depending on the preference of the surgeon. Care should be taken to avoid damage to the inferior alveolar nerve. The proximal fragment can be positioned with a gauze-packing instrument or forceps, after repositioning the distal fragment, placing the acrylic wafer and intermaxillary fixation.

A miniplate of appropriate design and length is bent to accommodate the anatomical contour and is fixed with 5 mm or 7 mm screws (**Fig. 22.9**). L-plates are found to be extremely useful for this purpose. If required, and if the anatomy allows, a second plate may be placed above the first. The surgeon, however, should be aware of the location of the inferior alveolar nerve near its entrance into the mandible. The buccal plate may be thin, which can give rise to damage to the nerve when screws enter the bony canal.

In this authors experience, one plate will suffice if only one side is treated in this way and the other side is treated with a sagittal split osteotomy, using the usual one-plate fixation.

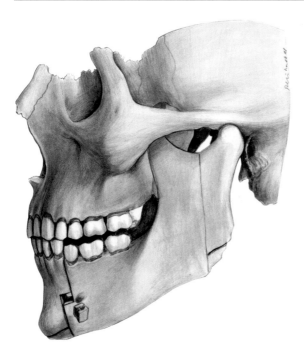

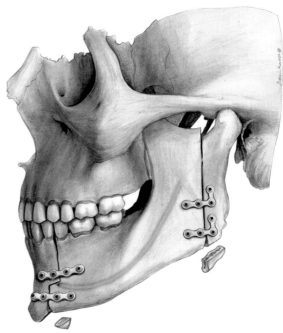

Fig. 22.8 Simultaneous osteotomies of the horizontal body and vertical ramus allow for cranial positioning of the premolar- and molar-bearing area of the mandible, in cases of posterior vertical open bite. Excess bone can be removed as indicated.

Fig. 22.9 Intermediate fragment positioned and fixed with appropriate miniplates.

Body (Step) Osteotomies

Introduction

Body osteotomies or ostectomies are particularly useful in cases where asymmetries in the horizontal part of the mandible require correction (Sandor, Stoelinga, and Tideman, 1982). They can also be used for patients who have teeth missing from the mandibular arch, thereby avoiding or minimizing the need for bridges, if setback osteotomies are performed. The best indications, however, are those cases in which the occlusal plane needs to be corrected because of reversed or extremely deep curves of Spee. In special cases, body osteotomies can be combined with vertical ramus osteotomies, such as the sagittal split osteotomy or intraoral vertical ramus osteotomy and extraoral vertical ramus osteotomy (Stoelinga and Leenen, 1992). They are also indicated where the surgeon may choose to do a body osteotomy on the one side and a ramus osteotomy on the other (see **Figs. 22.8**, **22.9**).

Body ostectomies anterior to the mental foramen are indicated in some edentulous patients with a reversed intermaxillary relationship caused by a combination of advanced alveolar resorption and a pre-existing hyperplastic mandibular body. A body osteotomy allows for correction of the anterior and transverse dimensions of the mandible in a controlled fashion. The mandible can be set back by taking out a planned amount of bone, while at

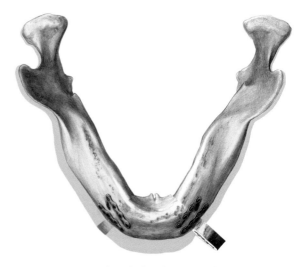

Fig. 22.10 Excision of a calculated amount of bone in the horizontal body allows for narrowing of the mandibular arch and relative setback of the chin.

the same time the transverse dimension can be reduced by inward rotation of the proximal fragments (**Fig. 22.10**).

Miniplates are ideal to fix the fragments rigidly in all body osteotomies, thus avoiding the need for intermaxillary fixation or splints.

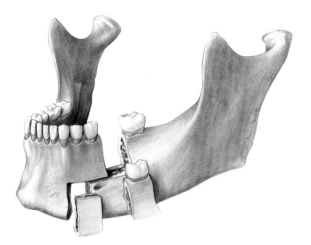

Fig. 22.11 Bone blocks removed to allow the mandible to be set back.

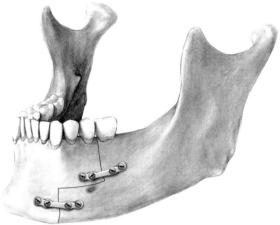

Fig. 22.12 Miniplate fixation using four-hole plates with a bridge.

Technique

The area where the osteotomy is to be performed is exposed through a mucoperiosteal incision and dissection. The design of the incision is largely defined by the anatomical situation, such as the presence of teeth. The mucoperiosteal dissection should also be performed on the lingual side to the level of the horizontal cut of the osteotomy. A stepped cut is made in the bone, avoiding damage to the inferior alveolar nerve. Where setback of the distal fragment is needed, the appropriate amount of bone is removed first, after which the horizontal bone cut is completed (**Fig. 22.11**). Following reposition of the distal and proximal fragments, the occlusion is secured using an acrylic splint and intermaxillary fixation.

A plate of appropriate length, which includes two holes in the proximal and distal segments, is selected and bent to fit the step in the bone contour. The plate is fixed with four screws of 5 mm or 7 mm length, below the mental foramen and mandibular canal (**Fig. 22.12**).

If the height of the mandible permits, a second plate is used and fixed above the level of the nerve. Care should be taken not to damage the apices of neighboring teeth. In those cases where application of a plate above the nerve is not possible, an arch bar should be used or an acrylic splint fixed to the lower teeth.

In body osteotomies in edentulous patients, there is no problem in using two plates on either side (see **Fig. 22.10**). However, attention should be paid to the course of the mandibular canal, so as to avoid penetrating it with the screws, which could cause nerve injury.

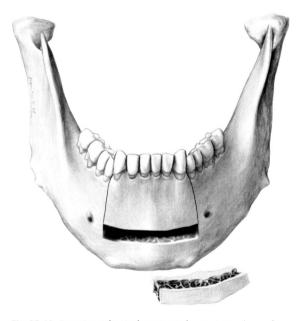

Fig. 22.13 Anterior subapical segmental osteotomy (according to Hofer) to correct supraposition of the lower anterior teeth.

Anterior Subapical Segmental Osteotomy

Introduction

This osteotomy, first introduced by Hofer (1942), is particularly suitable for correcting supraposition of the lower anterior teeth, but can also be used for advancement or setback in selected cases (**Fig. 22.13**). In most cases this osteotomy is performed in conjunction with ramus osteotomies to correct more complicated mandibular de-

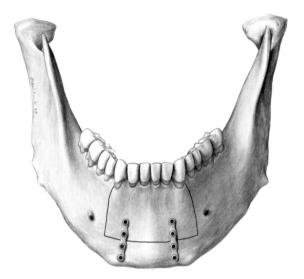

Fig. 22.14 Anterior subapical segmental osteotomy. Two four-hole plates, positioned vertically.

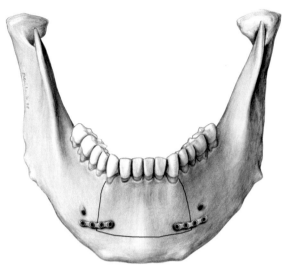

Fig. 22.15 Anterior subapical segmental osteotomy. Two four-hole plates, positioned horizontally.

formities. Stabilization of the anterior fragment is easily accomplished with miniplates, since muscular displacing forces tend to be minimal.

Technique

Following completion of the osteotomy, which is performed in the usual fashion, the fragment is maneuvered into place and temporarily secured with the aid of an acrylic splint. Intermaxillary fixation may be used at this stage, if necessary.

Two four-hole plates of any configuration may be used to stabilize the fragment, if placed in a vertical fashion (**Fig. 22.14**). However, this may not be feasible because of the presence of the roots of the anterior teeth. The plates may then be placed horizontally (**Fig. 22.15**), but this may cause the fragment to tilt. This can be counteracted, however, by a rigid orthodontic wire inserted postoperatively.

Genioplasties and Midline Symphyseal Osteotomies

Introduction

Genioplasties are widely used to correct chin abnormalities (Trauner and Obwegeser, 1957). Depending on the design of the osteotomy, the osseous chin can be moved in any direction and usually adequately fixed with wire osteosynthesis. Miniplates, however, can be extremely useful when augmentation is desired in a vertical dimension, or when extreme advancement is anticipated. In general,

an unstable symphyseal bone fragment can be adequately fixed with two miniplates.

Midline symphyseal osteotomies are sometimes performed to narrow or widen the lower dental arch. This, almost inevitably, has to be combined with bilateral ramus osteotomies to allow for these movements (**Fig. 22.18**). Narrowing of the mandible is fairly easy to achieve, since no muscle stretching is involved. A narrowing of up to 5 mm in the molar area is feasible, without too much tilting of the mandibular body. Widening of the mandible is much more difficult, since it involves stretching of the mylohyoid muscle. If anterior widening is desired, bone grafting is necessary to bridge the gaps. This procedure carries a considerable risk of periodontal damage. At present, widening of the anterior part of the mandible is usually achieved using osteodistraction techniques (see Chapter 28).

Miniplates are highly reliable in that adequate fixation of the fragments can be achieved, allowing for immediate release of intermaxillary fixation.

Technique

In genioplasties the fragment is held in place with bone clamps or forceps, and two four-hole plates of suitable length are selected to include two holes in the chinbone fragment and two in the body of the mandible. The best position is vertical (see **Fig. 22.16**) but, if anatomical circumstances preclude such a position, the plates may be placed in any other suitable direction and area, since displacing muscle forces are minimal.

The plates are bent to adapt to the anatomical situation and screws of 5 mm or 7 mm in length are used to fix the chin fragment. Existing gaps may be filled with either

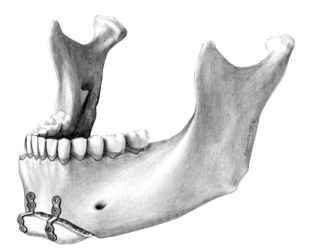

Fig. 22.16 Two four-hole plates are used to fix the advanced chin fragment.

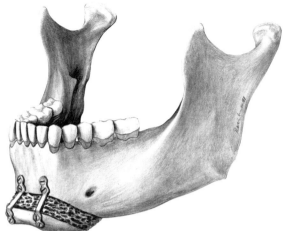

Fig. 22.17 Vertical lengthening of the chin requires grafting the gap. Miniplates are ideal to maintain the height gained.

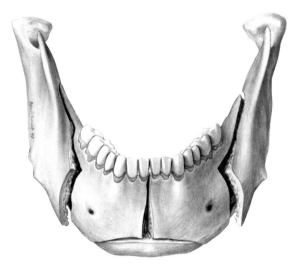

Fig. 22.18 Bilateral sagittal split osteotomy combined with a midline osteotomy to narrow the arch, and a genioplasty to advance the chin.

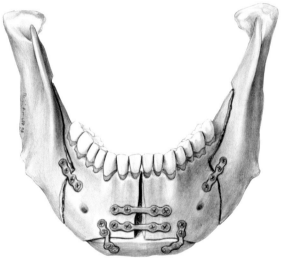

Fig. 22.19 Fixation of all fragments with appropriate mini-plates.

autogenous bone grafts or with allogenic material (see **Fig. 22.17**).

Midline osteotomies are best treated with two four-hole plates, according to Champys principles for treating symphyseal fractures. For this reason the proximal fragment is loosely fixed in intermaxillary fixation before the actual midline splitting is done. The bone cut is first made through the buccal cortical bone, between the roots of the central incisors. Below the level of the apices, the cut should also include the lingual cortex of the symphyseal body. Following insertion of an acrylic splint and loose intermaxillary fixation using 0.4-mm stainless steel wires—and accepting the fact that the occlusal fit will not be ideal at this stage—an osteotomy is used to complete the midline split by wedging and torquing this in-

strument. It is the intention that the lingual cortex of the alveolar part will now break. The two proximal fragments can then be maneuvered into their proper position and the intermaxillary fixation tightened. When narrowing the mandibular arch, the buccal gap will widen (**Fig. 22.18**). Two four-hole plates are adapted to the curvature of the buccal contour and fixed with 5-mm or 7-mm long screws (**Fig. 22.19**).

A genioplasty does not preclude the use of a midline osteotomy. In these cases it is recommended to carry out the osteotomy for the genioplasty first and then the midline split. Fixation, however, is first secured in the midline. The chinbone fragment is then fixed to the mandibular body (see **Fig. 22.19**).

23 Osteotomies of the Maxilla

Paul J. W. Stoelinga

Anterior Maxillary Segmental Osteotomy

Introduction

The anterior maxillary segmental osteotomy described by Wassmund (1935a) and Wunderer (1962) was one of the most frequently used osteotomies to set back the anterior segment of the maxilla in cases of dentoalveolar protrusion. With the increased cooperation between orthodontists and surgeons, the need for these osteotomies has been drastically reduced. Yet, there are still indications for performing an anterior maxillary segmental osteotomy, particularly when vertical movements are required or when asymmetries need to be corrected. Miniplates may play an important role in stabilizing the anterior segment.

Technique

Both the Wassmund and Wunderer approaches include a distally curved but basically vertical incision in the buccal vestibule. This usually provides sufficient access to apply a four-hole plate on each side to stabilize the fragment. Attention should be paid to the location of the root tips of the canines and bicuspids in order not to make burr holes in these roots. There is usually room for one plate on each side, which provides enough stability, particularly when an acrylic splint is wired in place (**Fig. 23.1**).

Posterior Maxillary Segmental Osteotomy

Introduction

The bilateral posterior maxillary segmental osteotomy, introduced by West and Epker (1972), to close the anterior skeletal open bite is rarely used anymore, because tilting osteotomies on a Le Fort I level have largely replaced this technique. The posterior maxillary segmental osteotomy, however, has several other indications. It may be used to close gaps in the alveolar process when teeth are missing, or to correct asymmetries in the arch form in any direction.

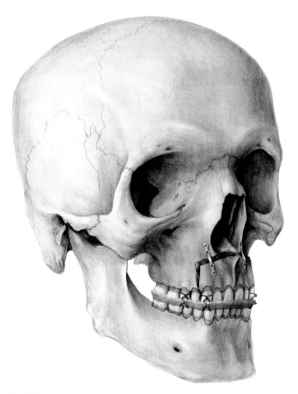

Fig. 23.1 Anterior segment secured by two four-hole plates and an acrylic splint wired to the maxillary teeth.

The technique is most useful, however, when the lesser fragment in patients with cleft lip and palate needs to be repositioned. Miniplates, but especially microplates, are almost indispensable for stabilizing the fragment.

Technique

The technique most commonly used entails a buccal mucoperiosteal pedicle as the main blood supply to the fragment. This implies that a relatively small vertical incision can be made which, of course, limits the access. After completion of the osteotomy through a palatal incision, the fragment is maneuvered into place and fixed to the main fragment using an acrylic splint. A suitable four-hole microplate is selected, which may be straight or L-shaped. In most cases only one microplate can be placed, fixed

The stability of Le Fort I osteotomies using wire osteosynthesis is adequate, particularly if advancement and intrusion is the main purpose. When extrusion is wanted, however, the stability is far from acceptable. Furthermore, it is difficult (if not impossible) to predict the extent of any relapse that will occur, even if bone grafts are used.

Miniplates and microplates have also proven to be highly successful in providing stability in cases of extrusion of the maxilla (Baker et al., 1992). This is particularly important when carrying out bimaxillary surgery, where postoperative positional changes of the maxilla can be detrimental to the final result.

Since the application of miniplates and microplates is simple and quick, a further advantage of using them to stabilize the fragment is a considerable reduction in operating time.

Technique

A Le Fort I osteotomy is performed in the usual fashion and the fragment is temporarily secured by intermaxillary fixation. The mandibular–maxillary complex can then be placed in the desired position, but attention should be paid to avoid pulling the condyles out of the fossae when rotating the mandible. If this happens it usually requires bone to be trimmed in the posterior area of the osteotomy. This mistake is particularly prone to happen when intrusion is the main objective.

The plates can best be fixed at the zygomatic buttress and alongside the piriform aperture, since the bone in these locations is usually thicker than in the canine fossa. Miniplates or microplates are bent to follow the curvature of the bone structures or to accommodate discrepancies that may exist in a transverse or anteroposterior plane. Two straight, four-hole or L-shaped plates on each side are usually sufficient to adequately stabilize the maxilla (**Fig. 23.3**). An additional plate, placed horizontally under the piriform aperture, may be necessary in the case of midline splits to adjust for transverse discrepancies. This plate can be bent under the nasal spine (**Fig. 23.4**). The same applies when simultaneous segmental osteotomies are performed in the bicuspid–molar area.

Bone grafts should be used when defects are apparent after repositioning of the fragment. This is particularly important when the maxilla is moved downward. The blocks are contoured to fit the gaps in the lateral sinus wall and preferably placed with their cortex toward the plates (**Fig. 23.5**). If necessary, a screw may be inserted in the free bone graft to help to stabilize the graft.

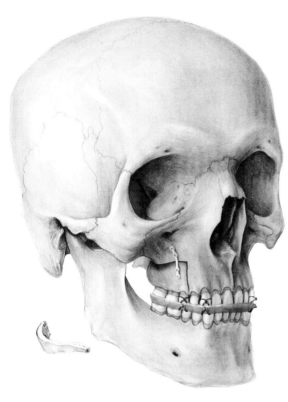

Fig. 23.2 Posterior segment secured with one four-hole microplate and an acrylic splint wired to the maxillary teeth.

with 4 mm or 6 mm long screws. Defects resulting from positional changes of the segment should be grafted, preferably using autogenous bone. One plate does not provide enough stability, but in combination with an orthodontic arch wire or acrylic splint, or both, stability is usually adequate (**Fig. 23.2**).

Le Fort I Osteotomy

Introduction

The Le Fort I osteotomy, first described by Wassmund (1935b) and later standardized by Obwegeser (1965) and Bell (1975), has become the most frequently used osteotomy in the maxilla. This osteotomy allows for almost any movement of the tooth-bearing area of the maxilla including advancement, caudal and cranial positioning, tilting, and rotation in a horizontal plane. All these movements can be achieved fairly easily, and often two or even more directional changes can be accomplished at the same time. Narrowing or widening of the arch can also be accomplished by extra palatal cuts. The only movement not easily achieved is a setback, since it implies cutting away bone in the tuberosity area or pterygoid plate.

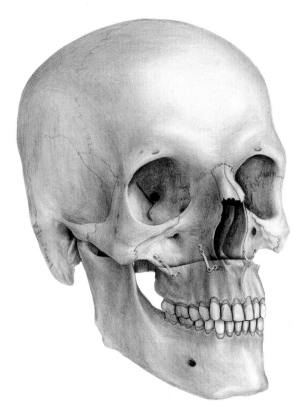

Fig. 23.3 Position of four L-shaped microplates with bridges to secure the maxillary segment.

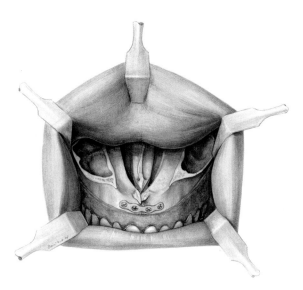

Fig. 23.4 Four-hole microplate bent around the nasal spine and fixed to maintain the transverse position of the expanded maxilla.

Quadrangular Osteotomy

Introduction

The quadrangular osteotomy, as introduced by Kufner (1960), is especially useful for patients with maxillary hypoplasia extending to the infraorbital and zygomatic area. Several modifications have been described, mostly related to the extent of the osteotomy in the lateral orbital wall and zygomatic area. The basic benefit from this osteotomy, however, is the improvement of infraorbital and malar projection when the whole zygomatic–maxillary complex is advanced, leaving the nose behind.

Miniplates and microplates will provide sufficient stability, if applied properly in strategic locations; additional intermaxillary fixation may be necessary for a few weeks because it is not always possible to achieve truly rigid fixation.

Technique

A modification developed by Stoelinga and Brouns (1996) is performed by an intraoral route. The nasal aperture, infraorbital rims and part of the lateral orbital wall with the zygomatic prominence are exposed via a vestibular incision, which is carried all the way to the back. The osteotomy runs to the infraorbital rim, although the bone cut runs around the infraorbital foramen, to prevent damage to the nerve. The lateral bone cut may be carried as far laterally as necessary, but should include the zygomatic bone. The extension in the lateral orbital wall depends on the needs of the patient. If that part needs to come forward as well, a coronal incision may be necessary to gain adequate access to this area (**Fig. 23.6**).

After advancement of the maxilla and temporary intermaxillary fixation, the mandibulary–maxillary complex is maneuvered into position. Bone grafts are contoured and used to bridge the gaps, particularly in the infraorbital region and the zygomatic and medial areas. An onlay graft is used to cover the infraorbital foramen, but care should be taken not to put pressure on the nerve. Fixation can be achieved by placing a four-hole plate in the zygomatic area, which crosses the gap on both sides (**Fig. 23.7**). If enough space is available, a second plate may be placed parallel to the first one.

There is not usually enough bone volume available to place another plate in, for instance, the medial area. The infraorbital "wing" is typically very thin, and the presence of the lacrimal duct precludes placement of screws in the lateral nasal wall. This often leaves the maxilla attached to only two or four plates in the posterior area, which theoretically may allow for a tilting movement. Intermaxillary fixation may therefore be necessary for a few weeks. The length of this period depends on the degree of mobility

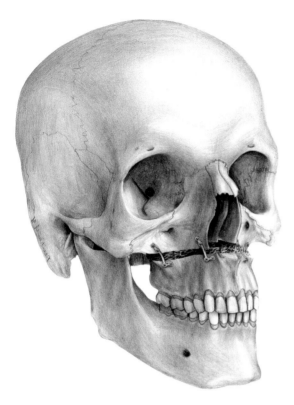

Fig. 23.5 Four four-hole plates to fix the extruded maxilla. An interpositional bone graft in place.

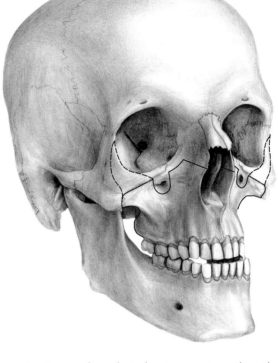

Fig. 23.6 Design of quadrangular osteotomy avoiding the course of the infraorbital nerve. The dotted line represents extension in the lateral orbital rim, for which a coronal incision is necessary.

shown by the maxilla. This should be monitored closely by clinical examination or cephalometric evaluation.

Le Fort II Osteotomy

Introduction

The Le Fort II osteotomy, introduced by Henderson and Jackson (1973), is designed to correct nasomaxillary hypoplasia or depressions resulting from trauma. Limited numbers of patients may benefit from this osteotomy but, when indicated, it serves its purpose well. It is particularly useful for patients suffering from Binder syndrome, and some cleft patients with a hypoplastic maxilla in conjunction with a depressed nasal bridge.

The best approach to the naso-orbital complex is achieved through a coronal incision. Plates used to fix the fragment, therefore, should be as small as possible, since their removal would require repeated coronal dissection. For this reason, and because the bone to be used for osteosynthesis is usually thin and prone to break when larger screws are used, microplates are the best solution.

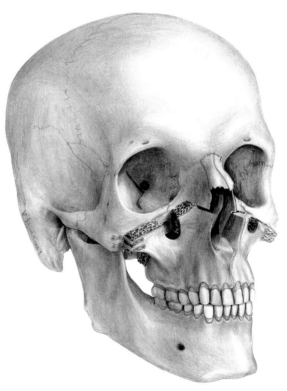

Fig. 23.7 One or two miniplates secured along the infrazygomatic crest on both sides provides sufficient stability.

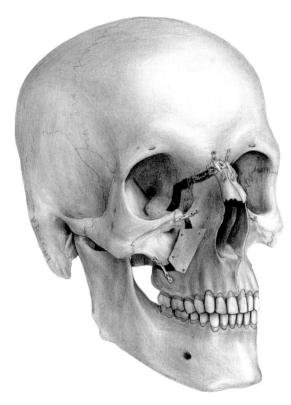

Fig. 23.8 Maxilla advanced according to the Le Fort II pattern. Microplates along the nasal bridge, infraorbital rim and infrazygomatical crest provide sufficient stability for the advanced maxilla. Corticocancellous bone grafts are necessary to fill the gaps.

Technique

Access to the nasomaxillary complex is gained through a coronal incision and dissection to the orbit and nasal bridge. An intraoral, vestibular incision will allow exposure of the infraorbital area and tuberosity. The infraorbital rim should be exposed through either a conjunctival or subciliary incision. After completing the bone cuts in the way described by Henderson and Jackson (1973), the nasomaxillary complex is mobilized and brought forward. When proper advancement has been achieved, intermaxillary fixation is applied and the mandibular–nasomaxillary complex is maneuvered into the desired position. Bone grafts are contoured and used to fill the gaps, especially in the nasal bridge area, the infraorbital rim and lateral sinus wall. In most cases it is necessary to use an onlay graft on the dorsum of the nose. For this reason careful subperiosteal–subperichondrial dissection should be performed, which may be carried as far distally as the tip of the nose.

An appropriate piece of cortical bone should be carved to fit the recipient site and inserted. Stabilization is achieved by fixing four-hole straight or L-shaped microplates along the nasal bridge and the infraorbital rims and,

if possible, along the infrazygomatical crest (**Fig. 23.8**). The plates should be bent to adapt to the curvature of the bone and the steps and can be fixed with 4 mm or 6 mm long microscrews.

At the end of the procedure intermaxillary fixation can usually be released, since four-point fixation will be adequate. Loose intermaxillary fixation with rubber bands may be used to guide occlusion if indicated.

Le Fort III Osteotomy

Introduction

The Le Fort III osteotomy (Gillies and Harrison, 1950; Tessier, 1967), performed through a subcranial route, has only limited applications. Patients with nasomaxillozygomatical hypoplasia or recession because of trauma may be candidates for this type of osteotomy. Mild forms of telecanthus or hypertelorism may also be treated using a modified Le Fort III osteotomy. This osteotomy may also be performed in conjunction with a Le Fort I osteotomy, if the hypoplasia in the dentoalveolar area is more pronounced than in the midfacial region. Miniplates and microplates may be used because usually relatively thick bone struts are available for screw fixation. Microplates, however, are preferred, because plate removal would almost necessarily imply exposure of the naso-orbital skeleton again, via a coronal approach. Miniplates tend to show through the relatively thin skin, whereas microplates can be left in place.

Technique

Just as in the Le Fort II osteotomy, access to the maxillofacial skeleton is achieved by a combination of a coronal incision and dissection and an intraoral vestibular incision. Through this route the whole nasomaxillozygomatical area can be adequately exposed. The osteotomy is performed as described by Gillies or Tessier, or modified in any way to meet the needs of the patient. Once the osteotomy is complete, the whole complex is gently mobilized and brought forward. Intermaxillary fixation is applied and the mandibular–maxillary complex is maneuvered into place. Corticocancellous bone grafts are contoured to fit the defects that are the result of the advancement of the fragment. In particular, the lateral orbital rim and nasal bridge form ideal areas for plate fixation (**Fig. 23.9**). Miniplates or microplates are selected and bent to fit the anatomical situation. If possible, four-hole plates are selected in either shape to accommodate the needs. Since at least a four-point fixation can be achieved, the fixation can be considered sufficiently rigid to allow for immediate release of intermaxillary fixation.

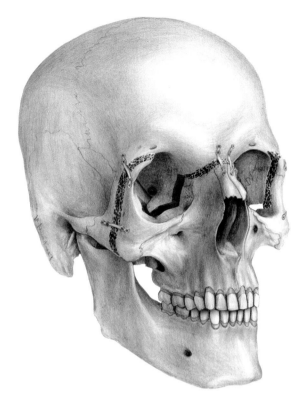

Fig. 23.9 Le Fort III osteotomy to advance the midface. Note corticocancellous bone grafts in the gaps of the lateral orbital wall and nasal bridge. Microplates along nasal bridge and lateral orbital wall provide sufficient stability.

Osteotomies in Cleft Lip and Palate Patients

Introduction

Maxillary osteotomies in cleft lip and palate patients are different in that scars limit the maneuverability of the fragments. The vascularization of the tooth-bearing area is also impaired both by scar tissue, because of previous operations, and anatomical aberrations inherent in the deformity. Several studies have shown that the stability of Le Fort I osteotomies using wire osteosynthesis is far from adequate. Segmental osteotomies as proposed by Tideman, Stoelinga, and Gallia (1980) appear to give rise to better results. This technique also allows for simultaneous closure of the alveolopalatal bony defect without putting the vitality of the fragments at risk.

At present, most patients with cleft lip and palate will undergo early secondary bone grafting at age 8–10 years. This allows eruption of the canine into the arch and orthodontic alignment of the teeth. Yet, in around 20% of such patients a Le Fort I osteotomy is indicated to correct a maxillary hypoplasia or misalignment of the dentoalveolar segments.

Stoelinga et al. (1987) pointed out that in most of these patients, whether they had early secondary bone grafts or not, segmental procedures are necessary. For reasons of safety a buccal mucoperiosteal pedicle is preferred over a palatal pedicle, because the latter is often scarred and thus less reliable as the only source of vascularization to the fragment. Only in cases of straight Le Fort I advancement without segmental procedures is a limited vestibular incision warranted.

Miniplates have proven to provide much better stability than wire osteosynthesis (Erbe, Stoelinga, and Leenen, 1996). They also allow for fixation of fragments to form a solid arch. Miniplates or microplates can easily be used to span the gaps in the alveolar region.

Technique

Unilateral clefts are treated by a Le Fort I approach to the major fragment and a segmental approach to the lesser fragment. The incision for the greater fragment may be made in the usual fashion, although the author prefers an incision along the gingiva in the anterior region (**Fig. 23.10**). This will facilitate closure around the cleft. The lesser fragment is approached as described for the posterior maxillary segmental osteotomy. Following mobilization of the fragments, an acrylic splint is wired into the upper arch, and temporary intermaxillary fixation is applied. The maxillomandibular complex is then maneuvered into position. Miniplates or microplates are used to fix the major fragment in the usual Le Fort I fashion. The lesser fragment is usually fixed with one, four-hole plate. In some cases it might be better to span the alveolopalatal cleft to help to maintain the fragment in position (**Fig. 23.11**). Bone grafts are used to bridge the gaps or to reconstruct the nasal floor and alveolus.

Bilateral clefts are usually approached by incisions along the clefts (**Fig. 23.12**). The anterior fragment is treated as in the Wunderer anterior maxillary segmental osteotomy, in that its buccal mucoperiosteal attachment remains intact. This allows adequate repositioning of the fragment, even in an anterior direction, up to approximately 8 mm. The two posterior fragments are approached as described for the lesser fragment in the unilateral cleft patient.

Following mobilization, an acrylic splint is wired into the upper arch and temporary intermaxillary fixation is applied. The maxillomandibular complex is rotated upward and fixed with two to four miniplates, depending on accessibility. The anterior fragment may be separately fixed to the two posterior fragments. Bone grafts are used to reconstruct the nasal floor and to bridge the gaps and fill the alveolar clefts.

In patients with either unilateral or bilateral clefts early release of intermaxillary fixation depends on the quality

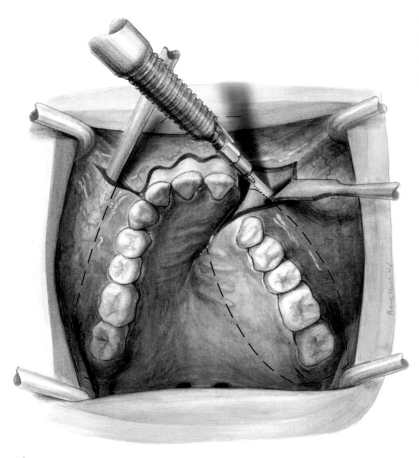

Fig. 23.10 Incisions to provide sufficient access to carry out Le Fort I osteotomy on the major fragment and segmental osteotomy on the minor fragment. Dotted lines represent the bone cuts.

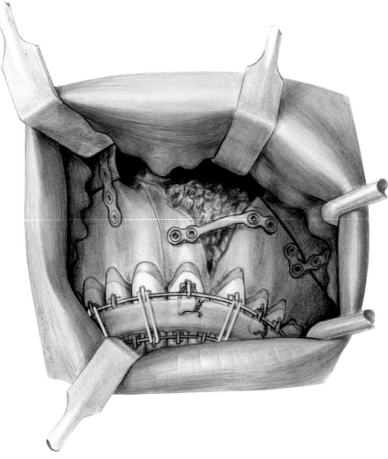

Fig. 23.11 Patient with unilateral cleft palate in whom maxillary segments have been secured with microplates. One plate is used to bridge the clefts, which adds to the stability of the transverse repositioning. Bone grafts are used to fill the gaps and the alveolopalatal cleft.

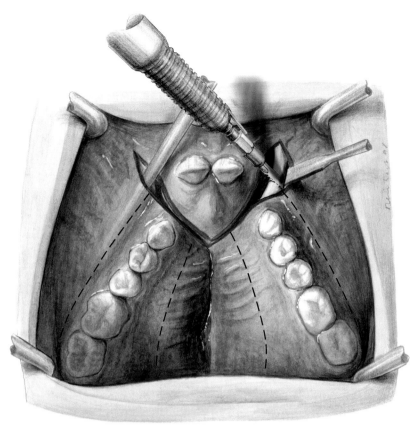

Fig. 23.12 Incision used to approach the bilateral cleft lip and palate. The two lateral fragments are approached through a tunneling technique.

of the fixation achieved. If only three plates are used in patients with unilateral clefts, this might be sufficient because the major fragment is usually adequately fixed. The acrylic splint in conjunction with the one plate will be enough to provide stability. In cases of bilateral clefts, in which there is not enough access to fix the posterior fragments with two plates each, fixation will probably not be rigid enough to allow for early release of intermaxillary fixation. In those patients a period of 4–6 weeks of intermaxillary fixation might be necessary to obtain a good result.

24 Orthognathic Surgery Distance Screws

Konrad Wangerin and Henning Gropp

Introduction

The simultaneous osteotomy of the maxilla and mandible, first described by Obwegeser in 1970, runs the risk of incorrect positioning of the maxilla, the mandible, and both condyles, if the opration is done without full supporting actions, including (but not limited to) an exact diagnosis, preoperative orthodontics, operation planning (method and simulation), and careful postoperative control. The use of miniplates and microplates in the midface and the mandible has led to greater convenience for patients; nevertheless, without the additional supporting activities referred to above the results will be dependent solely on the experience of the surgeon. Throughout the last quarter of the 20th century, significant developments in fields such as operation planning, operation simulation, and support skills and services have led to reproducible, lasting, and stable results from this operation.

The double-splint method (Lindorf, 1977) is frequently used to control the horizontal dimension during the step-by-step positioning of maxilla and mandible in reaching a neutral occlusion. Controlling the vertical dimension is done intraoperatively by direct measurements between screw holes above and below the Le Fort I osteotomy line, or indirectly with extraoral appliances (Speculand and Jackson, 1984; Neubert, Bitter, and Somsiri, 1988; Luhr and Jäger, 1994), or intraorally using positioning plates (Wangerin, 1990).

Technique

After preoperative orthognathic treatment, extensive clinical diagnosis, planning, and simulation of the operation are performed.

Clinical Diagnosis

First of all, the necessary clinical aesthetic parameters are considered and recorded, including the vertical facial symmetry that embraces the harmony of the three parts of the medial section of the face, the laugh line of the upper lip and the profile of the face. The stomatognathic system is evaluated, including the chewing function, tongue and mimic muscle activities, the condition of the teeth and the periodontium, and function of both temporomandibular joints.

Radiographic Diagnosis

A panoramic radiograph is taken to judge the position of the mandibular canal and the wisdom teeth, where present. A lateral cephalogram is made for the Bergen analysis (Hasund, 1974), which provides information about maxillary and mandibular growth. In cases of asymmetries of the face a posterior–anterior cephalogram is necessary to determine the skeletal dimensions of abnormal jaw growth. These analyses are the basis for planning the operation.

Model Diagnosis

The unstable malocclusion leads to an undefined position of the condyles (**Fig. 24.1**). Therefore, a check bite in centric occlusion is performed to put the condyles in a physiological position (**Fig. 24.2**). These condylar positions are monitored radiographically while using the check bite. Plaster models of the maxilla and mandible are made to analyze the orthodontically aligned upper and lower dental arches.

Planning

Cephalometric measurements on the lateral cephalogram determine the planned maxillary displacement. The aesthetic parameters are considered. The mandible is then placed in neutral occlusion to the maxilla. After analysis of the new facial profile a decision is made to determine the chin correction.

Simulation

The model of the maxilla is cut at the level of the Le Fort I osteotomy line. The model of the mandible is cut at the lower border of the mandible. By using the centric check bite, which is equivalent to the first splint, these separate

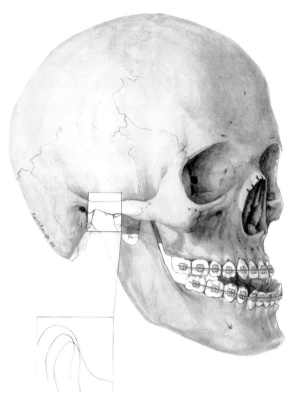

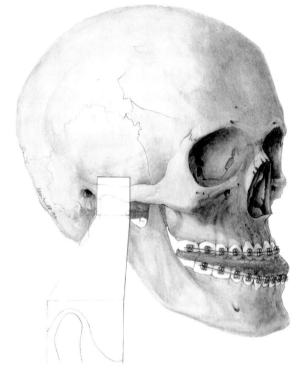

Fig. 24.1 Unstable class III malocclusion and anterior open bite with continuously changing occlusal contacts, intensified during orthodontic movement of the teeth, and permanently changing positions of both mandibular condyles.

Fig. 24.2 Preoperative normal positioning of both mandibular condyles by an occlusal splint, which determines the maxillo-mandibular relation.

models are arbitrarily mounted in an individual articulator system, for example, a SAM articulator, so that they are level with an upper plane corresponding to the lower border of the mandible. Thus both jaws can be shifted in their proper planes. Subsequently the maxillary model is loosened from the upper plane and fixed with glue in the new position. The second splint is prepared in this relationship.

The mandibular model is then loosened from the lower plane and brought into a neutral occlusal relationship to the maxilla. The mandibular model is glued to the lower plane, the difference in height being filled with plaster. The third occlusal splint is prepared.

If maxillary advancement is not possible, as for example in a case of extreme class III malocclusion with a deep bite of the upper frontal teeth, a fourth splint to spread the dental arches must be prepared first to perform this simulation.

Surgery

The maxilla is exposed from the piriform aperture to the maxillary tuberosities by a buccal marginal rim incision. In the mandible the buccal and lingual parts of the angles of

the mandible are exposed by incising the gingiva from the premolars to the anterior edge of the ascending ramus, and by separating it from the inserting masseter muscles and the pterygoid muscles. The first splint is inserted, the condyles are placed in the physiological position, and intermaxillary fixation is applied using rubber bands or wire ligatures.

Two rigid titanium positioning plates are bent to fit the distance from the body of the zygoma to the buccal surface of the mandible on either side, without tension (**Fig. 24.3**). They are fixed with two monocortical screws on each end and immediately removed. Their purpose is to enable the centric condyle–fossa relationships to be maintained during the operation.

Intermaxillary fixation is released and the first splint is removed. A Le Fort I osteotomy is performed and the maxilla is completely mobilized. The second splint is inserted and the mobile maxilla is fixed to the intact mandible by means of rubber bands (**Fig. 24.4**). The maxillomandibular complex can now be rotated cranially by a rotational movement in both temporomandibular joints (**Fig. 24.5**). The new position of the maxilla is controlled by the positioning plates which, refixed to the buccal surfaces of the mandible and after rotation of the maxillomandibular complex, rigidly fix the maxilla to the zygoma

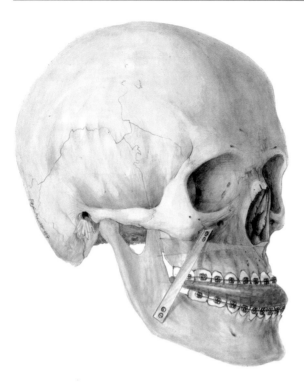

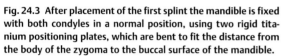

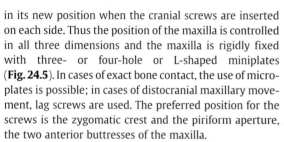

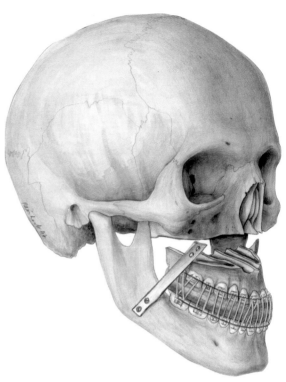

Fig. 24.3 After placement of the first splint the mandible is fixed with both condyles in a normal position, using two rigid titanium positioning plates, which are bent to fit the distance from the body of the zygoma to the buccal surface of the mandible.

Fig. 24.4 After Le Fort I osteotomy, total mobilization of the maxilla, placement of the second splint and fixation of the maxilla to the mandible, the maxillomandibular complex is autorotated, until the cranial plate holes correspond to the screw holes in the body of the zygoma. Control of the new position of the maxilla in three dimensions is possible.

in its new position when the cranial screws are inserted on each side. Thus the position of the maxilla is controlled in all three dimensions and the maxilla is rigidly fixed with three- or four-hole or L-shaped miniplates (**Fig. 24.5**). In cases of exact bone contact, the use of microplates is possible; in cases of distocranial maxillary movement, lag screws are used. The preferred position for the screws is the zygomatic crest and the piriform aperture, the two anterior buttresses of the maxilla.

The positioning plates, intermaxillary immobilization, and splint can now be removed. Subsequently, the sagittal splitting of the mandibular rami is performed (**Figs. 24.6, 24.7**). After mobilization of the osteotomized mandibular body the third splint is inserted and wired to the maxilla. The mobile mandible is moved to fit the splint and fixed to the maxilla by rubber bands. The rigid positioning plates are reinserted to ensure correct positioning of the condyles by connecting the buccal surfaces of the mandible with the zygoma. By means of three or four positional screws placed transbuccally into the mandible, the condyles are kept in their physiological position (**Fig. 24.8**). It is possible to use an angular screwdriver for the intraoral approach without an extraoral buccal stab incision. Miniplates on the buccal aspect of the mandible can be used to fix the sagittal osteotomies.

In cases where a patient has a cleft lip and palate, the use of positioning plates is not recommended because of the risk posed by the disturbed blood supply to the maxilla. In these cases the very limited bone exposure through the vestibular approach is not suitable for placing positioning plates.

Once intermaxillary fixation is removed, the new temporomandibular joint function is finally controlled by using the third splint for 6 weeks.

Skeletal Stability

One year postoperatively, perfect vertical and horizontal skeletal stability after correction has been reported in class III cases (Hoffmeister and Wangerin, 1995). In class II cases, the maxilla is stable but a horizontal mandibular relapse of 0.7° is seen, because of the high tension of the surrounding soft tissue. Open bite is corrected in all cases by maxillary osteotomy. In all class III cases with open bite, a stable horizontal dimension was seen but also a vertical maxillary relapse of 2.7°, probably caused by the preoperative orthodontic treatment or a pathologic tongue function. In class II cases with open bite, correction of the open bite was stable in all cases, but there was a

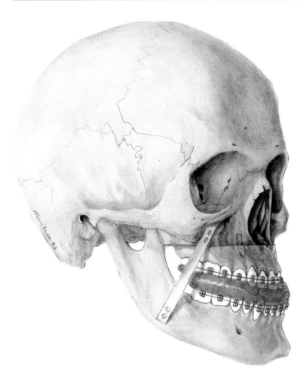

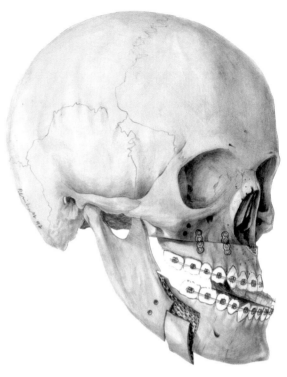

Fig. 24.5 The maxilla is fixed in the planned new position by placement of plates at the zygomatic crests and piriform rims. The open bite is corrected and the maxilla is advanced in the planned position.

Fig. 24.6 Sagittal splitting of the ascending mandibular rami with removal of the buccal cortical plate and placing the mandible in the planned position, guided by the third splint.

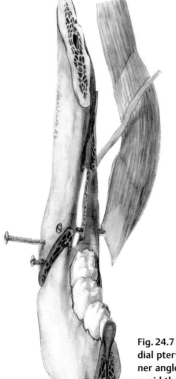

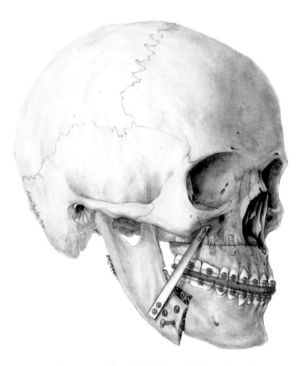

Fig. 24.7 Loosening of the medial pterygoid muscle at the inner angle of the mandible to avoid the relapse movement of the mandible.

Fig. 24.8 After using the third splint and after physiologic repositioning of both mandibular condyles, fixation of the mandible by means of transbuccally placed position screws is performed.

small horizontal and vertical maxillary relapse. The probable explanation is that the change of maxillary position in two directions, rotation and advancement, seems to be a less stable movement. In these cases Wangerin and coworkers considered using a bone graft from the hip. If an open bite alone was corrected by maxillary osteotomy, there was an amazing skeletal stability after 1 year (Hoffmeister and Wangerin, 1995). Reoperation in 2% of patients was necessary because of bad splits, temporomandibular joint problems, or malocclusions.

Because of the good results achieved by this method, Hoffmeister and Wangerin (1995) have extended the indications for bimaxillary surgery to include correcting low false positions of the maxilla and mandible. Around 80% of class II and class III orthognathic surgery cases can be corrected by bimaxillary osteotomies.

When only mandibular surgery is indicated, the positional screw technique can also be performed. Before sagittal split osteotomy is performed, mandibulomaxillary position plates are applied with the splint in a centric position and are taken out immediately.

After osteotomy, the mandible is brought into the class I position using a second splint and intermaxillary fixation is undertaken. The position plates are applied and positional screws inserted. Once the position plates are removed, the planned mandibular position and occlusion are confirmed.

25 The Adjustable Miniplate for Sagittal Split Ramus Osteotomy

Ulrich Joos

Introduction

After sagittal split osteotomy, osteosynthesis for stabilization of the fragments is usually performed by means of rigid or semirigid fixation to avoid maxillomandibular fixation. Sometimes, this leads to malpositioning of the fragments with resulting "immediate relapse" or disturbances of the temporomandibular joints. Therefore, the split-fix plate with a glider was developed, which allows three-dimensional adjustment, even after fixation of the fragments. The configuration of the system avoids intraoperative dislocation of the mandibular condyle. The method was used successfully in 40 patients, of whom 27 had mandibular retrognathism and 13 had mandibular prognathism. In particular, there has been no evidence of resorptive changes. There were no postoperative complications (Joos, 1998).

Method

The plate is designed for use with the 2 mm osteosynthesis system, and has two holes at each end of the plate for final fixation. Instead of being solid, the middle of the plate has two horizontal struts (**Fig. 25.1**). This gives the plate a maximum bending moment edge-strength of 520.2 Nmm and a surface elasticity of 5.4 N. The plate has a remarkably high torsional strength of 469 Nmm. The elasticity of the adjustable sagittal ramus osteotomy plate and a 2-mm mandibular plate shows comparable edge and torsional values, whereas the adjustable plate is about three times more flexible when bent along its flat surface. To adjust the fixation, a small mobile clamping element compresses the two struts of the bone plate to the underlying bone, allowing temporary rigid fixation. Using the adjustable clamping element, sagittal and vertical corrections of the position of the anterior segment are possible by loosening the screw that fixes the clamping element to the bone.

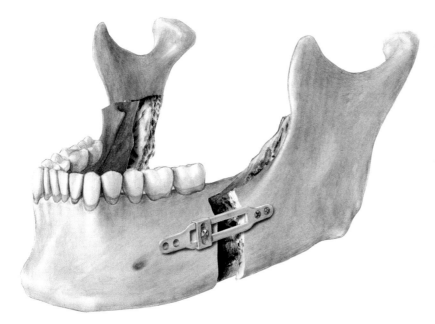

Fig. 25.1 Three-dimensional correction of the split-fix plate after fixation by two screws in the proximal segment. The adjustable clamping element is in position. The clamping element holds the proximal and distal segments safely in place. After the mandible has been correctly positioned, the two distal screws are placed monocortically into the bone plate and the clamping element is then removed.

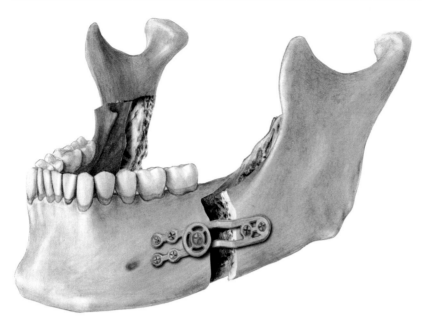

Fig. 25.2 A modification of the adjustable miniplate.

Technique

After the sagittal split osteotomy is complete, maxillomandibular fixation is secured. The split-fix bone plate should be positioned so that there is a sufficient amount of bone plate resting on the lateral cortex of the anterior segment to accommodate the clamping element. A hole of 1.5 mm diameter is drilled through the anterior extension of the proximal segment to accommodate the bone plate. The plate is secured to the proximal segment with a screw 6 mm long and 2 mm in diameter. The second hole is drilled through the proximal segment and a second screw is inserted to secure the bone plate rigidly. The proximal segment is then manipulated into its correct position and a 1.5-mm hole is drilled into the lateral cortex of the distal segment between the two struts of the plate. The clamping element is then placed over the hole and a 6-mm long screw is used to "clamp" the bone plate to the outer cortex of the distal segment.

The same procedure is carried out on the opposite side. The maxillomandibular fixation is then released and the occlusion verified. If the mandible does not rotate passively into the proper relationship with the maxilla, the adjustable clamping element can be loosened, the proximal segment repositioned, the clamping element retightened, and the occlusion re-evaluated. Once the proper occlusion has been established, the patient is placed back into maxillomandibular fixation and the two distal screws are placed monocortically into the bone plate. After placement of the two screws into the distal segment, the clamping element is removed.

A modification of the adjustable miniplate has been developed (**Fig. 25.2**). After application of these miniplates an evaluation of the function of the mandibular joint did not reveal any restriction. On the contrary, with Angle class II malocclusion, function of the mandibular joint could even be improved (Kleier et al., 1998).

26 Craniofacial Surgery

Hermann F. Sailer

Hypertelorism

The surgical correction of hypertelorism, perhaps the most breathtaking procedure seen in modern surgery, was developed by Paul Tessier (1967, 1972).

In principle, the operation consists of the cutting out of the orbits from the anterior and medial cranial fossae and medially rotating the upper midface with the orbital contents.

A coronal and a median transnasal and transfrontal approach is used to expose the anterior half of the skull, the supraorbital rims, the whole nasal skeleton, the lateral orbital rims and walls, the zygomatic complex, and the infraorbital area as far as possible from the temporal access. Often a transconjunctival approach (Sailer, 1977, 1978) is used for better control of the median and lower orbital wall. The inner canthal ligaments are exposed and preserved and the periorbital tissues carefully stripped off the bone on all four sides of the orbit. The infraorbital area and the canine fossa is approached via an upper vestibular incision.

With the aid of preoperative planning using computed tomographic scans, three-dimensional imaging, stereolithography models, and the necessary clinical data (Sailer and Grätz, 1995), the craniotomy and osteotomy lines are outlined with a Toller burr (**Fig. 26.1**).

A simulation of the operation with the aid of a stereolithography model should always be performed. After the craniotomy, a supraorbital bandeau is removed and the anterior skull base, the crista galli, and the anterior olfactory nerve filaments are exposed. First the interorbital bone and most of the nasal skeleton are removed (**Fig. 26.2**), then gradually the bone around the olfactory nerve filaments (using magnifying loops) and the inter-

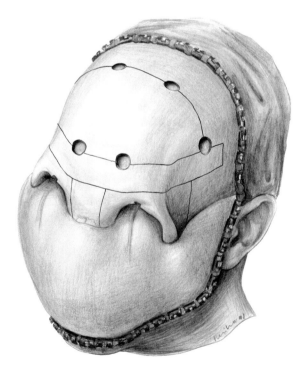

Fig. 26.1 Hypertelorism procedure. The osteotomy lines and burr holes are outlined.

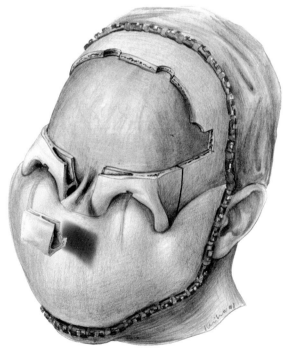

Fig. 26.2 After craniotomy and removal of the frontal bone the interorbital bone structures including the nasal ones are removed and the olfactory filaments carefully preserved when removing the anterior part of the cribriform plate.

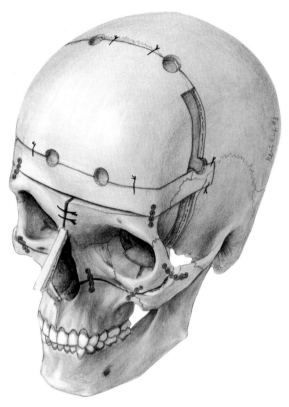

Fig. 26.3 After median rotation of the orbits with the aid of two wires in the glabela region the orbital structures are fixed by microplates and titanium wires and all defects bridged by lyocartilage and lyobone. A piece of calvarial bone is taken (left side) for reconstruction of the nose.

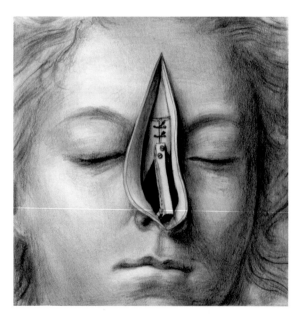

Fig. 26.4 Finally, the nasal frame work is reconstructed using a piece of calvarial bone which is fixed by mini screws to the glabela area. The surplus skin in the nasal and frontal area is removed (Rosalba Carriera, *Self-portrait*, ca. 1710/1720, Kupferstichkabinett, Berlin).

orbital ethmoidal cells are removed (Sailer and Landolt, 1987a, b).

The osteotomies through all orbital walls are performed behind the greatest diameter of the orbital contents; sometimes it is necessary to connect the osteotomies of the median orbital wall and the orbital floor via a transconjunctival approach (Sailer, 1978). The zygomatic complex is divided transversely, in an infraorbital direction (**Fig. 26.3**). The zygomatic osteotomy is completed below the infraorbital foramen into the piriform aperture beneath the lower turbinate, using an intraoral upper vestibular approach. A triangular piece of bone above this osteotomy is removed from both sides of the piriform aperture. Both orbits are gently mobilized by finger pressure and by the use of broad chisels placed into the lateral orbital osteotomy.

Now, >two wires are placed within the glabela region and both orbits gently pulled and pressed together. The fixation of the supraorbital bandeau to the orbits and the calvaria is done mostly with titanium wires. A few miniplates can be used, preferably at the lateral orbital rim, in the zygomatic area for fixation of the lyophilized bone grafts (Sailer, 1992), and in the infraorbital region (**Fig. 26.4**).

In children we prefer to use resorbable plates and screws, because contour corrections are necessary later, which would require removal of often-osseointegrated titanium plates, causing loss of bone. The defects in the cranial base and orbital walls are bridged by lyophilized cartilage slices (Sailer, 1992). The nasal frame work is reconstructed by an L-shaped strut of calvarial bone, which is fixed firmly to the glabela region by two miniscrews (see **Fig. 26.4**).

At the end of surgery the surplus skin in the frontal and nasal area is excised along the median transnasal–transfrontal incision.

Correction of Craniosynostosis

The correction of the fronto-orbital area in a syndromal or nonsyndromal craniosynostosis condition is based on the work of Tessier (1967) and Marchac et al. (1974). The most common fronto-orbital corrections have to be performed in scaphocephaly, frontal plagiocephaly, trigonocephaly, and brachycephaly. The principles of correction of occipital scaphocephaly and occipital plagiocephaly (Sailer and Landolt, 1991) are described later.

Craniosynostosis corrections are usually performed during the first years of life when skull growth is fast. Clinical experience has shown that metallic plates on outer skull surfaces disappear in the intracranial direction by outer bone apposition and inner calvarial resorption. Finally, the plates and screws are lying on top of the dura and screws can penetrate into it. For this reason metallic plates on the growing skull have to be removed approx-

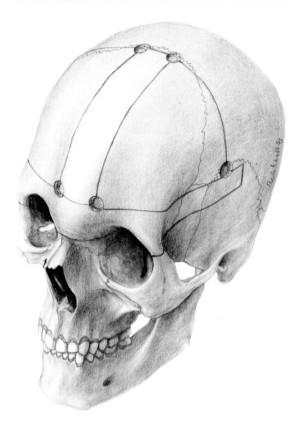

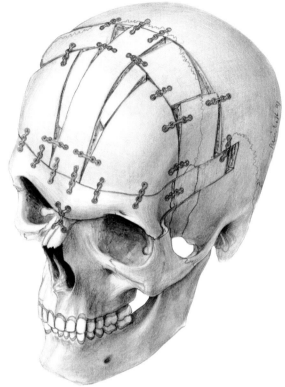

Fig. 26.5 Fronto-orbital correction in trigonocephaly (as modified by Sailer). The osteotomies are arranged so that the sinus system is protected by a strip of bone in the median skull area.

Fig. 26.6 The fronto-orbital bandeau is bent with a bone forceps so that the supraorbital rims are advanced and more prominent. This bandeau is fixed by microplates. The median bone strip is fixed to the supraorbital bandeau and the parietal bone by titanium wires or microplates. The median bone strip determines the curvature of the forehead and also the height of the anterior skull. Defects in the calvaria are closed by lyophilized bone or cartilage.

imately 6 months after surgery—or resorbable plates and screws should be used. From our point of view, titanium miniplates should always be removed (Rosenberg et al., 1993) because a metallosis is possible.

We started the application of resorbable osteosynthesis materials in infant craniofacial surgery 20 years ago (Illi et al., 1989), and developed several materials for the cranio-maxillofacial region (Haers et al., 1998; Haers and Sailer, 1999; Sailer et al., 1998).

We consider this technique nowadays to be state of the art (Sailer, 2000) in pediatric craniofacial surgery.

Fronto-Orbital Corrections

The correction of a trigonocephaly condition is described as a typical example of fronto-orbital osteotomies. The aim of the procedure is to advance the supraorbital rims and the lateral forehead areas, in particular, to achieve a rounded natural skull form (**Figs. 26.5, 26.6**).

After the coronal incision the forehead, the supraorbital rims and the nasal structures (without detaching the inner canthal ligaments) are all exposed and the craniotomy and a supraorbital bandeau are outlined (see **Fig. 26.5**). For safety reasons, burr holes are placed laterally, away from the expected course of the superior sagittal sinus system (see **Fig. 26.6**). Usually, six burr holes are made, though sometimes a maximum of eight is necessary. The most important part is the fronto-orbital bandeau; the osteotomies run over the fronto-nasal suture, along the anterior part of the orbital roof, through the zygomaticofrontal suture and from there far backward within the frontal, sphenoidal, temporal, and parietal bones, depending on the direction of the chosen osteotomy (see **Fig. 26.5**).

The fronto-orbital bandeau is totally removed and fashioned according to the desired plan. First, the inner cortex of the glabela region is cut vertically to allow the supraorbital rims to be bent outward easily. Then, with a bone forceps, the lateral supraorbital area and the finger-like extension of the bandeau are bent to the planned shape. The supraorbital bandeau is fixed to the nasal structure by a titanium microplate (Champy et al., 1977), or titanium wiring, or the smallest resorbable plates available. The disadvantage of some resorbable plates is that they are bigger than corresponding titanium plates and can disturb the aesthetics of the frontonasal angle until resorption is completed.

The fingerlike posterior extension can be fixed to the parietal bone in the desired position using titanium wires, direct screws, microplates, or resorbable osteosynthesis material (see **Fig. 26.6**).

The position of the fronto-orbital bandeau determines the width of the skull form and the angulation of the fronto-nasal region. The enlargement of the cranial width can now be seen by the space between the brain and the new position of the fronto-orbital bandeau.

A median strip of bone is fixed above the sagittal sinus system by wires or resorbable plates (see **Fig. 26.6**). This bone strip defines the curvature of the forehead and the height of the skull. On both sides of the median bone strip the rest of the calvaria is now reconstructed as symmetrically as possible.

Fixation is done by titanium wires, microplates, or resorbable plates. If the skull bones are very thin, only wires can be used. Screws that are too long have to be cut to avoid trauma to the dura. Because the volume of the skull will be larger, calvarial defects are always present. These defects are closed using either lyophilized bone (homologous calvarial bone or sternum) or, most often, lyophilized cartilage slices. It is well known that this kind of cartilage (Sailer, 1983) is transformed into the patient's own bone (Sailer, 1992).

Occipital Corrections

In severe cases of occipital scaphocephaly or plagiocephaly a correction is necessary for aesthetic and functional reasons. In occipital scaphocephaly, the patient cannot lie on the occiput and the head is always falling sideways. In occipital plagiocephaly the patient always lies on the flat area of the head. The head cannot take a natural position during sleeping, which may also cause further functional problems of the vertebra, growth impairment, etc. A special technique has been developed for surgical correction of occipital craniosynostosis (Sailer, 1991; Sailer et al., 1998).

During surgery the patient is lying face downward to allow easy access to the posterior part of the skull. A coronal incision is made from ear to ear in an undulating way and the whole posterior part of the skull is exposed, down to the nuchal musculature. The osteotomies and the craniotomy are outlined so that a median bone bandeau is created that has the sagittal suture line in the center (**Fig. 26.7**). Usually eight to ten burr holes are necessary for the bilateral craniotomy.

Correction of Occipital Scaphocephaly

In a scaphocephalic condition the posterior skull form has to be made shorter, higher, and wider (see **Fig. 26.7**). This is accomplished by first shortening and bending the me-

dian bandeau, which is the key structure in the corrections of occipital craniosynostosis, as the fronto-orbital bandeau and the anterior median bone strip are for anterior craniosynostosis operations. The median sagittal bandeau is segmented for this purpose and is stabilized by multiple titanium plates, or the largest resorbable miniplates to give maximal stability, because the child will immediately lie on the occiput after surgery. The bandeau puts a moderate pressure onto the posterior cerebral structures. By doing this, the brain widens bilaterally and vertically. The median bandeau must be firmly fixed to the occipital and parietal bones. It is the structure that has to carry most of the weight of the head immediately after surgery. The lateral parts of the skull are bent so as to achieve a symmetrical head form.

Correction of Occipital Plagiocephaly

In an occipital plagiocephalic condition the aim is to create a round symmetrical skull form to allow the child to lie comfortably on the occiput. Again, a median sagittal bandeau is the key structure to achieve this. The plagiocephaly is always corrected bilaterally, diminishing the intracranial volume on the "normal" side and allowing cerebral expansion on the affected side. In occipital plagiocephaly the median bandeau is usually turned through 180°, bent according to the desired form of the occiput and again stabilized and fixed in this form by resorbable miniplates. Then the missing bone structures are brought into position as symmetrically as possible on both sides. Osteosynthesis is done by resorbable miniplates and wires, as described above (see **Fig. 26.7**).

Patients operated on by using the median bone strip method clearly demonstrated better aesthetic and functional results than patients operated on without the median bone strip method (Sailer et al., 1998).

High Midface Osteotomies

High midface osteotomies include frontofacial advancement, the pure Le Fort III osteotomy, the combined procedure of Le Fort III plus Le Fort I osteotomy, and the Le Fort III minus Le Fort I osteotomy. Combinations of these with correction of hypertelorism have been described (Sailer and Grätz, 1995).

Before miniplate osteosynthesis of the frontofacial area was used, there was a tendency to perform osteotomies of bigger units such as the frontofacial osteotomy in one block, the facial bipartition procedure (Obwegeser et al., 1978) and the pure Le Fort III osteotomy. These blocks could be stabilized by bone grafts and wiring. Thanks to rigid fixation it is now possible to stabilize smaller anatomical units using miniplates and microplates. This allows the position of every anatomical structure to be individually determined by segmental osteotomies, without the risk of relapse (Sailer, 1985; Sailer and Obwegeser, 1983). Use of miniplates and microplates in craniofacial

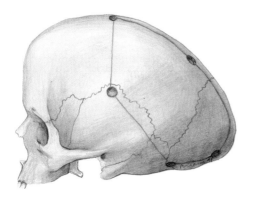
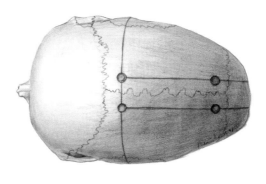
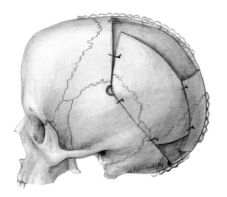
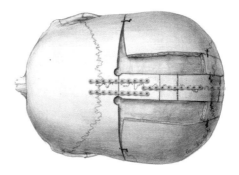
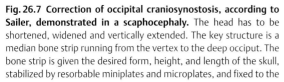

Fig. 26.7 Correction of occipital craniosynostosis, according to Sailer, demonstrated in a scaphocephaly. The head has to be shortened, widened and vertically extended. The key structure is a median bone strip running from the vertex to the deep occiput. The bone strip is given the desired form, height, and length of the skull, stabilized by resorbable miniplates and microplates, and fixed to the parietal and occipital bone by plating. The residual bones are fixed on both sides of the median bone strip as symmetrically as possible. Residual defects are closed by lyophilized bone or cartilage. Immediately after surgery the patient can lie on the reconstructed occiput. The same procedure is used in occipital plagiocephaly.

surgery also allows reduction of the use of autologous bone grafts. If additional bone is necessary, homologous lyophilized bank bone in combination with miniplates and microplates can totally replace autologous bone in craniofacial surgery (Sailer, 1992).

Segmented Frontofacial Advancement Including Le Fort III plus Le Fort I Osteotomy in Two Parts

This procedure exemplifies several high midface osteotomies in one operation. The procedure should not be performed before adolescence (Sailer and Landolt, 1991).

The indication for this procedure is usually a syndromal craniosynostosis, like the Apert and Crouzon syndromes, with retrusion of the forehead, the infraorbital bony structures and the tooth-bearing part of the maxilla; the most striking symptom in these cases is the exophthalmos. Most of these patients show also a very high palate with narrow maxillary arches and an open bite.

The segmental frontofacial advancement procedure (**Figs. 26.8–26.10**) is performed using the "sun glass osteotomy" (Sailer and Landolf, 1991); within the lateral

orbital rims and lateral orbital walls a bony pillar is preserved on both sides from where the osteotomies of the orbital roof and the orbital floor are performed. The pillars serve as reference points for measuring the different movements and as fixation points for microplates and wires. The intraoperative timing demands that the osteotomy and mobilization of the midface be performed first by a Le Fort III osteotomy.

After full mobilization of the midface is undertaken, a Le Fort I osteotomy can be performed and the tooth-bearing part of the maxilla mobilized using broad chisels. The palate can also be split parasagittally, to correct narrow arches.

Intermaxillary fixation is applied, followed by positioning of the zygomatic complex and infraorbital region on each side. Asymmetries of the infraorbital areas can be corrected by a paramedian splitting of the nasal bone, which allows for easier tilting of the zygomas according to need (see **Figs. 26.8–26.10**). The zygomatic bones are now fixed to the zygomatic arches, in combination with lyophilized bank bone, with miniplates, and to the lateral pillars using microplates.

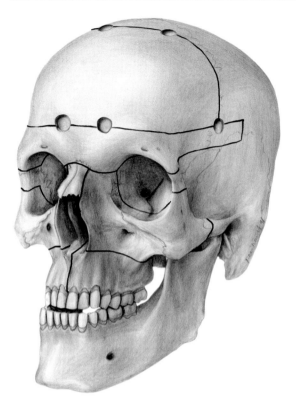

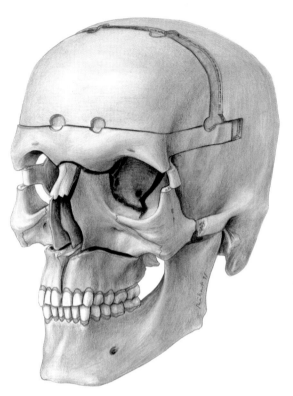

Fig. 26.8 Osteotomy lines for segmented frontofacial advancement including Le Fort III plus Le Fort I osteotomy. This is indicated for severe forms of syndromal craniosynostosis and permits forward-positioning of the whole midface and fronto-orbital area.

Fig. 26.9 All anatomical key structures of the midface and the forehead are mobilized. Note the paramedian nasal osteotomy which allows tilting of the infraorbital structures and of the zygomas, independent of each other.

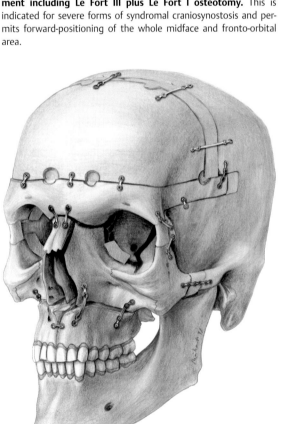

After this, the intraoral fixation of the maxillary halves takes place, again using miniplates and lyophilized bank bone. The nasal bones have not been fixed at this stage. The craniotomy is performed once the midfacial structures are stabilized.

This particular intraoperative sequence is necessary, because it would be very difficult to mobilize the midface after craniotomy. The fronto-orbital bandeau is then osteotomized (as described earlier for isolated craniosynostosis) and advanced according to the preoperative plan, the lateral orbital pillars allowing exact measurement of the movements of the upper and lower segments and also the fixation of these structures by microplates. The calvarial bone is then placed into position to achieve the best possible form of the forehead and calvaria. The defects within the calvaria are closed by either using lyophilized bank bone or cartilage.

Two vacuum drains are inserted, and the coronal suture is closed using subcutaneous Dexon stitches and stapling of the incision line.

Fig. 26.10 Stabilization by the use of miniplates and microplates. The bony defects are bridged by lyophilized homogenous bank bone and cartilage.

27 Application of Resorbable Plates, Screws, and Pins for the Treatment of Midface and Condylar Neck Fractures and Correction of Craniosynostoses

Klaus Louis Gerlach and Uwe Eckelt

Introduction

Different chapters of this book describe applications of various mini/microplate and -screw systems that guarantee in nearly all cases a secure and successful bone healing of osteotomized or fractured bone segments, in mandibular and midfacial fractures as well as in orthognathic procedures. Plates and screws are generally made of titanium, and until now these have been regarded as the "gold standard."

Some disadvantages have become apparent, however, such as interference with later diagnostic or therapeutic radiological investigations (e. g., computed tomography, magnetic resonance imaging), under-the-skin palpable plates, growth inhibitions of craniofacial bones in infants followed by passive migration, loosening of screws, hot and cold irritabilities, and, not least, secondary intervention to remove osteosynthesis materials. These considerations have led to the development of biodegradable osteosynthesis materials as possibilities for more than three decades (Kulkarni et al., 1971; Champy et al., 1993; Gerlach, 2000).

The major advantages of biodegradable osteosynthesis devices are that functional stress is gradually transferred to the bone as it remodels and matures, and the material hardly ever requires surgical removal.

Among the various resorbable polymers used for this purpose, semicrystalline poly-L-lactide (PLLA), amorphous poly-D,L-lactide (PDLLA), polyglycolide (PGA) and their copolymers (P[L/LD]LA and PLGA) are the most important and commonly used.

The mechanical characteristics, the biocompatibility, and the duration of biodegradation vary among the different systems available. These depend upon the polymers or copolymers used, their amount of crystallinity, and their molecular weight. The methods used to produce and form the materials, for example self-reinforced techniques (SR), the sterilization process, the amount of materials used, and the perfusion of tissues overlying the material once implanted also differ according to the system.

Polylactic acid (PLA), which is the most often used, has two enantiomeric forms, L-lactic acid and D-lactic acid. Whereas in L-lactide identical polymer chains can be tightly packed, which makes these polymers partially crystalline, adding D-isomers into an L-isomer-based polymerization system balances the tightening of the packing

and, depending of the amount of D-lactide, reduces the crystallinity or results in an amorphous copolymer. Although both PLLA and PGA are highly cristalline, their co-polymer, for example with a PLLA:PGA percentage ratio of 82:18, is amorphous.

The mechanical characteristics are especially improved by an increase of the molecular weight, but on the other hand these properties prolong the duration of biodegradation.

At present numerous different systems are clinically available. These are, however, characterized by the polymer used or their respective polymer compositions; also by differing physical properties, biological compatibilities, and absorption times resulting in persistence lasting between 1 year and more than 5 years (Buijs et al., 2006). Moreover, the primary and continuous tension or bending strength, and especially the stiffness, are much lower with all available systems compared with conventional materials made from stainless steel or titanium (Daniels et al., 1992). The application is therefore especially recommended for the stabilization of sections of the face that are not strongly load-bearing (midface and cranium), and exceptionally in growing patients. The following discussion focuses particularly on our own experiences with a system made from poly-D,L-lactide.

Resorb-X

The source material is 50 : 50 poly-D,L-lactic acid (PDLLA), from which pins, micro and mini osteosynthesis screws are produced using an injection molding process. The osteosynthesis plates and meshes are pressed and milled from granulated polymer. Prior to sterilization, the plates have a molecular weight (M_w) of 200 000 g/mol, a melting point of 120°C (248°F), a tensile strength of approximately 60 MPa, and a bending strength of 120 MPa. The material is gamma-sterilized with an overall dose of 25 kGy.

After in-vivo examination, a slight decrease of the bending strength of 15 % was observed within 6 weeks postimplantation; thereafter a rapid falling off of the mechanical properties occurred (Heidemann et al., 2003a).

The complete degradation of this material had been shown in different examinations. Under in-vitro conditions, the PDLLA rods had disintegrated almost completely 52 weeks after incubation and could be identified only as flaky residues in Ringer solution. Following implantation of PDLLA specimens into the back muscles of rats, the specimens were macroscopically invisible after 52 weeks (Heidemann et al., 1996, 2002a, 2003a), with complete resorption from the extracellular space after 72 weeks, as determined by light-microscopical examination (Gerlach, 2000). In addition, Resorb-X plates and screws were applied to the femoral bones of rabbits. Complete degradation and drill-hole ossification could be verified after 14 months in these cases (Heidemann et al., 2003b). These resorption differences may be due to the different implantation sites.

The degradation process of the PDLLA after clinical application could be traced through ultrasound imaging and X-ray examination to determine the ossification of the bore holes. A complete degradation could be observed between 24 and 30 months.

In regions where the bone is covered only by thin soft-tissue layers (especially in the periorbital region), transient swelling of the osteosynthesis material can occur in some cases. However, the patients involved did not feel any impairment as a result of the painless swelling. Since the extent of the swelling depends on the initial thickness of the osteosynthesis plates, the plate thickness was reduced from 1.5 mm to 1.1 mm during the course of the study, without compromising the plates' mechanical properties. When using these thinner plates, the swelling is hardly noticeable—even in the periorbital region (Heidemann and Gerlach, 2002c, 2002b).

Principles of Osteosynthesis

An essential condition for a secure osteosynthesis with plates/meshes and screws is the exact adaptation of the plates on the osseous surface after repositioning of the fragments. Incongruities as a result of a plate not lying directly on the bone while screwing in the screws lead to dislocation of the fragments or to a fracture of the plate.

Customary metallic plates can be bent easily into any forms with the help of various bending pliers However, plates or meshes made from polymers can be formed only after heating them above the glass transition temperature (from 45 to 70°C). For this purpose the material can be immersed in a special heated, sterile water bath for approximately 10 seconds. Alternatively, an air-heating device, a countering pen/forceps, or a heat package may be used. Afterward the material is malleable and can be adapted on the bone surface. After cooling-off or hardening at room temperature for roughly 8 to 10 seconds, the plate or mesh is prepared for fixing to the bone. Previous adaptation of a metal foil from slightly pliable metal (template) to the osseous contour is also to be recommended; the plates/meshes are subsequently adapted in the water bath directly to this prepared template. Re-

peated heating and fresh bending are also possible, and previously heated plates can be shortened with an edging instrument as required or the mesh can be adapted.

To perform the osteosynthesis, the prepared plates or the adapted mesh are placed on the reduced fragments so that at least two perforations exist on every fracture side to accommodate the fixing screws. With a drill, the diameter of which corresponds to the width of the screw core, bore holes are prepared through the preformed holes of the plate, or even through the plate or mesh itself perpendicular to the surface of the bone. In the following procedure another preparation of the drilling canal with a tapper is necessary, so that in the following procedure the screws can be tightened by the plate holes in the bone. During screw tightening, large torsional forces develop along the long axis of the screw, which can shear off the screw head. Therefore, tightening of the screw should be completed when it has made contact with the plate. In the case of breakage of a screw, a new hole can easily be drilled through the broken screw and a new screw inserted.

These drawbacks can be avoided by using, as an alternative, ultrasonic pin fixation with the Sonic Weld System (Pilling et al., 2007b). Resorb-X pins (2.1×4 mm) are inserted with the aid of ultrasound. Following conventional hole drilling (diameter 1.6 mm) the pins are inserted using a special applicator with the aid of ultrasound (capacity 20 W). In contrast to fixation with conventional screws, no time-consuming thread cutting is required. No screwdriver is necessary and no screw-head fracture can occur. Due to the ultrasound application, the pin is melted into the bone trabeculae and welds together with the plate. This process fixes the plate or mesh (thickness 0.3, 0.6, and 1.0 mm) on the bone fragments. Fixation of the first mobile fragment in particular is facilitated.

In conventional fixation by means of a screw, its stability in the surrounding bone is based on the interlinkage of the profiles of screw and thread cut into the drilled hole. In contrast, the pin inserted by using ultrasound obtains its stability by filling the cavities in the trabecular bone structure opening by the hole-drilling, and by fusion with the osteosynthesis material (**Fig. 27.1**). In addition, the pins are welded to the plate or mesh (Pilling et al., 2007a).

Mechanical testing in animal experiments evaluated the tensile and bending strengths of bone welding pins compared with resorbable screws (Pilling et al., 2007b). The study showed advantageous characteristics of the pin osteosynthesis. However, in contrast to conventional resorbable screws, bone-welding pins develop thermal energy during the ultrasound application. An important aspect of interest is the reaction of the soft and hard tissue to this thermal stress. Clinically, no signs of inflammation or pin-loosening could be observed (Eckelt et al., 2007b), and histological examinations in animal studies showed no signs of foreign body reaction or thermally induced necrosis (Mai et al., 2007).

Midface Fractures

For the osteosynthesis of midface fractures, in particular cheek bone, frontal bone, and Le Fort I fractures, the plates/meshes and screws are very well appropriated. The operative procedure, such as the surgical approach and repositioning of the fragments, completely corresponds to the treatment of fractures as described in Chapter 19. To stabilize cheekbone fractures, plates can be placed at the lateral orbital rim and at the infra-orbital edge; they can be applied just as well at the crista zygomatico alveolaris. In each case at least two screws should be applied lateral to the fracture line (**Fig. 27.2**). At the Le Fort I level and for treatment of frontal bone fractures the use of a suitably cut and formed mesh is very advantageous (see **Figs. 33.3, 33.4**).

In a pilot study 50 patients with cheek-bone fractures had been treated; the follow up checks were performed at 2- to 6-month intervals up to 30 months after the operation (Heidemann and Gerlach, 2002b). Wound and fracture healing were uneventful in all cases; no second operation was necessary.

The PDLLA degradation process as well as increases and decreases in the polymer volume could be documented by ultrasound imaging. Up to the eighth postoperative month, ultrasonography detected no changes in the osteosynthesis plates. Thereafter, the plates began absorbing water resulting in the plate interior becoming increasingly hypodense, with blurring of the outer plate contours. The maximum plate thickness was reached 14 months after the operation and remained constant for approximately 4 months. Afterward, plate thickness decreased (Heidemann and Gerlach, 2002c). Thirty months after the operation, the plates were neither palpable nor sonographically traceable any longer. For 20 patients reexamined for between 30 and 41 months, the X-rays taken showed complete ossification of the drill holes.

Screw-shaft fractures occurred at a rate of less than 5 % of cases. This complication is avoided when using the Sonic Weld System.

Condylar Neck Fractures

While fractures of the mandibular body in adults, as a rule, should be immobilized with titanium miniplates, there is an indication, especially in cases of deep condylar neck fractures, to perform the osteosynthesis with absorbable material after repositioning of the fragments (Heidemann and Gerlach, 2002b).

The potential use of osteosynthesis plates and screws made of resorbable PDLLA (Resorb-X) was demonstrated by Rasse et al. (2007) after creating deep condylar neck fractures in 12 sheep followed by repositioning of the small fragment and performing an osteosynthesis using,

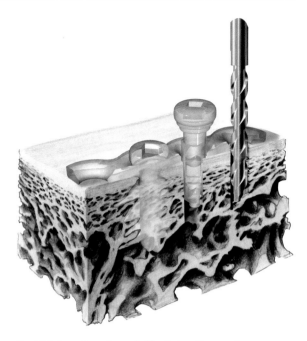

Fig. 27.1 Insertion of resorbable pin by ultrasound.

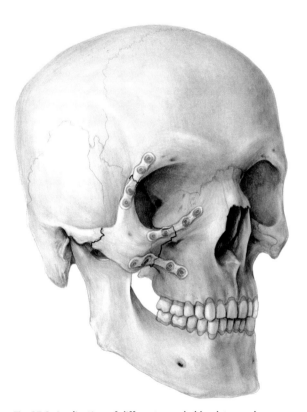

Fig. 27.2 Application of different resorbable plates and screws at the lateral orbital rim, the infraorbital edge, as well at the crista zygomatico alveolaris.

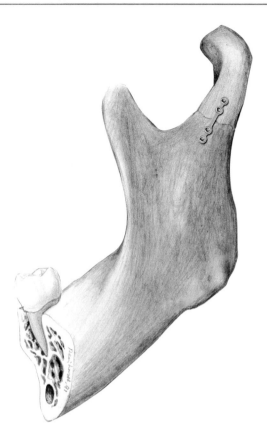

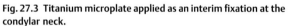

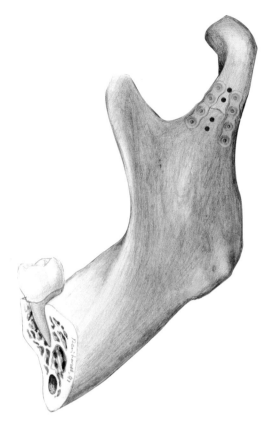

Fig. 27.3 Titanium microplate applied as an interim fixation at the condylar neck.

Fig. 27.4 Resorbable plates anterior and posterior at the condylar neck. The titanium microplate is removed.

in each case, two plates and eight screws. Postoperatively the animals received normal food; the healing of the fractures was uneventful in all cases with one exception, as one sheep died. During a 12-month follow-up, after 6 months primary bone was recognized; no material-related inflammations could be ascertained.

For clinical use a perioperative intermaxillary fixation is recommended. The periangular surgical approach described in detail in Chapter 5 (see **Fig. 5.17**) allows a good representation of the fracture site. After repositioning of

the small fragment and performing an intermaxillary fixation, a titanium microplate is applied as an interim fixation of the fragments. This microplate should be localized centrally. Next, a resorbable plate anterior and posterior, respectively, can be applied (**Figs. 27.3, 27.4**). Following secure fixation with pins, the temporarily applied microplate is removed prior to closure of the wound. Due to the oblique insertion of the pins, sometimes pins with a length of 6 or 7 mm are recommended.

Craniosynostoses

Application of the resorbable material to the fixation of osteotomized parts of the cranial vault as well as the supraorbital bandeau in infants (en grove technique) is particularly ideal. The surgical action corresponds to the description given in Chapter 26. Especially on the cranial vault, the surgical action is facilitated and requires less time due to the use and application of larger meshes and pin-fixation by ultrasonography.

Clinical application (Eckelt et al., 2007a) revealed that this produced the same stability as conventional resorbable osteosynthesis fixation by means of screws. In particular, the 1-mm thick resorbable mesh produced excellent stability intraoperatively. Easy adaptation of the warmed Resorb-X mesh and fixation by means of pins rendered osteosynthesis much easier than had been the case earlier with conventional screws, and allowed optimal configuration of the cranial vault (**Fig. 27.5**).

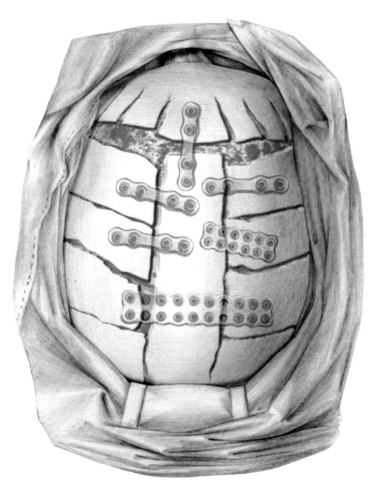

Fig. 27.5 Application of 1-mm thick resorbable meshes and plates. Pin fixation was performed by ultrasound.

28 Drill-free Screws

Klaus Louis Gerlach and Wolfgang Heidemann

Introduction

In craniomaxillofacial surgery, the use of self-tapping bone screws is now virtually universal in osteosynthesis to stabilize most skeletal and mandibular fractures and deformities. The requirement of drilling a pilot hole to use conventional self-tapping screws is a time-consuming extra step, which has some potential disadvantages. These include damage to nerves, tooth roots or germs, thermal bone necrosis, screw stripping due to an overdrilled pilot hole especially in thin cortical or soft cancellous bone, drill bit breakage, improper drill-bit size selection and, finally, the extra cost of single-use drill bits.

Normally, self-tapping screws (Champy et al., 1976b) have asymmetric threads with sharp edges to the screw shaft. The surface of the threads is nearly perpendicular to the direction of pull-out force, to provide maximum load transmission. The thread spirals around a cylindrical core with a pitch (the distance between the threads) of 0.75 mm or 1 mm. A cutting flute is engraved at the leading end of the threaded portion of the screw (**Fig. 28.1**).

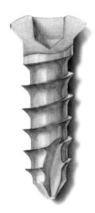

Fig. 28.1 Technical design of a self-tapping screw.

Technique

After drilling a pilot hole with a comparable diameter to that of the screws core, the sharp flute cuts the bone in preparation for the threads further along the screw's shaft, as the screw is turned (**Fig. 28.2**).

Inserting drill-free screws without the need to drill pilot holes beforehand was made possible by changing the tip of the screw. The pointed screw tip with its thread is comparable in design and function to a corkscrew. Here, in contrast to self-tapping bone screws, the threads are spiraled along a cone-shaped axis of rotation up to the tip of the screw. Again, the thread pitch is 0.75 mm or 1 mm. An additional cutting flute cuts part of the bone like a chisel and acts as a channel for the removal of bone chips produced at the cutting site. The threads cut into the bone must not be broken or compressed. After drill-free screws are inserted, bone dust accumulates around the screw head (**Figs. 28.3, 28.4**).

Drill-free screws are available in both micro (1.5 mm) and mini (2 mm) diameters. In a comprehensive experimental trial Heidemann et al. (1996) compared different

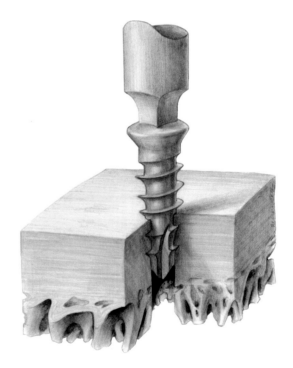

Fig. 28.2 Self-tapping screw. Insertion and tightening into the bone after preparation of a pilot hole

parameters (such as insertional, maximum torque, and, especially, the pull-out force) of common, titanium self-tapping microscrews and miniscrews with drill-free screws of the same size. Test materials included mandibular cortical bone of pigs and, to enable a statistical comparison between the parameters of the screws used, hardwood and PVC as a homogenous substance with constant material qualities.

Depending on the thickness of the test material, the measured pull-out force of drill-free screws was found to lie between 70% and 104% of that of self-tapping screws. The maximum torque in bone and wood was comparable with that of common self-tapping screws (Heidemann and Gerlach, 1998; Heidemann et al., 1998a, 1998b).

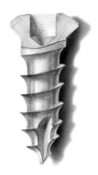

Fig. 28.3 Technical design of a drill-free screw.

The results of the experimental evaluations suggested that drill-free screws should be used in bones with a thin cortical layer, up to 2–3 mm thick. In a first clinical pilot study, the use of 1.5-mm drill-free screws, especially for osteosynthesis of segmented parts of the midface (Le Fort I, II, and III osteotomies), in orthognathic surgery and also in traumatology, gave excellent results. The use of drill-free screws is therefore recommended for the fixation of bone fragments in the entire midface and, with some reservations, in the cranial and periorbital regions.

Although the use of drill-free screws in bone segments in orthognathic surgery is almost without problems, in traumatology their use in fixation of small pieces of bone is sometimes difficult. Here it is advisable to put a small hook behind the bone to resist the pressure of the screw and screwdriver on the bone. Once the bony surface is perforated by the tip of the screw, the thread cuts itself into the bone and continuous insertional torque pulls it into the bone, in a corkscrewlike manner.

The use of drill-free screws in the mandible is limited to children up to 13 years of age and, in adults, to application in the paramedian regions only. For treatment of mandibular angle fractures, the dense bone structure and the thickness of the cortical layer in the osteosynthesis area along the oblique line will occasionally require the use of a drill as a guide pin.

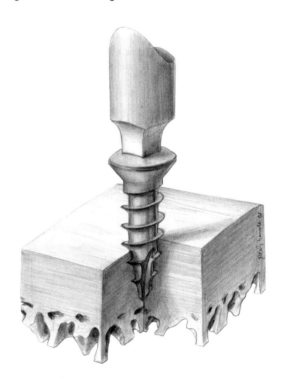

Fig. 28.4 Drill-free screw. Insertion and tightening into the bone without previously preparing a hole.

29 Reconstructive Preprosthetic Surgery and Implantology

John I. Cawood

Introduction

Reconstructive preprosthetic surgery can be defined as the restoration of oral function and facial form, rendered deficient through loss or absence of teeth and related structures, by a combination of surgical and prosthetic means. Nowadays the application of endosteal implants has extended the scope and effectiveness of reconstructive preprosthetic surgery (Cawood and Stoelinga, 1996). Of the many variables that govern the use of such implants the availability of sufficient bulk of bone is the most important. There is a progressive reduction in the residual alveolar ridges, following the loss of teeth, due to alveolar bone resorption, which occurs relatively rapidly in the first year after tooth loss and then continues at a slower rate for many years (Tallgren, 1972). This process occurs to a greater extent in the mandible compared with the maxilla and leads to a quantitative and qualitative reduction of the alveolar bone.

Cawood and Howell (1988) analyzed patterns of alveolar resorption and described a pathophysiological classification of alveolar resorption, which is accepted internationally (**Figs. 29.1, 29.2**).

When considering reconstructive preprosthetic surgery of the edentulous jaw, it is important that the clinician fully understands the anatomical consequences of reduction of the residual ridges. Based on a classification of the edentulous jaws, changes in the relationship of the jaws to each other, in muscle relations and function, in the oral mucosa and in facial morphology have been measured relative to the stage of resorption of the edentulous jaws (Cawood and Howell, 1991).

Anatomical Consequences of Jaw Atrophy

Interarch Changes

With progressive resorption from class I to class VI there are three-dimensional changes in jaw relations. Anteroposteriorly the mandibular and maxillary arches become shorter. Transversely, due to the pattern of resorption, the maxillary arch becomes progressively narrower while the mandibular arch becomes progressively broader. Vertically the interarch distance increases, although this is counteracted to some extent by the vertical shortening of the lower face caused by the autorotation of the mandible producing a more prominent chin and prognathic jaw relationship (**Figs. 29.3–29.5**).

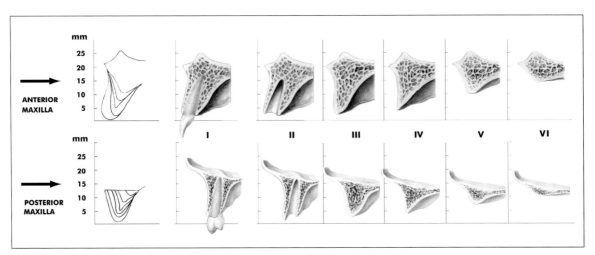

Fig. 29.1 Modified classification of edentulous jaws (maxilla).
Class II, post dental extraction; class III, broad alveolar process; class IV, narrow alveolar process; class V, flat ridge (loss of alveolar process); additional class VI, no ridge (total loss of alveolar process).

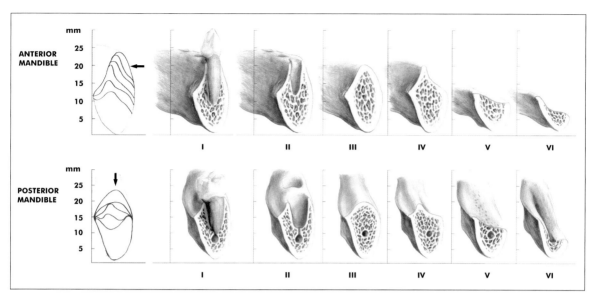

Fig. 29.2 Classification of edentulous jaws (mandible). Class II, post dental extraction; class III, broad alveolar ridge;class IV, knife-edge alveolar ridge; class V, flat ridge (resorption of alveolar process); class VI, submerged ridge (resorption of basal process).

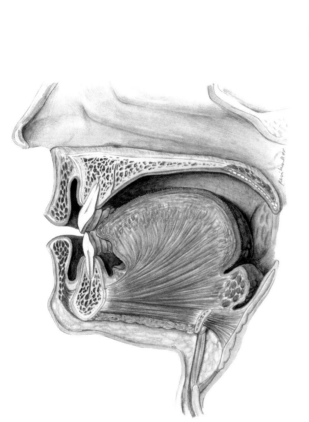

Fig. 29.3 Dentate jaw. Normal dental, jaw and soft tissue relationships.

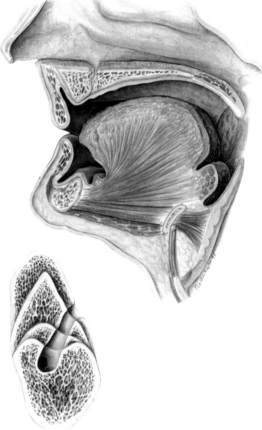

Fig. 29.4 Edentulous jaw. Encroachment of lips, tongue, and floor of mouth associated with jaw atrophy. Cross-section of the mandibular body in the foramen mentale region (resorption of alveolar process and change of the position of the mental foramen).

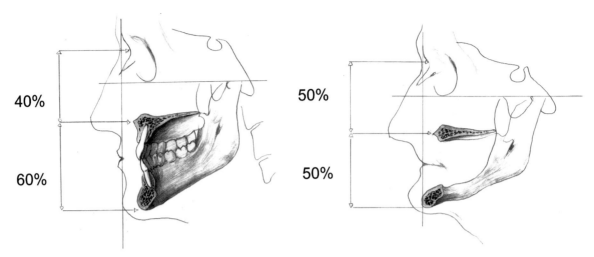

Fig. 29.5 Consequences of jaw atrophy. Decreased lower face height, relative prognathism, and collapse of lower facial soft tissue are shown.

Muscle Changes

The attachments of the circumoral musculature and that of the floor of the mouth delineate the extent of the vestibular and lingual sulci. With the continued loss of alveolar bone from class I to class VI these muscles become progressively more superficial (**Fig. 29.6**).

Mucosal Changes

In the edentulous jaw the mucosa covering the residual ridge comprises partly keratinized attached mucosa and partly unattached mucosa. With the resorption of the alveolus, the quantity of both attached and unattached mucosa diminishes significantly. In the mandible, as a result of alveolar bone loss, the inferior alveolar canal becomes relatively superficial (**Fig. 29.7**). In the dentate mandible the blood supply is principally centrifugal, arising from the inferior alveolar artery and periodontal arcades. However, in the edentulous mandible the blood supply is principally centripetal, arising via the subperiosteal plexus of vessels (**Fig. 29.8**).

Facial Changes

Watt and MacGregor (1976) liken the circumoral and facial musculature to a curtain draped between the maxilla and mandible. Loss of the anterior dentition results in loss of the "dental bulge" and causes a shortening of the buccinator muscle and consequent distortion of the facial curtain (see **Fig. 29.9**). The muscles of facial expression decussate to form the modiolus and also intersect directly with the fibers of the orbicularis oris muscle. With tooth loss and reduction of the residual ridge there is hypotonia

of the orbicularis oris muscle and the muscles of facial expression. The position of the modiolus changes, being pulled inward and backward, resulting in contraction of the orbicularis oris muscle and distortion of the muscles of facial expression (**Figs. 29.9–29.11**). The distortion of these muscle groups culminates in an alteration in facial form causing decreased nasolabial and paranasal support, narrowing of the width of the commissure, decreased show of the vermilion margin, loss of labiomental support, decrease in lower face height, and increased prominence of the chin (**Fig. 29.11**).

Awareness of the pattern of resorption of the edentulous jaws and associated soft-tissue changes enables clinicians to anticipate and possibly avert future problems.

Pre-implant Surgery

The successful application of endosteal implants depends on favorable anatomical form and environment, biocompatibility, and favorable biomechanical conditions.

The availability of sufficient bulk of bone and a healthy soft-tissue environment are the most important of the many variables that govern the success of endosteal implants. If such conditions do not exist, adjunctive surgical procedures such as osteotomy, bone grafting, and vestibuloplasty should be undertaken. The object of pre-implant surgery is to restore a favorable interarch relationship, creating a healthy environment to allow placement of endosteal implants of maximal size at optimal axial inclination with optimal load distribution and optimal aesthetics. Pre-implant surgery is indicated where there has been atrophy of the jaws, congenital deformity of the jaws, or after bone loss resulting from traumatic avulsion or as a result of tumor ablation.

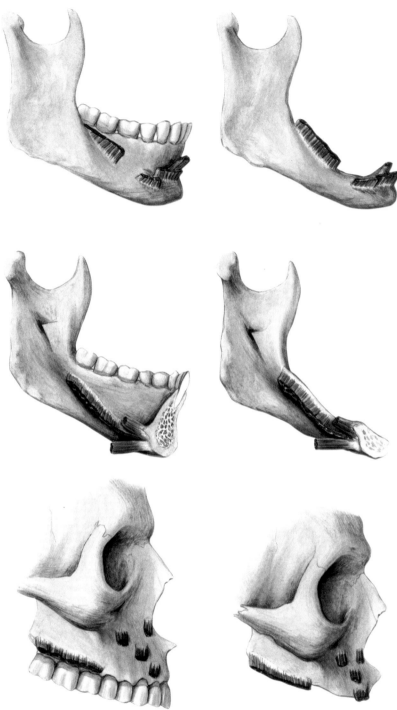

Fig. 29.6 Consequences of jaw atrophy. The attachment of the circumoral and floor-of-mouth musculature delineates the extent of the vestibular and lingual sulci. With continued loss of alveolar bone from class I to class VI these muscles become progressively more superficial.

Improvements in both surgical technology and surgical techniques have increased the predictability of pre-implant surgery and also reduced morbidity of such surgery. Technological advances include improved imaging techniques, dedicated instrumentation, and developments of biomaterials, such as bone substitutes, bone plates, and screws, and membranes for guided tissue regeneration.

Advances in surgical techniques include osteoplasty, such as manipulation of bone by either expansion or compression, or by augmentation utilizing onlay, inlay, or interpositional bone grafts. Application of miniplate or microplate osteosynthesis, position screws, and lag screws has further enhanced the predictability and effectiveness of pre-implant surgery. Osteosynthesis ensures stable fixa-

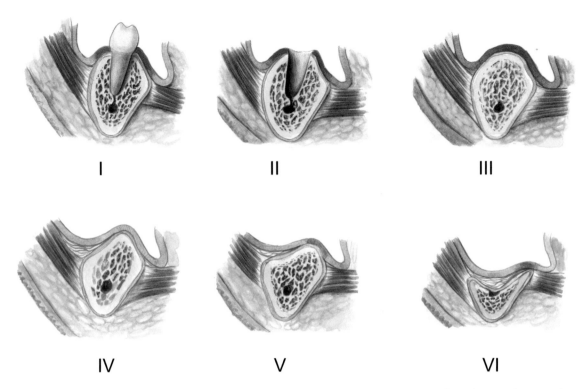

Fig. 29.7 Consequences of jaw atrophy (posterior mandible). Progressive reduction of residual ridge from class I to class VI results in decreased attached mucosa and in muscle encroachment. The inferior alveolar canal becomes more superficial.

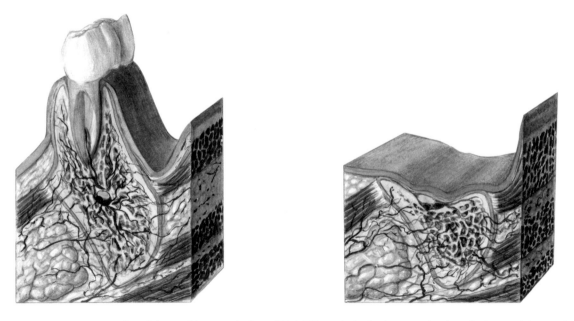

Fig. 29.8 Consequences of tooth loss and jaw atrophy (mandible). This results in alveolar resorption, loss of sulcus, and decreased and altered blood supply (centrifugal in the dentate jaw, centripetal in the edentulous jaw).

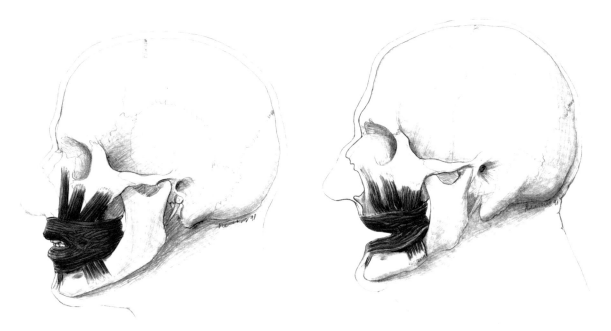

Fig. 29.9 "Dental bulge." Tooth loss results in loss of the "dental bulge" causing distortion of the circumoral musculature.

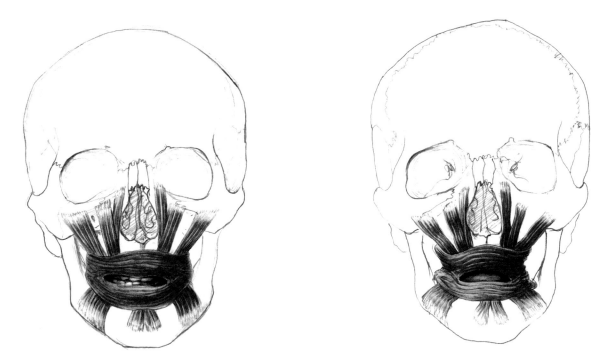

Fig. 29.10 Consequences of jaw atrophy on circumoral musculature. This results in circumoral hypotonia, contraction of orbicularis oris muscle, and distortion of muscles of facial expression (elevators and depressors).

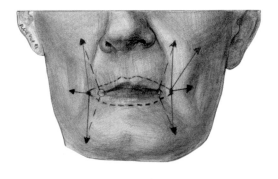

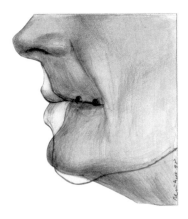

Fig. 29.11 Consequences of jaw atrophy on facial form. These are circumoral hypotonia, distortion of elevator and depressor muscles, narrowing of commissural width, decreased show of ver-milion margin of lips, obtuse nasolabial angle, loss of labiomental support, decreased lower face height, and increased chin promi-nence.

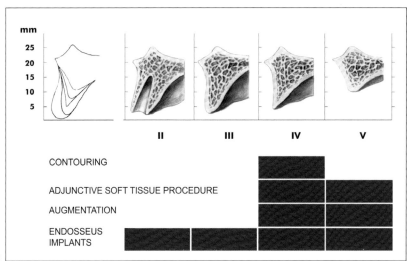

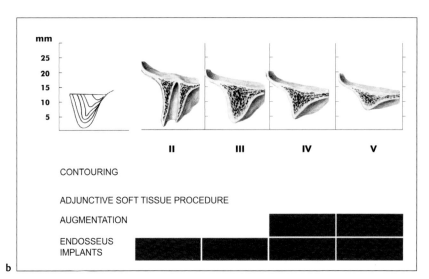

Fig. 29.12 a–d Scheme for pre-implant surgery based on the Cawood and Howell jaw classification. a Anterior maxilla. **b** Posterior maxilla.

Fig. 29.12 c, d ▷

tion of osteotomized bone segments and bone grafts, a prerequisite for predictable bone healing (Hayter and Cawood, 1996).

A scheme for pre-implant surgery based on the Cawood and Howell classification of the edentulous jaw has evolved (**Fig. 29.12a–d**). In her study Longman noted that the most frequently encountered patterns of jaw atrophy are class IV in the maxilla and class V in the mandible (**Figs. 29.13, 29.14**).

interarch relationship with the mandible and an increase in the vertical interarch distance. Bone volume is further decreased due to encroachment of the maxillary sinuses.

The deficiencies in bone volume and interarch discrepancies can be corrected utilizing bone grafts (onlay, inlay or interpositional) sometimes in combination with an osteotomy.

Class IV Maxilla

In the anterior maxilla the direction of bone loss is horizontal, with progressive loss of bone on the labial and buccal aspects. This converts the broad class III ridge, which provides adequate height and width of residual bone to accommodate endosteal implants, into a knife-edge class IV ridge, which has adequate height but inad-

Atrophic Maxilla

Atrophy of the edentulous maxilla results in three-dimensional changes in shape. The maxilla becomes shorter in anteroposterior and vertical dimensions and narrower in the transverse dimension. This results in an unfavorable

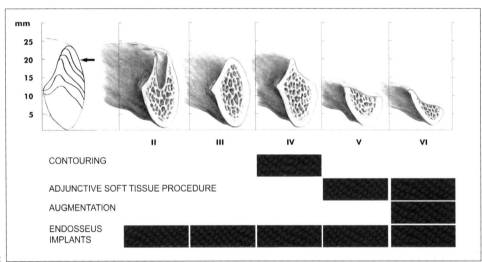

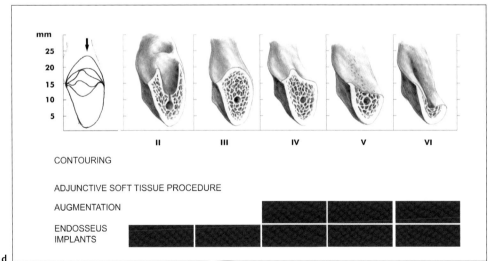

Fig. 29.12 c, d (cont.) c Anterior mandible. **d** Posterior mandible.

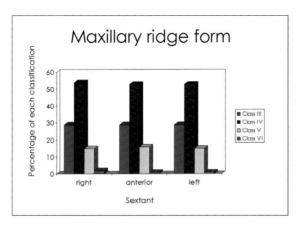

Fig. 29.13 Incidence of maxillary alveolar atrophy.

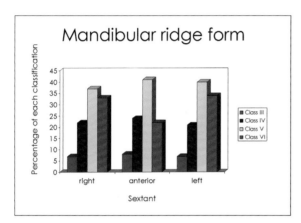

Fig. 29.14 Incidence of mandibular alveolar atrophy.

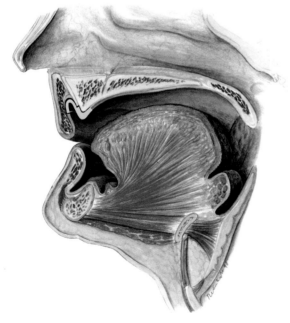

Fig. 29.15 Outline of modified Edlan flap.

equate width of residual bone. Placement of endosteal implants in the edentulous maxilla is often restricted because of lack of available bone. Exposure of the underlying anterior maxillary bone frequently reveals a ridge form that is adequate in height but too narrow to accommodate endosteal implants. A horseshoe-type osteotomy, extending from the ridge crest into the floor of the nose, has been developed, which allows advancement of the outer cortex to restore lost facial form and placement of an interpositional bone graft and endosteal implants to restore lost function (Richardson and Cawood, 1991).

Anterior Maxillary Osteoplasty to Broaden the Narrow Maxillary Ridge

Patient Assessment
This procedure is indicated in patients with a class IV maxillary anterior ridge. In assessing the width of the ridge, clinical examination may be misleading, as the knife-edge nature of the ridge may be masked by relatively thick submucosa on the palatal aspect. A lateral radiograph of the maxilla will show the outline of the bone in the midline. Reformatted axial computed tomograms can be useful to demonstrate ridge form and also the presence of intervening cancellous bone between the labial and palatal cortical plates, which is essential for this technique.

Operative Technique
A horseshoe-shaped incision is made in the labial mucosa, and a mucosal flap dissected to a point a few millimeters below the crest of the ridge. The periosteum is then incised and the dissection continued subperiosteally, onto the palatal aspect of the ridge, to expose the crest (**Fig. 29.15**). Crestal irregularities are eliminated and cancellous bone is exposed between the cortical plates to allow the crestal osteotomy cut to be made. This cut extends obliquely from the crest of the ridge to the floor of the nose (**Fig. 29.16**). It is extended laterally in the premolar region through the buccal plate. The anterior nasal spine is removed and the anterior part of the nasal septum detached from the segment to be mobilized (**Fig. 29.17**). The labial segment is then mobilized and stabilized with microplate osteosynthesis (**Figs. 29.18, 29.20**). An interpositional bone graft of particulate cancellous bone is inserted (**Figs. 29.18, 29.19**). The mucosal flap is then positioned to cover the graft and the repositioned labial segment, and sutured without tension. The mucosal defect on the inside of the upper lip heals by secondary intention. Endosteal implants are placed at a second operation 3 months later, following healing and incorporation of the bone graft (**Fig. 29.21**). In the event of a narrow V-shaped ridge form of the anterior maxilla, this technique can be modified to increase the transverse width of the maxilla as well. This is achieved by dividing the anterior segment into two or three separate pieces. The

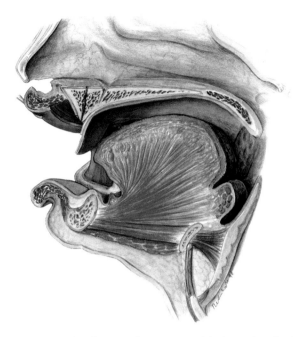

Fig. 29.16 Edlan flap raised to maintain labial, nasal, palatal blood supply. Position and direction of osteotomy cuts from crest of ridge to nasal floor.

Fig. 29.17 Anterior segment mobilized.

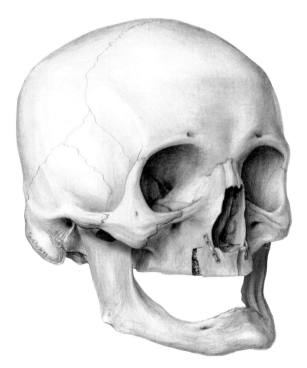
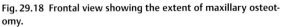

Fig. 29.18 Frontal view showing the extent of maxillary osteotomy.

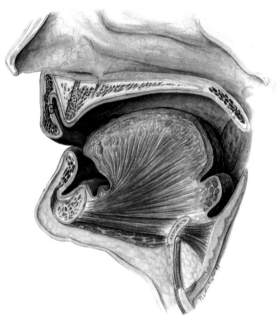

Fig. 29.19 Interpositional bone graft in situ.

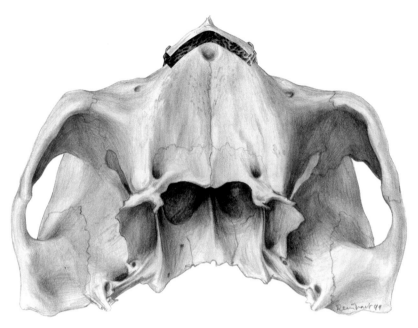

Fig. 29.20 Axial view showing maxillary osteoplasty with interpositional bone graft and stabilization of osteoplastic flaps with microplate osteosynthesis.

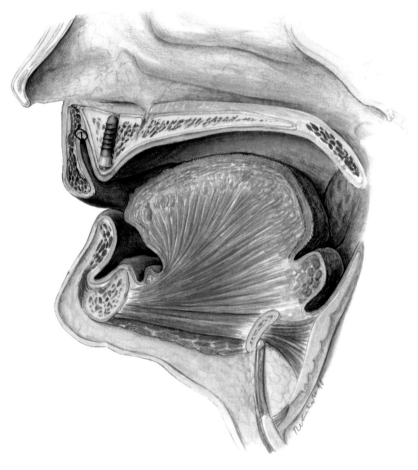

Fig. 29.21 Subsequent placement of endosteal implants into augmented maxillary ridge (implants are placed as a secondary procedure).

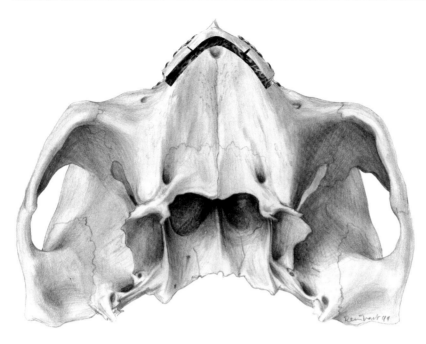

Fig. 29.22 Anterior maxillary osteoplasty. Multiple segments are stabilized with microplate osteosynthesis to expand the narrow V-shaped ridge at the same time as broadening the narrow ridge.

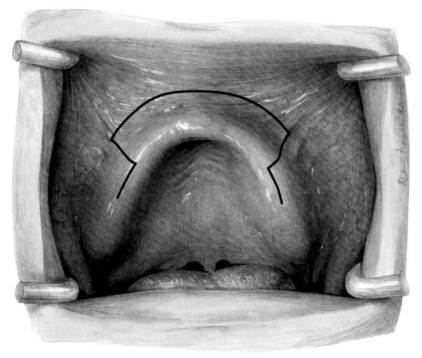

Fig. 29.23 Combined anterior maxillary osteoplasty and "sinus lift" procedure. Position of mucosal incisions.

osteotomized segments can be rigidly stabilized with microplates and screws (**Fig. 29.22**). This procedure can also be combined with the "sinus lift" to allow placement of endosteal implants both anteriorly and posteriorly (**Figs. 29.23–29.25**).

Where there is fusion of the cortical plates, that is to say no intervening cancellous bone, the osteoplasty and interpositional bone graft technique is contraindicated. In

these cases augmentation of the maxilla can be accomplished using block cortical cancellous grafts stabilized with position screws or with lag screws.

Alternatively, augmentation of the class IV maxilla can be obtained with an onlay veneer graft harvested either from the mandibular ramus or from the iliac crest, depending on the extent of the defect. It is possible to remove most of the buccal cortex of the mandibular hor-

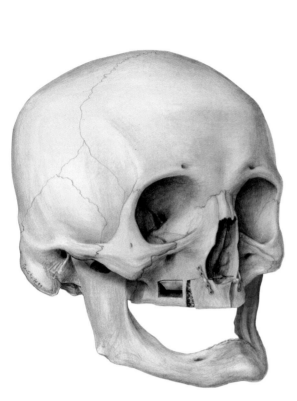

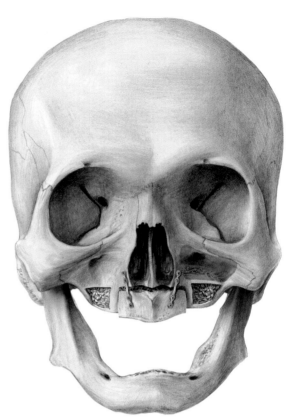

Fig. 29.24 Combined anterior maxillary osteoplasty and "sinus lift" procedure. Position of osteotomy cuts.

Fig. 29.25 Combined anterior maxillary osteoplasty and "sinus lift" procedure. Frontal view of augmented areas.

izontal ramus, which provides enough bone to augment the anterior maxilla. To avoid micromovement of the graft during the healing process, two lag screws are placed in each segment to stabilize the graft (**Figs. 29.26, 29.27**).

Class V Maxilla

Reconstruction of the class V maxilla requires a block cortico-cancellous bone graft to restore both the height and width of the deficient alveolus (saddle graft). For large defects bone is usually harvested from the iliac crest. Lag screws are used to stabilize the graft to the recipient site (**Fig. 29.28**).

Class VI Maxilla

Resorption of the maxillary alveolar process eventually leads to a relatively posterior and cranial position of the maxilla, resulting in a reversed intermaxillary relationship and increased vertical intermaxillary distance. Reconstruction of the class VI maxilla aims at restoration of the interarch relationship and augmentation of the alveo-

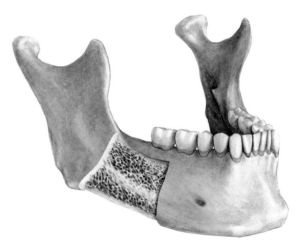

Fig. 29.26 Buccal bone available for veneer graft.

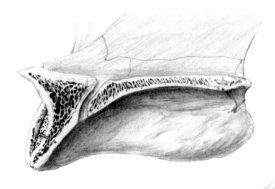

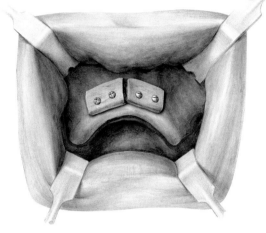

Fig. 29.27 Veneer graft to augment the class IV maxilla.

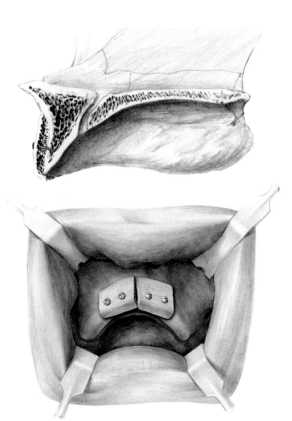

Fig. 29.28 Saddle graft to augment the class V maxilla.

lar bone to provide support for the collapsed facial musculature.

A revolutionary method to treat the class VI maxilla was described by Sailer (1989). He proposed a Le Fort I osteotomy in which the maxilla is repositioned forward and downward at the same time. Cortical cancellous block bone grafts are placed in the floor of the maxillary sinuses and in the floor of the nose. The caudal segment and bone grafts are stabilized with miniplate osteosynthesis and endosteal implants inserted simultaneously. Cawood and Stoelinga (1994) described a two-stage procedure to augment the atrophic maxilla, involving a Le Fort I osteotomy and interpositional bone graft using particulate cortical cancellous bone (to take advantage of the more rapid vascularization and increased osteogenic potential of particulate cancellous bone over block cortical cancellous bone grafts) (**Figs. 29.29, 29.30**). Following healing of the bone graft, endosteal implants are inserted in an optimal position using a surgical guide (**Fig. 29.31**).

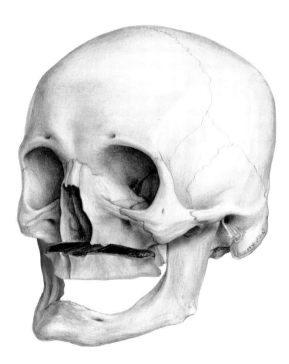

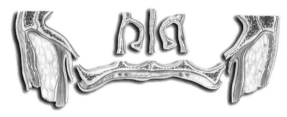

Fig. 29.29 Le Fort I osteotomy of class V maxilla.

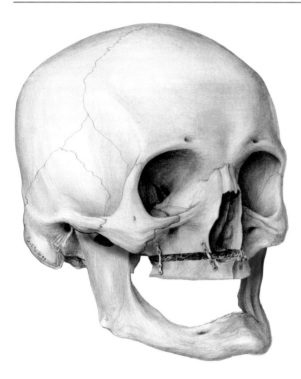

Fig. 29.30 Augmentation of class V maxilla with interpositional bone graft following Le Fort I osteotomy with inferior and anterior repositioning of the caudal fragment.

Atrophic Mandible

Unlike the maxilla, which is composed of trabecular bone predominantly with a thin cortex, the mandible has a thicker cortical layer, similar to a long bone. This provides superior support for endosteal implants, particularly in the anterior mandible. Following tooth loss and aging, the blood supply of the edentulous mandible differs from that of the dentate mandible. In the dentate mandible of the younger patient, blood supply is mainly centrifugal, that is to say it arises from the inferior alveolar artery and periodontal arterial arcades (see **Fig. 29.8**). The blood supply to the edentulous mandible in the older patient is mainly centripetal, being derived via the subperiosteal plexus (see **Fig. 29.8**). Therefore, when carrying out preprosthetic surgery of the edentulous mandible, raising of the mucoperiosteum must be performed carefully to avoid damaging the periosteal layer and ischemic necrosis of the underlying bone.

Class II and Class III Mandible

Endosteal implants can be inserted into the class II and III mandible with minimal pre-implant surgery being required. However, it should be noted that any surgical interference with the inferior alveolar nerve may lead to sensory alteration and loss.

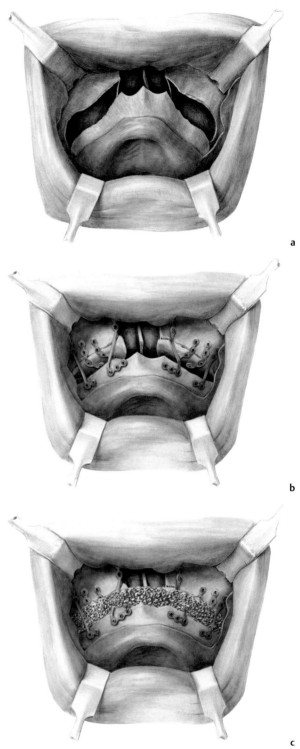

Fig. 29.31 Le Fort I osteotomy of class VI maxilla. Surgical access, stabilization of caudal segment, and interpositional bone graft (particulate cancellous bone).

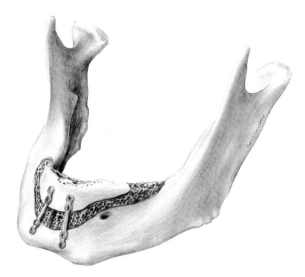

Fig. 29.32 Mandibular augmentation with interpositional graft and stabilization with osteosynthesis plate.

Class IV Mandible

In the class IV anterior mandible, contouring to remove a narrow ridge or onlay bone grafting may be required, to obtain sufficient bone bulk to accommodate endosteal implants.

Class V Mandible

In the anterior mandible, bone grafting is not usually required as there is sufficient residual bulk of bone to provide implant anchorage. However, where the soft-tissue environment is unfavorable, either an interpositional bone graft or onlay bone graft may be required to prevent unfavorable soft-tissue encroachment, which would interfere with prosthetic function.

Class VI Mandible

To obtain sufficient volume of bone to place endosteal implants and provide optimal biomechanical function and soft-tissue support, either an interpositional bone graft or onlay bone graft is usually indicated (**Fig. 29.32**).

Oral Rehabilitation

Current management of oral cancer following tumor resection includes reconstruction of the surgical defect with free vascularized flaps and rehabilitation of oral function with the aid of endosteal implants. The choice of flap for reconstruction influences the use of implants, and further soft-tissue surgery is frequently required to enhance the success of oral rehabilitation.

30 Bone Graft and Membrane Stabilization in Implantology

Franz Haerle and Hendrik Terheyden

Introduction

Localized repair of severe ridge defects for implant placement using autogenous bone grafts is a very well accepted method (**Fig. 30.1**). The iliac crest is the most common donor site in maxillofacial reconstruction for the repair of large defects. For the repair of localized severe alveolar defects alternative donor sites such as the mandibular symphysis (Misch, 1992), the oblique line (coronoid) as described by Schliephake (1995, 1996), and the maxillary tuberosity (Moenning and Graham, 1986) are also useful. In small defects, bone augmentation can be performed by guided bone regeneration under membranes. Larger defects require bone grafts, often in combination with membranes or titanium mesh. The fixation of the bone grafts by membranes, titanium mesh, or screws is important for incorporation without resorption. Membranous bone grafts seem to show less resorption than endochondral bone grafts (Smith and Abramson, 1974; Zins and Whitaker, 1983) and revascularize more rapidly (Kusiak, Zins, and Whitaker, 1985).

Technique

The bone grafts are harvested from the chin region in one or two complete blocks, or from the oblique line (coronoid) in one or two complete blocks, by the use of an oscillating blade or a Lindemann burr and chisels. When the bone is harvested from the maxillary tuberosity, chisels are used. In all techniques it is possible to obtain some cancellous bone chips, which can be used to fill any residual defects. Bone dust and fillings can be retrieved by use of a bone collector in the suction unit, and these can be placed into small gaps.

If possible, the use of bone from the maxillary tuberosity and the oblique line is preferable. Vitality tests on anterior teeth following mandibular symphysis bone grafts have been found to be negative in up to 20% of the teeth tested (Lindquist and Obeid, 1988). Pulp response studies after symphysis bone grafts have shown a high frequency (12%) of pulp canal obliteration (Hoppenreijs, Nijdam, and Freihofer, 1992).

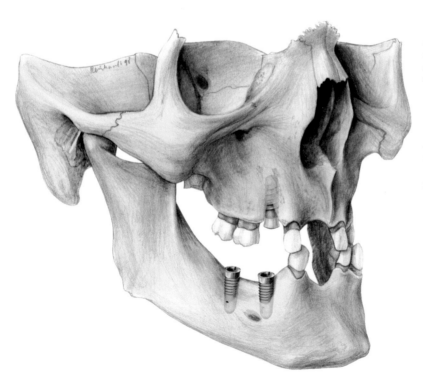

Fig. 30.1 Typical bone defects in implant dentistry. In the premolar region of the right maxilla: facial bone dehiscence of a primary stable ITI implant. In the incisor region of the right maxilla: bone atrophy causes a sharp narrow ridge. In the incisor region of the mandible: vertical and transverse atrophy causes a severe defect. In premolar and molar regions of the right mandible: facial bone dehiscence of two primary stable Camlog implants causes a sharp narrow ridge.

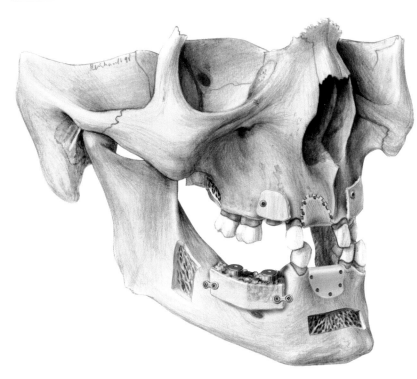

Fig. 30.2 Fixation devices for intra-oral bone grafts (donor and recipient sites). In the premolar region of the right maxilla: a corticocancellous graft from the maxillary tuberosity fixed with a mini lag screw. In the incisor region of the right maxilla: lateral augmentation of a sharp ridge with primary implant insertion using a titanium grid fixed by miniscrews. Cancellous chips and bone fillings harvested by a bone collector from the suction unit are used as a space filler. In the incisor region of the mandible: vertical and transverse augmentation with a corticocancellous block and chips and from the linea obliqua, using a membrane with pin fixation. Second stage implant insertion required. In the premolar and molar region of the right mandible: lateral ridge augmentation with primary implantation using a block and cancellous chips from the mandibular symphysis fixed with microplates.

In the recipient site the bone grafts can be anchored by titanium microscrews, resorbable screws and pins (see Chapter 27), microplates, mini lag screws or nails. The use of a membrane appears to give the best results. Perforation of the underlying alveolar bone with a small drill increases the availability of osteogenic cells from the bone marrow, accelerates revascularization, and improves osseous union (**Figs. 30.2–30.4**). In severe defects of the alveolar crest it is better to perform bone transplantation and implant insertion in a two-stage procedure. If the implant can be stabilized in the desired position, bone transplants can be used to cover any defects. In all situations a stable fixation of grafted bone on the bone to be augmented is important (ten Bruggenkate et al., 1992). The resorption usually does not exceed 1 mm in height. If the screw head after surgery is at the level of the bone transplant, on screw removal usually only the head of the screw is found exposed. An unloaded healing period of 6 months is recommended (Jovanovic and Spiekermann, 1992).

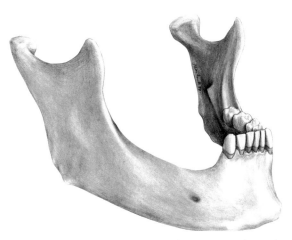

Fig. 30.3 Transverse atrophy causes a sharp narrow ridge in the right mandible.

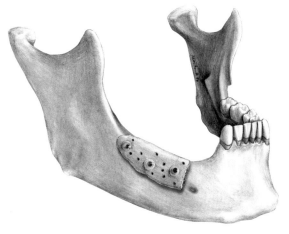

Fig. 30.4 Lateral augmentation of the mandible: a corticocancellous block from the linea obliqua of the left mandible as fixed with Resorb-X pins.

31 Alveolar Bone Distraction

Johannes Hidding and Joachim E. Zoeller

Introduction

Diminished vertical height of the alveolar ridge often leads to loss of vertical dimension of the face, which causes impaired masticatory function and poor facial aesthetics. The alveolar ridge reduction may be caused by traumatic injury, tumor resection, and bone destruction with periodontosis, or general atrophy accompanying tooth loss or old age. In many of these cases, dentures cannot be worn due to lack of mechanical retention. Alternatively, dental implants have been inserted in such situations, where a sufficient amount of bone is available. In order for dentoalveolar implants to be successful, however, a minimum height and width of bone is required.

Where too little bone is available, the alveolar ridge is often augmented using techniques such as guided bone regeneration, onlay grafts, or implantation of alloplastic material. Bone grafts, however, involve an increased surgical risk and consequently a high complication rate. Donor site morbidity and considerable resorption of the grafted bone occur within the year following the procedure (Chiapasco, Zaniboni, and Rimondini, 2007). In light of these problems, several groups have been developing new techniques of vertical alveolar ridge augmentation based on the principles of callus distraction established by the Russian orthopedic surgeon, Gavriel Ilizarov (1989a, b), who pioneered the reconstruction technique of distraction osteogenesis for managing a variety of limb deformities.

The initial work on alveolar ridge distraction was done in dog experiments by Block, Chang, and Crawford (1996), who demonstrated histological evidence of regenerated bone formation during alveolar ridge distraction.

Since 1996 our medical team at the University of Cologne has also been working on alveolar ridge augmentation with the vertical distraction osteogenesis technique. Using the Ilizarov protocol as a basis, we have applied this technique for vertical augmentation of both the dentulous and edentulous alveolar process.

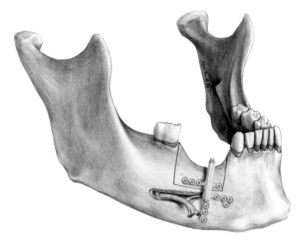

Fig. 31.1 **Osteotomy of the segmental cranial part of the toothless bone.** The distractor has been inserted.

Technique

In edentulous parts of the mandible after segmental resection in tumor surgery or trauma loss, reconstruction by vertical distraction can be used instead of bone transplantation (**Fig. 31.1**). After osteotomy the segmented cranial part of the toothless bony gap of the mandible is mobilized. The vascular supply of this segment is dependent on the preservation of the alveolar attachment and the lingual or the palatal mucoperiosteal flap. Afterward the distractor can be inserted (see **Fig. 31.1**) and the bony segment is stabilized for 7 days. The regimen for callus distraction is 0.5 mm, twice each day. In compromising tissues with scaring or after radiotherapy less activation is recommended (Amir et al., 2006). Within 10 days a previously estimated vertical increase of 10 mm can be obtained. Four weeks later, mineralization of the new bone in the distracted gap can be seen to be starting (**Fig. 31.2**), as well as reunion of the transported bone in the alveolar ridge. Early mineralization studies suggest that insertion of dental implants is possible after 3 months (Yamamoto et al., 1997).

In tooth-bearing areas of the mandible, vertical bone distraction of the alveolar ridge to transport tooth-bearing segments is also possible. This is used in cases such as a

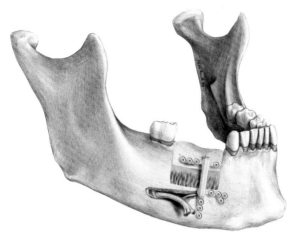

Fig. 31.2 Four weeks after bone distraction, mineralization of the new bone in the distracted gap has begun.

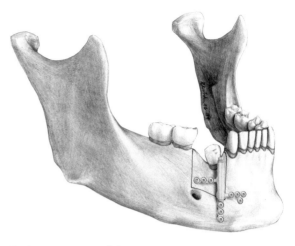

Fig. 31.3 Osteotomy of the segment, with the ankylosed tooth and insertion of the distractor.

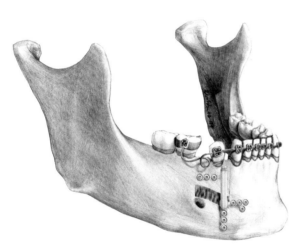

Fig. 31.4 Mineralization of the new bone is seen 4 weeks after insertion of the bone distractor and bone distraction. To prevent relapse, a bracket stabilization with an orthopedic wire is performed.

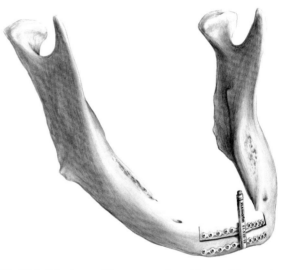

Fig. 31.5 Osteotomy of the segmental cranial part of the toothless bone in the severely resorbed mandible in the interforaminal region.

local open bite, because of vertical undergrowth of the alveolar ridge or the articular process. Sometimes ancylotic teeth are responsible for local undergrowth. In these cases we consider a segmental osteotomy. First the segment with the ancylotic tooth is osteotomized with a Lindemann burr in the outer cortical layer and finished with a reciprocating saw, via a vestibular approach. The lingual cortical layer is separated by feeling the top of the saw and guiding it with the index finger in the mouth floor, preventing any damage of soft tissues, especially nerve structures. After complete osteotomy and mobilization of the segment, the distractor is inserted and the segment stabilized for 7 days (**Fig. 31.3**). An increase of 10 mm is achieved in the segment (**Fig. 31.4**). After 2–3 weeks the distractor should be removed to mold the weak callus formation according to the floating bone concept

(Hoffmeister, Marcks, and Wolff, 1998), and to allow fine correction of the bony segment by an orthodontist.

To prevent relapse, bracket stabilization with an orthopedic wire is performed. During distraction the vitality of the mobilized tooth can remain intact and damage of neighboring teeth should be avoided. One month after distraction, bony structure and mineralization in the distracted gap region is seen (see **Fig. 31.4**).

An important indication for vertical distraction of the alveolar crest is the severely resorbed mandible, especially in female patients from 45 to 60 years of age. Instead of inserting short implants with described complications (Binger et al., 1999), we recommend distraction osteogenesis in the interforaminal region (**Fig. 31.5**) and 3 months later implantation of regular implants in a well prepared implant bed.

Clinical Aspects

In clinical practice distraction osteogenesis of the alveolar crest is a safe procedure with few complications. Conditions for excellent results are a sufficient matrix of the transported segment with adequate height and breadth, creating a good soft-tissue formation of the alveolar crest in addition to gaining attached gingiva. The attachment success of fixed gingiva in our study group was 3 to 4.5, depending on different regions of the alveolar process.

Yamamoto et al. (1997) reported stable bone formation in the distraction gap after 3 months. They found new bone in canine maxillae 4 weeks after bridging the distraction gap, and after 8 weeks the border between the original and regenerated bone was difficult to distinguish. Histologically, the matured, regenerated bone was visible in the gap, which was filled with a network of lamellar bone.

Distraction osteogenesis now provides the possibility for almost unlimited new bone formation. Because of early mineralization, dental implants can be inserted into the new bone after 3 months. In addition to the vertical increase of bone a simultaneous gain of soft tissue is apparent such that a complete histogenesis of the alveolar ridge can be seen, as well as bone transport and osteogenesis. In the consolidation period of 3 months before implant placement there is a continuous bone resorption that should be considered in advance. The resorption rate varies from 10% to 20% so that overdistraction is indicated (Kanno et al., 2007). Clinically, there is an important advantage of distraction osteogenesis over augmentation procedures, because of noticeably less resorption (Chiapasco, Zaniboni, and Rimondini, 2007).

To improve distraction results, we increased the frequency and reduced the rate of activation and found considerable better results of bone quality. This could be approved in animal studies in the so-called dynamic distraction (Kessler, Neukam, and Wiltfang, 2005), where a continuous hydraulic pressure provokes distraction. Another procedure to stabilize the callus formation, especially in compromised irradiated bone, is the callus massage (Lazar et al., 2005). With repeated, stepwise compression and distraction there is a positive effect on the consolidation of the regeneration.

Table 31.1 Complication rates for the vertical distraction osteogenesis technique in a study group of 362 patients

Minor complications:	Dehiscence	21/362
	Tilting of the segment	12/362
	Infection	8/362
	Nerve disturbances	5/362
	Incomplete success during distraction	4/362
	Implant loss	7/699
Major complications:	Fracture of the mandible	1/362
	Necrosis of segment	1/362
	Fracture of activating rod	1/362

Complications

Complications are rather few and the overall success rate is nearly 90% (Mazzonetto et al., 2007). We distinguish between major and minor complications (see **Table 31.1**). Major complication obviously means failure of the procedure (Perdijk et al., 2007) and minor complications required immediate intervention but had no effect the final result. In our study group of 362 patients there were only three cases with major complications (0.8%) and 50 patients with any kind of minor complication (13.8%). The most important fault was a nondislocated fracture of the angle of the mandible requiring osteosynthesis.

Most of these failures occurred in the posterior mandible.

Conclusion

Compared to conventional techniques of bone transplantation, vertical distraction osteogenesis promises some further important advantages.

Callus distraction in toothless bony gaps:
- no bone harvesting
- no donor site morbidity
- distraction of vascularized bone
- less resorption comparable to augmentation
- minimal risk of infection
- early mineralization of new bone
- implantology in juvenile growing bone formation after 3 months
- shortening of entire treatment time

Callus distraction of tooth-bearing segments:
- therapy of local open bite
- safe blood supply to the segment
- teeth vitality can remain intact
- hardly any periodontal problems

Vertical distraction osteogenesis is a safe and predictable procedure in the reconstruction of atrophic or traumatic loss of the alveolar crest as well as in therapy of orthognathic disorders. To obtain good clinical results, the dimensions and size of the distractor should be in accordance with segment volume (Hidding, Zöller, and Lazar, 2000). Permanent preservation of alveolar bone depends on functional load with dental implants.

32 Mandible Alveolar Bone Reconstruction by Endodistraction

Christian Krenkel

Introduction

Traditionally, for functional rehabilitation of severely atrophic edentulous mandibles, short implants with long abutments are used. Another possibility for treatment is bony reconstruction by bone transplantation. Recently, distraction osteogenesis has offered a third option for reconstruction of the alveolar process. The simple principle is based on the natural healing process of fractured or split bones to grow together by osteogenesis, and is called callus distraction (Ilizarov, 1989). Other common distraction appliances are fixed to the bones with two plates, and there is a need for bulky rods projecting outward into the oral cavity. The endodistraction screw sits in a tap-hole in the body of the mandible and is combined with a hollow implant and tap, which is anchored to the osteotomized superior segment of the bone and rests on a metal shoulder of the endodistraction screw. The endodistraction screw appears up to 10 mm beyond the inferior border of the mandible, hidden in the soft tissues of the chin. This distance corresponds to the possible amount of distraction osteogenesis. By turning the endodistraction screw, the hollow implant together with the osteotomized bone is lifted up step by step; the osteotomy gap increases, and distraction osteogenesis begins.

The main indication for this technique is a mandible classified as Cawood 5 or 6 (Cawood and Howell, 1988). The best anatomical predisposition for distraction osteogenesis is in the anterior aspect of the mandible, because of its good blood supply from the Tsusaki vessels on the lingual side (Tsusaki, 1955), which are terminal branches of the sublingual arteries (Krenkel et al., 1985).

Materials and Method

The endodistraction method for vertical callus distraction osteogenesis is a single device, which allows callus formation to be realized in every desired height, width, and direction. For planning the correct vector of the distraction osteogenesis, we use lateral transcranial X-ray and simple drawings according to the ideal position of the intended dentures. Our reference plane is the inferior border of the mandible, which is reliable also during the operation. With the help of an angle-measuring device

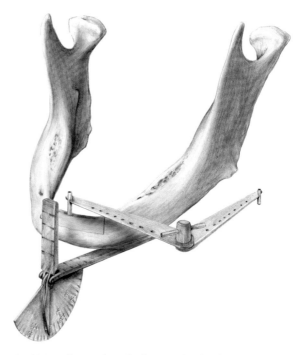

Fig. 32.1 **Drilling in the right direction for the planned vector of distraction osteogenesis is performed with a Josef calibrator (Padgett, Germany, Nr. P690).**

according to Josef (**Fig. 32.1**) during the operation, we choose the right angulation for the tap-hole of the endodistraction screw in the basal arch. The marking is then performed, exactly in the midline of the alveolar crest. First a 2-mm diameter hole is drilled in the desired direction, through and beyond the basal arch. Then supraperiosteal dissection is performed from the vestibule of the mouth, and the mental nerves are identified. This is followed by the planning and marking of the osteotomy. A hole is traced and drilled in the edges of the osteotomy. The osteotomy itself can be performed either by a sagittal microsaw or by piezosurgery with ultrasound (**Fig. 32.2**). The 2-mm hole in the osteotomized upper segment is widened for the hollow implant. After this, the 2-mm hole in the basal arch is tapped for the endodistraction screw. Then follows the tapping (left-hand tap) for the hollow implant in the osteotomized upper segment. The endodistraction screw is inserted through the larger tap

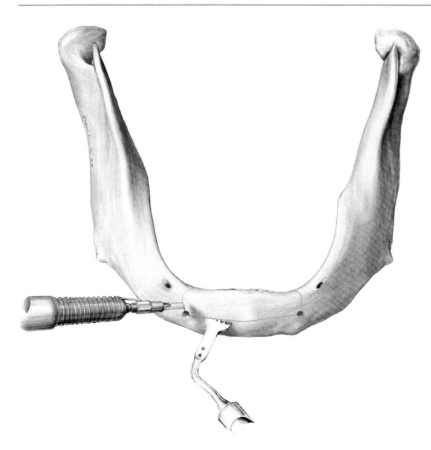

Fig. 32.2 Osteotomy of the transport segment by means of a sagittal microsaw or by piezosurgery with ultrasound. The osteotomy lines are first marked on the mandible by pen from the drill holes at the edges up to the alveolar crest, preserving the gums for blood supply and fixation of the transport segment.

hole of the upper segment into the tap in the basal arch, until the metal shoulder appears within the osteotomy gap. After this, the hollow implant is placed in the upper segment (left-hand tap) and tightened until it rests on the metal shoulder of the endodistraction screw within the osteotomy gap. A primary gap up to 3 mm is helpful for starting callus formation—according to the findings of Zöller (2002) (**Fig. 32.3**). A cover-screw subsequently blocks the system for 1 week before the distraction begins. The endodistractor allows the patient to control the daily callus formation. The surgeon simply instructs the patient, in front of a mirror, how much and how long he or she has to turn the distraction screw with a special key. Twisting up the endodistraction screw on a daily basis—increasing from 0.25 mm to 3 × 0.25 mm according to the actual width of the distraction gap—enables distraction osteogenesis to take place in an almost painless manner. After 3 weeks of distraction, 13 mm height of additional new bone can be achieved (**Fig. 32.4**). In cases of a sharp alveolar crest, an "overdistraction" is required for gaining not only satisfactory height, but also width for the following implants. After a retention time from approximately 4 months, four interforaminal implants are usually inserted, and connected by a temporary bridge for temporary dentures with soft underlining (**Fig. 32.5**). Osseointegration takes place within 5 months. The bioengineered spongy

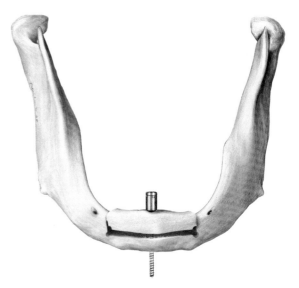

Fig. 32.3 Transport segment during the first retention time (1 week after the osteotomy) with a primary gap of 2–3 mm for starting callus formation. The distraction screw may project up to 15 mm into the soft tissues of the chin, and its oversize in relation to the actual height of the ridge would determine the amount of bone that would be gained by distraction. The distraction screw and the hollow implant are safeguarded during the retention time by a cover screw.

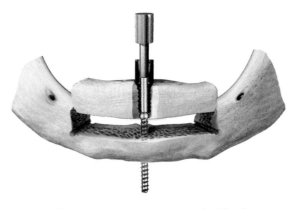

Fig. 32.4 The transport segment at the end of the distraction time, 3 weeks after the osteotomy with the newly formed callus formation. Using a special key within the hollow implant, the distraction screw is twisted up by the patient, 0.25 mm a day and more, up to the desired height, following an individual distraction protocol.

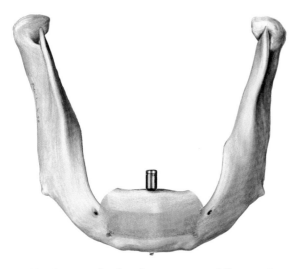

Fig. 32.5 Four months after the osteotomy and the second retention time the callus formation is calcified and the endodistractor can be removed and replaced by four interforaminal dental implants.

bone provides additional stable anchorage for dental implants.

Indications

The minimally invasive endodistraction implant guarantees stable, bioengineered, mature bone of predictable height in the required vertical direction without utilization of additional bone substitute materials (Krenkel et al., 2007). In the lower jaw, the preferred region is in the midline, due to the superior quality of bone and minimal

damage to nutrition because of the absence of nutrient foramina. In the lateral aspect of the jaws, endodistraction implants can also be used in the premolar region in an eccentric fashion, minding of course the mental nerve or the maxillary sinus. Needless to say, the endodistractor allows a callus to form also in a gap between teeth, using a smaller device. Furthermore, the endodistractor can be applied—in several sizes and with some additional devices—in almost any facial region.

Discussion

With the endodistraction technique one can easily choose any vector and the amount of distraction, according to the treatment plan, with only one device. Running in the center of the bone with central loading, fractures of this device are not expected. A new oral vestibule is re-established. The upper part of the device, with the cover screw on top, resembles the abutment of an implant and disturbs neither the lips nor tongue. Removal of the endodistraction implant is simple and almost painless, and can be performed with superficial mucosal anesthesia, because the endodistraction device does not become integrated into the bone. Because the majority of patients with early loss of teeth and high atrophy of jaws suffer from severe trismus, for psychological reasons a case history is important before starting the treatment. Warning must be given, when using a temporary prosthesis during retention time, because this can have negative effects on the endodistraction device and the distracted bone. There is no urgent reason for providing a temporary denture during retention time, because the re-established bone with gums provides a natural support for the lower lip, which appears natural when speaking, in spite of the patient not wearing a denture. Sometimes, the ends of the endodistraction screw are initially visible through the skin, which appears to be a problem. The gently positioned, smooth ends of the endodistraction screw glide within the tissues and never cause necrosis or pain. It is a great advantage that the endodistraction screw is safeguarded in a sterile pocket in the chin; in this way we can avoid the conventional bulky rods reaching out into the oral cavity, which is not a sterile area. After distraction begins, the tip of the endodistraction screw disappears within a short time, but has never proved porblematic for patients. After applying the dentures fully supported by implants, the new functional loading, together with shortening of the prosthesis in the molar region new bone formation, is recognized on top of the alveolar channel. In the event of the endodistraction device becoming loose during the latency period, an emergency hollow implant is provided for further fixation of the osteotomized segment. Pitfalls, like a fatigue fracture of the body of the mandible, which can occur in the middle of the latency period, are less dangerous for patients. An operation and osteosynthesis are not necessary, because the bulky distraction callus already formed bridges the fracture ends. Conservative treatment with antibiotics and soft diet is sufficient, and after fracture healing the implants can be placed in the usual way.

Summary

The endodistraction technique has its primary indication in the high atrophic mandible. Further indications are the local, high atrophic alveolar crest and the atrophic single tooth gap in both jaws. In cases of tumor treatment involving resection of the alveolar process, the reconstruction of alveolar bone and gums is a potential indication. The technique can also be applied for secondary reconstruction of the alveolar crest in totally resected mandibles after reconstruction by iliac crest, scapula, or fibula, to obtain better preconditions for the implantological and prosthetic rehabilitation. Further indications may also be maxilla, zygoma, and the extreme hypoplastic chin. Endo-distraction, with its alternative way of working compared with devices of microplate design, is characterized by the following features and benefits: one "single-screw" device in the middle of the bone; no adaptation work during fixation; only one device for all directions and heights; no tilting problems; and no second operation to remove the device.

33 Mesh Fixation of Bone

Bodo Hoffmeister

Introduction

Different osteosynthesis techniques can be applied to fix bone grafts when reconstructing the mandible. This chapter looks at titanium mesh, which adds to the osteosynthesis techniques described in previous chapters and completes the spectrum of available fixation methods.

Lambotte published an article in 1913, describing the treatment of a median mandibular fracture using a plate, which identifies the basic principles for mesh osteosynthesis. Boyne (1969) first used titanium mesh for mandibular reconstruction; later Hauenstein and Steinhäuser (1977) reported on technical advantages and clinical experiences. The titanium mesh was originally developed for mandibular reconstruction in combination with cancellous bone chips (Boyne, 1969). The idea was to replace the mandible by a U-shaped titanium mesh filled with autologous iliac crest spongiosa (Steinhäuser, 1982; Dumbach and Steinhäuser, 1983; Dumbach, 1985; Dumbach et al., 1994). A range of titanium meshes has been developed, based on those used by earlier workers, and are available in a selection of different sizes.

Wolff et al. (1996) reported on 24 cases of mandibular reconstruction using a fibula free flap with microsurgically anastomosed vascular pedicles. He observed one broken plate and one infection at the osteosynthesis line.

Individual patient requirements determine which size of titanium mesh to use. For mandibular reconstruction, the 2 mm system is the osteosynthesis material of choice. In special cases where free bone of the alveolar crest, or other bone graft, is to be fixed on the mandible to reconstruct the alveolar ridge, the 1.5 mm system is useful (**Figs. 33.1, 33.2**).

Further development of mesh fixation concerning the principles of three-dimensional fixation of the bone using titanium mesh has been introduced by Farmand (1991, 1995). He developed three-dimensional osteosynthesis plates for multipurpose use.

Mesh systems are valuable in that they give the surgeon the opportunity to construct a plate according to the individual needs of the patient. With a special instrument, the mesh cutter, custom plates can be produced to meet the specific demands presented by the particular part of the facial skeleton to be reconstructed.

Custom-made osteosynthesis plates can satisfy the surgeon's individual needs for different approaches. Excel-

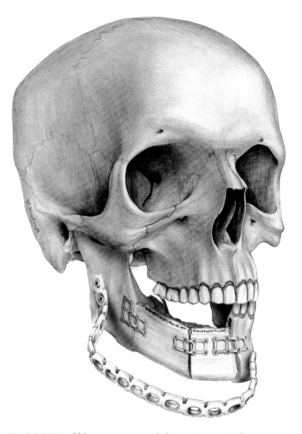

Fig. 33.1 Mandible reconstructed by microsurgically anastomosed iliac crest flap using 2 mm titanium mesh. Note the temporary fixation of the ascending rami during the osteosynthesis of the iliac crest flap.

lent results have been achieved using titanium mesh systems in the reconstruction defects of the facial skeleton during tumor surgery. Titanium mesh is ideal for use in the lateral orbit, or other bony structures of the facial skeleton, in interdisciplinary treatments for craniofacial tumors involving the neurosurgeon and the ophthalmologist (**Fig. 33.3**). This mesh reconstruction of the skeletal parts gives the patients an acceptable aesthetic and functional outcome. In interdisciplinary treatment of craniofacial tumors, a mesh system is nearly always used as the osteosynthesis material for reconstruction of the resected bone.

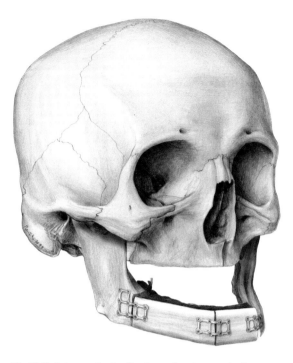

Fig. 33.2 Osteosynthesis fixation of microsurgically anastomosed fibula flap to reconstruct the mandible. This is a case of osteoradionecrosis following irradiation for oral cancer.

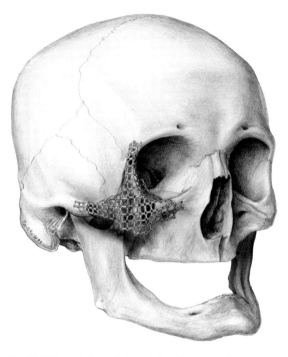

Fig. 33.3 Bony defect of the midfacial skeleton due to tumor involvement of the zygoma. The facial skeleton was reconstructed by using pre-bent titanium mesh. In such cases there is nearly always an acceptable aesthetic and functional outcome.

Indications

As well as for reconstructive surgery, particularly of the mandible, mesh fixation of bone is also indicated in other fields of maxillofacial surgery, such as:

- traumatology—repair of bony defects; osteosynthesis in comminuted and multiple fractures
- orthognathic surgery—fixation of the maxilla after Le Fort I osteotomy (**Fig. 33.4**); fixation of osteotomized bone segments after genioplasty (**Fig. 33.5**); and
- reconstructive surgery after tumor operations

Traumatology

In the treatment of midfacial and mandibular fractures, the usefulness of miniplates or microplates in some midfacial regions is obvious. In a very few cases the application of titanium mesh in different sizes may be helpful. In some cases of severely comminuted fractures of the facial wall of the maxillary sinus, a micromesh can re-establish the normal size of the maxillary sinus. In addition, if osteosynthesis is required for badly comminuted fractures of other midfacial regions, even in the mandible, the bone pieces generally can be collected and fixed using titanium mesh. Removal of the material can be performed up to 1 year postoperatively.

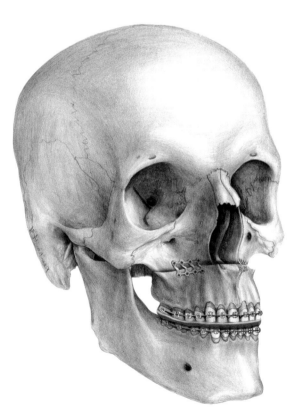

Fig. 33.4 Titanium mesh fixation after Le Fort I osteotomy in orthognathic surgery. Titanium mesh plates are easy to bend and easy to fix.

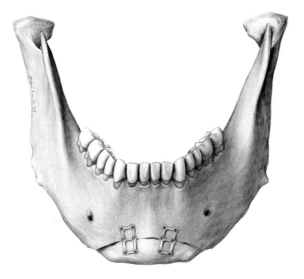

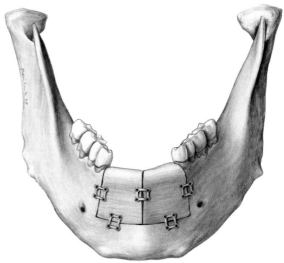

Fig. 33.5 Genioplasty with chin reduction and osteosynthesis using titanium mesh. Titanium mesh is very easy to bend and may be precisely applied to the individual situation.

Fig. 33.6 Reconstruction of the alveolar crest of the mandible in the frontal region after tumor resection and postoperative irradiation. Note the fixation of the iliac crest graft. Due to the monocortical application of the screws and mesh osteosynthesis, it is not always necessary to remove the material when titanium dental implants are used.

Orthognathic Surgery

The titanium mesh system represents an additional osteosynthesis material that is very useful in orthognathic surgery for fixation of the maxilla after Le Fort I osteotomy. The mesh is easy to bend and very easy to apply. Some surgeons prefer 1.5 mm osteosynthesis systems for maxillary fixation during orthognathic surgery.

In addition to maxillary fixation with titanium mesh, osteosynthesis in genioplasties including chin reduction and chin augmentation can be performed.

In some cases of sagittal split osteotomy with complications due to the osteotomy (bad split), titanium mesh plates are very helpful for a stable osteosynthesis. The possibility of individually adapting the mesh plates to the cortical bone may be an advantage in these cases.

Surgical Applications

Titanium mesh has proved very useful because the surgeon can customize plates to suit any particular case.

In addition to its use in routine orthognathic surgery, titanium mesh can be used in managing complications such as "bad" mandibular sagittal split. The versatility of the material allows customizing at surgery, and application to provide secure fixation of the bone part, leading to uneventful healing and an acceptable outcome.

The titanium mesh system can be used to reconstruct the bony continuity of the mandible using microsurgically anastomosed bone flaps, for example, from the fibula, the iliac crest, or other sites. The preferred flap for mandibular bone reconstruction is currently the fibula transplant (see Chapter 36).

The osteosynthesis used is monocortical osteosynthesis, as described in previous chapters. In some cases parts of the mandible can be fixed before resection, using reconstruction plates to stabilize the ascending ramus and both condylar processes (see **Fig. 33.1**). Irrespective of the size and shape of the tumor during resection, this bridging plate device will stabilize the residual mandible. Harvested bone can be placed in the gap, trimmed, shaped into the proper position, then fixed using 2 mm titanium mesh with a minimum of four screws at each osteotomy site. After fixation the reconstruction plate must be removed, then the microsurgical anastomosis can be performed. This surgical procedure results in the proper position of the ascending rami as well as a mandibular shape similar to that of the original.

One advantage which titanium mesh offers over reconstruction plates is that the mesh used as described allows functional loading of the transplanted bone, which aids healing and re-establishment of mandibular continuity.

In most cases monocortical osteosynthesis should not hinder the proper insertion of dental implants, when these are necessary. There should be no difficulty in removing the titanium mesh after 1–1.5 years, should the patient's prosthetic restoration or dental implants require this (**Fig. 33.6**).

The general principles of mandibular osteosynthesis with miniplates should be followed to avoid pitfalls with these osteosynthesis procedures, in particular:

- be careful not to put titanium mesh around the lower border of the mandible, because strain interaction will lead to plate fractures
- avoid sharp edges which could perforate the mucosal layer

Intermaxillary fixation is not required when using this mesh osteosynthesis technique in mandibular reconstruction.

Conclusion

To summarize, the major advantage of mesh osteosynthesis systems in reconstructive surgery of the maxillofacial region lies in the ability to customize the material, in size and in shape, during surgery. This gives the surgeon the opportunity to perform reconstruction in a moderate amount of time and with reasonable stability.

34 Mandibular Reconstruction with Free, Nonvascularized Bone Grafts

Hans-Dieter Pape and Klaus Louis Gerlach

Introduction

The first free transplantations of autologous bone for reconstruction of the mandible were performed by Lexer, who, in 1907, used bone from the tibia and, in 1908, part of a rib (Reichenbach and Schöneberger, 1957). Various techniques of reconstruction have since been developed.

The functional integration of a free bone transplant into the local bone structures is of the greatest importance to a successful outcome. This ensures that physiological stress factors can influence early remodeling of the transplanted bone. The quality of the bone transplant, the stability of bone fixation, and the condition of the surrounding soft tissue are critical to the success of the transplantation. Experience has shown that the iliac crest is the ideal bone for reconstruction of the jaw. Rib transplants are mainly used as substitutes for the neck and head of the condyle and for reconstruction of children's jaws.

Reconstruction is usually performed using an extraoral approach. In cases of benign tumors a primary reconstruction directly following resection is possible. This can be done intraorally, if the size and location of the tumor allow it. In malignant tumors bone reconstruction is generally performed as a secondary operation after 1 year free from recurrence.

Technique

Wire was the most frequently used osteosynthesis material for the fixation of an iliac crest transplant until 1975. Even today, parallel or crossed double-wiring with 0.5 mm soft steel wire is a reliable method of simple fixation, but it requires intermaxillary fixation for approximately 8 weeks because of its limited stability (**Fig. 34.1**).

Intermaxillary immobilization is unnecessary if bridging plates are used. This type of plate (e.g., AO, Osteo, Synthes, etc.) has to be fixed to the stumps of the mandible with at least three screws (**Fig. 34.2**). These screws have to be long enough to be bicortical. The plates assure complete stability of even large transplants. However, the large plate systems (Luhr, 1976; Reuther, 1979; Schmoker, von Allmen, and Tschopp, 1982; Raveh 1990) do have the problem of their large size, which results in considerable tension on the surrounding soft tissue, with a risk of dehiscence. Additionally, the revascularization of the transplant is delayed by the large area of contact with the plate. Strong plates have a high degree of inflexibility, which results in an insufficient transfer of function to the transplant. This effect, called "stress protection," leads to progressive sponginess of the bone and, if the plate is not removed, to marked atrophy after 5–6 months. Early re-

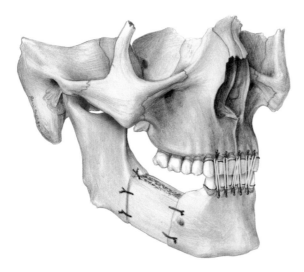

Fig. 34.1 Wire fixation of the graft and intermaxillary fixation of the mandible.

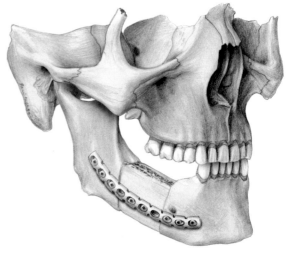

Fig. 34.2 Reconstruction of the mandible with a free graft fixed by a compression plate.

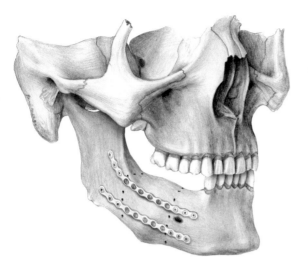

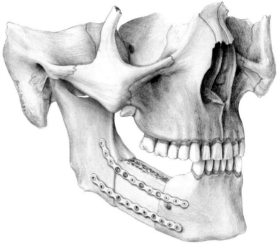

Fig. 34.3 Mandible with a benign tumor in the right molar area with bore holes in the resection lines. Two titanium reconstruction miniplates have been adapted and provisionally fixated on both sides.

Fig. 34.4 The same mandible as in Fig. 34.3 after resection of the tumor segment. Reconstruction with a free bone graft fixated with the two titanium reconstruction miniplates.

moval is necessary so that the bone can reconstitute itself under normal physiological loads.

The successful use of miniplates in fracture treatment led to the development of a titanium reconstruction miniplate, which has the same small size as the fracture plate but an increased thickness of 1.27 mm (Schmid and Pape, 1991; Pape et al., 1993; Pape, Gerlach, and Schippers, 1994). It is necessary to use these as double bridging plates. In all cases of primary reconstruction, the titanium reconstruction miniplate should be adapted and temporarily screwed to the surface of the unresected mandible, prior to ablation. If the length of the transplant is identical to the length of the resected bone, it is possible to reconstruct the mandible in its original anatomical form (**Figs. 34.3, 34.4**). It is recommended that the plate be fixed at each end with at least three and not more than five screws. The screws are of the same size as those used for fracture plates, but they should, of course, be longer for bicortical fixation. For the fixation of the free bone transplant it is sufficient to use one screw in every second plate hole.

In those cases where only a small part of the condylar head is available for fixation, narrow reconstruction plates are particularly useful (**Fig. 34.5**). If the entire ramus including the articular head has to be replaced, the titanium reconstruction miniplates should not simply be fixed to the stump of the jaw with the adjoining transplant, but should be long enough to fix nearly the entire length of the transplant (**Fig. 34.6**). This is not only to increase the stability of the transplant during the process of rebuilding, but also to ensure the transfer of functional stimuli to the whole transplanted bone. Clinical experience has shown that, even in such difficult cases, intermaxillary fixation is not necessary.

The application of two titanium reconstruction miniplates confirms the assumption that the early transfer of function to the transplant reduces the risk of atrophy and encourages stability (Pape, Gerlach, and Schippers, 1994).

As an alternative to fixation with plates, a preformed tray of titanium mesh can be used. This is also fixed with three screws to the stumps of the mandible and, because of its special shape, can be filled with cancellous and pieces of cortical bone (**Fig. 34.7**). Within 3–6 months the bone fragments will rebuild the missing part of the mandible in the form of the titanium tray (Boyne, 1969; Dumbach et al., Dumbach 1994). Removal of the mesh is complicated as some areas become integrated with the bone.

If narrow bone transplants can be placed on the buccal side of a mandible stump, lag screw fixation is a good alternative. In such cases the outer cortex of the stump has to be removed. Two lag screws are used to achieve a stable fixation for the transplant to the lingual cortex of the stump. Reconstruction of the articular surface with a rib transplant is an example of this technique (**Fig. 34.8**).

Irrespective of the method of osteosynthesis used, reconstruction of the mandible requires special care. The transplanted graft should not have any sharp bone edges under the surface of the mucosa. Direct and good contact between the graft and the stumps of the mandible is always necessary. Any spaces between the buccal cortex, caused by convex bending of the graft, should be filled with cancellous chips. Sufficient stability of the graft must be the goal whenever any kind of osteosynthesis is used.

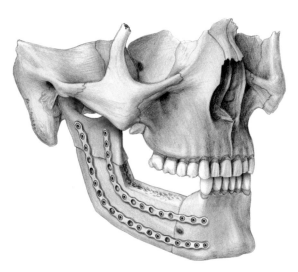

Fig. 34.5 Secondary reconstruction of the mandible from the canine to the condylar neck. Fixation of the graft with two titanium reconstruction miniplates.

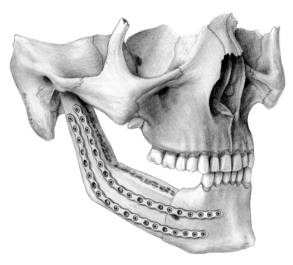

Fig. 34.6 Reconstruction of the mandible from the premolar region to the fossa articularis. The two titanium reconstruction miniplates extend nearly the entire length of the transplant.

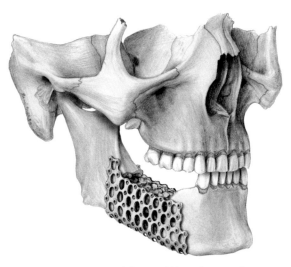

Fig. 34.7 Reconstruction of the mandible with a tray of titanium mesh filled with bone.

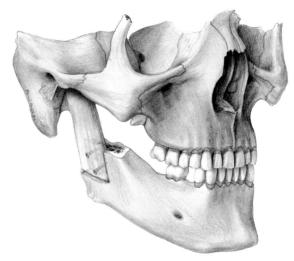

Fig. 34.8 Reconstruction of the articular process with a costochondral graft fixed with two lag screws at the stump of the mandible, after removal of the buccal cortex.

35 Intraoral Distraction Osteogenesis of the Mandible and the Maxilla

Konrad Wangerin, Henning Gropp, Winfried Kretschmer, and Werner Zoder

Introduction

The principle of distraction of the upper and lower extremities was developed by Ilizarov (1988) in the former Union of Soviet Socialist Republics between 1950 and 1985. In the late 1980s miniaturized distractors were manufactured in Western Europe for use in hand surgery. Ilizarov and McCarthy exchanged ideas during a visit to New York, resulting in the first-ever distraction of malformed mandibles using transbuccally fixated hand-surgery distractors. McCarthy's publication in 1992 sparked off an extensive search for distraction indications and frantic development of a variety of distractors for use in the craniofacial area of the skull. As well as multidimensionally adjustable equipment for extraoral use, more comfortable, enorally applied distractors were also developed, and these are used today in distraction of all parts of the craniofacial skeleton.

Publications on enoral mandibular distraction first appeared in the mid-1990s (Wangerin and Gropp, 1994; Diner et al., 1996). In 1995 Cohen and coworkers first treated a severe craniofacial microsomia by simultaneous distraction of the maxilla, the orbita, and the mandible using two distractors. Chin and Toth (1996) distracted the maxilla first, shortening the activation pin which perfo-

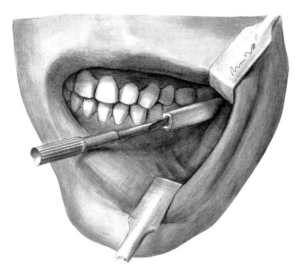

Fig. 35.1 Demonstration of a horizontal mandibular distractor, activated by turning the screwdriver anticlockwise.

rated the cheek as soon as possible after rapid maxilla advancement, thus avoiding scarring. Chin (1999) developed the equipment further to enable hidden Le Fort III distraction.

Enoral distraction methods do not restrict the quality of life, they avoid scar formation in the cheek areas, they have the advantage of being invisible during use, they are easy to use (**Fig. 35.1**), and can be retained for unlimited periods. The sole existing disadvantage, the unidirectional distraction, was offset by Triaca et al. (1998) who developed multiaxial mandibular distractors. Enoral distraction in the craniofacial skeleton has now become a gold standard.

Mandibular Distraction in Congenital Malformation or Acquired Deficiency

Indications for distraction are all syndromes with mandibular malformation. A major symptom is airway obstruction in severe cases of mandibular retrognathia. Deglutition problems may also be caused by malformation of the mandible. Another indication is speech impairment due to a reduced oral cavity size (Wangerin, 2005).

The development of distraction first broke the unspoken law that osteotomies should not be performed before bone growth is complete. Enoral distraction is possible even in small children from the age of 3–4 years. Prerequisite is a sufficient thickness of cortical bone surrounding the mandibular body, necessary to fix the distractor miniscrews.

Acquired shortening of the mandibular body, ascending mandibular ramus, and condylar process can also be considered indications for distraction. These alterations may be caused by trauma or rheumatoid degeneration of the condyle; they may also be the result of bone infections or tumor resection. They occur mainly in adults, and distraction therapy is especially effective in the ascending ramus. In the past the only solution was to reconstruct the ramus–temporomandibular-joint unit by means of costochondral graft, a procedure that was not always successful, showing acceptable results in only one-third of cases. Distraction is less complicated, more comfortable for the patient and has a very high success rate. Prerequisite for a successful treatment is the postopera-

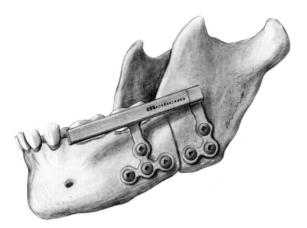

Fig. 35.2 Horizontal mandibular distractor in neutral position fixed to the mandible buccally parallel to the occlusal plane with monocortical 5 mm or 7 mm miniscrews.

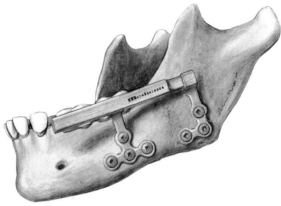

Fig. 35.3 Situation after horizontal distraction of the mandibular body to compensate for mandibular bony deficit.

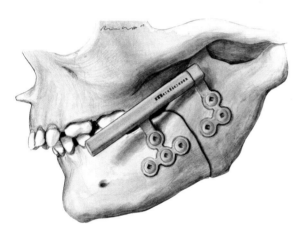

Fig. 35.4 Horizontal mandibular distractor situated at an angle to the occlusal plane to lengthen the mandibular body and the ascending ramus.

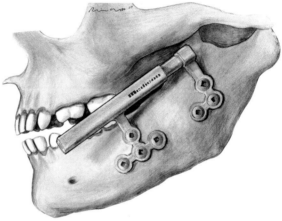

Fig. 35.5 Oblique distraction: the result is an enlarged mandible with an open bite.

tive integration of an interocclusal acrylic splint for 6 months to retain the resulting open bite until the ossification is complete.

Body Deficiency

Indication

A mandibular body which is simply too short is rare. It can occur unilaterally or bilaterally, in most cases in conjunction with a deficit of the ascending mandibular ramus. To reduce symptoms such as obstruction of the respiratory tract, difficult ingestion, or speech impairment, in some cases it is necessary to initially lengthen the mandibular body. This is often a prerequisite for a later, second distraction to elongate the likewise shortened ascending mandibular ramus.

Surgical Technique

Under general anesthesia or local analgesia, a posterior buccal vestibular mucoperiosteal incision is made, followed by subperiosteal exposure limited only to the buccal surface of mandibular angle region, while preserving the periosteal attachment to lingual surface. A horizontal mandibular distractor 20 mm or 25 mm in length is inserted and fixed monocortically onto both sides of the planned osteotomy by means of one miniscrew per side, thus defining the direction of distraction. In most cases distraction runs parallel to the occlusal plane (**Figs. 35.2, 35.3**), less commonly obliquely, so that the distraction results in an open bite (**Figs. 35.4, 35.5**). In cases of severe unilateral hemifacial microsomia it may at times be necessary to pre-bend the distractor miniplates to change distraction direction (**Figs. 35.6–35.9**) and to alleviate facial asymmetry. In such cases all the drill holes are bored in advance and the osteotomy is then marked with the

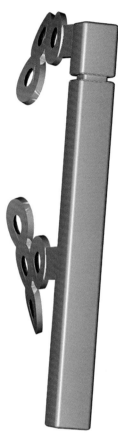

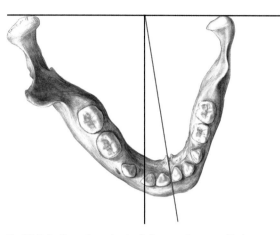

Fig. 35.7 Rudimentary shorter left ascending mandibular ramus with a noticeable midline shift to the left.

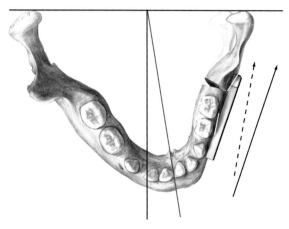

Fig. 35.6 Pre-bent miniplates on a horizontal mandibular distractor used to laterally shift a rudimentary condylar process, which extends into the oral cavity.

Fig. 35.8 After retromolar diagonal mandibular osteotomy. Fixation of the distractor with pre-bent miniplates and resulting lateral shift of the shortened left condylar process. The original distraction direction has changed (unbroken arrow).

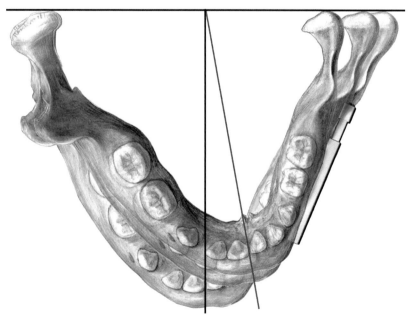

Fig. 35.9 Distraction results in expansion of the mandible on the left side and positioning of the mandibular midline in the correct midline position.

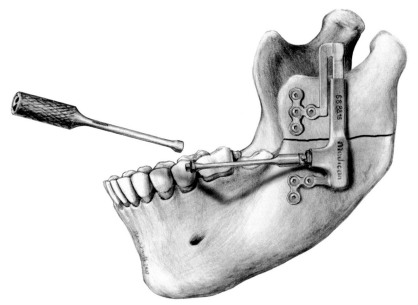

Fig. 35.10 Congenital malformations of the mandible often show a deficit in the ascending mandibular ramus; the most common distraction is therefore extension of the ascending ramus. The vertical mandibular distractor is fixed to the buccal side. The distraction cylinder marks the direction of distraction. This must be carefully planned in each individual case. The distraction is rerouted by means of a gear mechanism, so that the activation rod (which is jointed to make it flexible) comes easily to rest in the floor of the mouth.

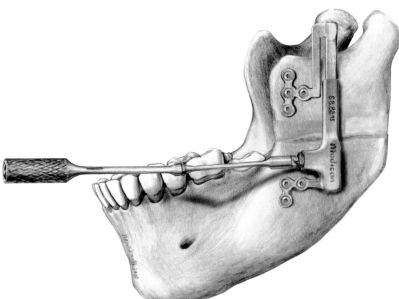

Fig. 35.11 Distraction has lengthened the ascending ramus. If the osteotomy is situated in the area of cancellous bone, bone growth is unlimited. A lateral open bite results in the nonocclusal area, which will have to be supported by an interocclusal splint for 6 months.

Lindemann burr. The distractor is removed and the osteotomy performed.

It is important to expose the inferior alveolar nerve and completely split the mandible. This split should be checked, especially toward the medial periosteally covered mandibular surface. During the active bone growth period there is always a risk of just a greenstick fracture occurring. The distractor is then reinserted and fixed permanently onto both sides of the osteotomy with monocortical screws of 5 mm or 7 mm in length. A test distraction should be performed, so that any unforeseen problems can be dealt with. Ultimately, the incision is closed with resorbable sutures.

Ramus Deficiency

Indication

If the mandibular body is long enough, many cases with a deficiency of the ramus require vertical distraction. In our patients this is the type of distraction we performed most often during the last decade (Kuder, 2006) (**Figs. 35.10, 35.11**).

In these cases planning the distraction vector is a prerequisite for successful treatment. Based on cephalometric analysis of the lateral X-ray the vector can be defined and transferred during the operation. In individual cases we checked the distractor position intraoperatively by vector determination pins or by radiographic verification. In other severe cases of hemifacial microsomia, operation planning was performed with the aid of computed tomography (CT) and stereolithography and the complete surgical procedure was simulated on a model skull. During this procedure the fixation plates of the distractor were pre-shaped, ensuring high accuracy when intraoperatively positioning the equipment.

The operative approach is identical to that in the horizontal mandibular area. Distraction is easily performed by patients themselves: with the aid of a mirror the patient uses a screwdriver to turn the activation pin in the mandibular vestibule. It can be pulled out at the end of distraction for total submergence of the device and to avoid infection in the distraction area (**Fig. 35.12**).

Combinations

The close connection between horizontal and vertical distraction in the mandible has already been described in the sections on body deficiency and ramus deficiency. Depending on primary presentation and the extent of the bony defect, procedures are planned individually for each patient. In the majority of cases horizontal distraction is performed first to relieve primary symptoms, which can be done by the age of 3 or 4 years according to the severity of the respiratory obstruction. In the early teenage years, vertical distraction is performed to develop a bony mandibular angle. In a case of a severe bilateral facial cleft with extreme mandibular retrognathy we performed two horizontal distractions 1 year apart, concluding therapy with a bimaxillary osteotomy at the end of skeletal maturity. Facial asymmetries caused by unilateral hemifacial microsomia in combination with mandibular retrognathia were treated with a combination of horizontal and oblique mandibular distraction, and ultimately corrected by bimaxillary osteotomy (Wangerin et al., 2006).

When indicated, these procedures can be undertaken in a consecutive manner 1 year apart.

Distraction in Orthognathic Surgery

Conventional osteotomies in orthognathic surgery do have anatomical and physiological limits. Certain relapse tendencies after jaw repositioning cannot always be completely avoided. The risk of a relapse grows as the magnitude of acute surgical movement increases.

Distraction, however, can keep such relapses to a minimum because advancement of the jaw, or parts of the jaw, is performed gradually, in multiple daily increments, and retention time is unlimited as the distractor is worn enorally.

Distraction enables advancement over longer distances than with conventional osteotomy. Chin and Toth (1996)

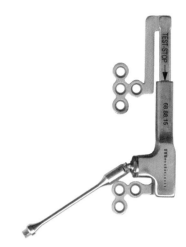

Fig. 35.12 The new modification of the vertical device allows the mobilization of the activation pin after the end of distraction. The total submergence avoids infection of the distraction region.

provided convincing evidence of this. The advantages of distraction methods in comparison to conventional osteotomy can be seen in mandibular or maxillary advancement or in transversal expansion of narrow mandibles or maxillae.

Mandibular Retrognathia

Indication

An indication for parallel mandibular distraction is mandibular retrognathia with angle class II malocclusion. Parallel positioning of the distractors is necessary to avoid an increase in intercondylary distance (**Figs. 35.13, 35.14**). The prerequisites here are full skeletal growth and normal position of the maxilla. In comparison to routinely performed bilateral sagittal splitting of the mandible, it appears that gradual daily advancement of the mandibular body lacks harmful effects on the function of the mandibular joints, which are endangered by a possible malposition of the articular disk. Gradually stretching the suprahyoid musculature and the soft tissue surrounding the mandible reduces any sensation of tension, a problem which occurs especially in older patients. Retromolar diagonal osteotomy of the mandible during distraction does not damage the inferior alveolar nerve, providing another advantage over conventional sagittal splitting, a method which cannot completely eliminate nerve damage.

A final advantage of this method is the close cooperation with the orthodontist who can carry out the distraction and define the extent of distraction to fit in with his or her orthodontic treatment plan. Dental or skeletal relapses have not been noted in these cases up to now.

It should be mentioned that a deep bite provides the best occlusal results, as distraction in these cases always

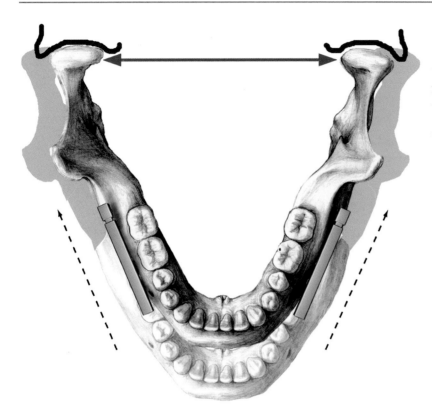

Fig. 35.13 When fitted bilaterally, horizontal distractions in the mandible lead to an enlarged intercondylar distance. This is acceptable in cases of joint malformations and in cases of severe mandibular retrognathia before the end of bone growth; it is not, however, suitable for correction of dysgnathia in adults.

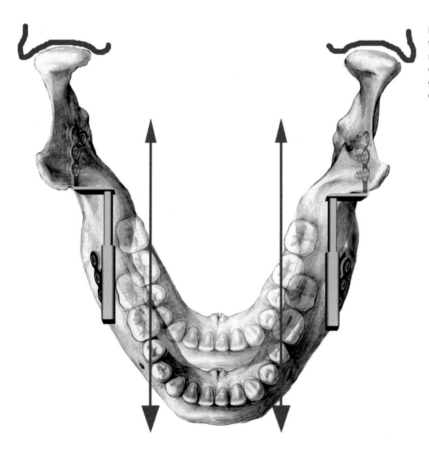

Fig. 35.14 Angled distractors, positioned on the buccal side of the mandible, allow parallel distraction of the mandibular body without greatly affecting the temporomandibular joints.

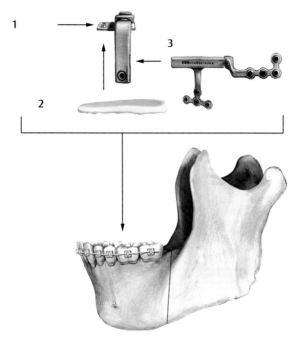

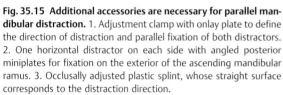

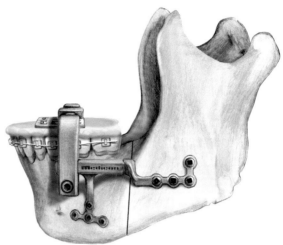

Fig. 35.15 Additional accessories are necessary for parallel mandibular distraction. 1. Adjustment clamp with onlay plate to define the direction of distraction and parallel fixation of both distractors. 2. One horizontal distractor on each side with angled posterior miniplates for fixation on the exterior of the ascending mandibular ramus. 3. Occlusally adjusted plastic splint, whose straight surface corresponds to the distraction direction.

Fig. 35.16 The onlay plate of the adjustment clamp is fixed onto the surface of the plastic splint, thus defining the direction of distraction. The plastic splint is fixed circularly onto the brackets with wires.

has a tendency to form an open bite. In such cases the use of the "floating bone principle" (Hoffmeister et al., 1998) is possible to achieve a neutral occlusion: overcorrection into an edge-to-edge bite, removal of the distractor 1 week after distraction is finished, and insertion of loose elastics to slowly close the bite.

Surgical Technique
Planning

Operation planning takes place with the aid of cephalometric analysis and definition of the distraction vector, which should run parallel to the occlusal plane. A plastic splint is manufactured on a plaster-cast model of the mandible, with occlusal adjustment of the fitting surface, and the upper side corresponding to the direction of distraction. An adjustment clamp is fixed onto the plastic splint with screws, into which the distractors are inserted parallel to each other. A complete simulation on a stereolithographic model is even more accurate (**Figs. 35.15–35.17**).

Operation

Under transnasal intubation anesthesia, a posterior buccal vestibular mucoperiosteal incision is made approaching the height of the external oblique ridge on both sides of the mandible, followed by subperiosteal exposure of the

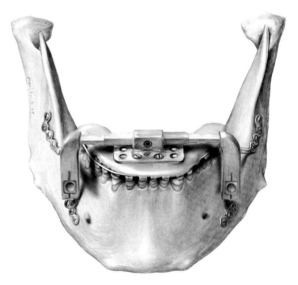

Fig. 35.17 The vertical parts of the adjustment clamp retain both distractors parallel to one another. By pushing both vertical clamp elements together in the middle of the clamp, the distractor miniplates come to rest in the planned position on the buccal side of the mandible. They can then be fixed into place with screws.

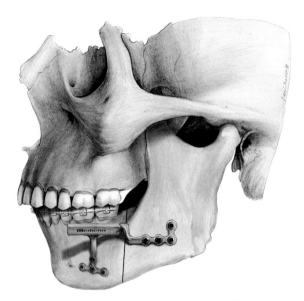

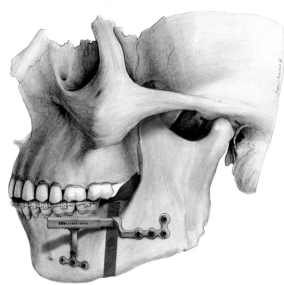

Fig. 35.18 Start position through deliberate mandibular distraction to correct a class II malocclusion and mandibular retrognathia.

Fig. 35.19 Parallel distraction of the mandible in class I occlusion.

buccal aspect of the mandibular angles and the front of both ascending rami. Occlusal application of the plastic mandibular splint follows and the adjustment clamp is used to define the vector. The parallel position of the distractor is fixed onto the splint with screws. The ends of the clamp pass around the side of the lower dental arch, and both oblique distractors are inserted and fixed parallel to one another. The miniplates of the distractors, which were pre-bent during the operation simulation, are now fitted and the distractors fixed with one screw each on both sides of the planned osteotomy line. All the screwholes are drilled in advance and the osteotomy line is marked. The splint is then removed along with the adjustment clamp and the distractors. The horizontal retromolar osteotomy is now performed and the inferior alveolar nerve is identified and secured. Both distractors are inserted, at this stage without the adjustment clamp, and screwed loosely into place. To ensure a parallel position of the distractors, the adjustment clamp is reinserted with the plastic splint. Both distractors are then fixed by tightening all the screws. The adjustment clamp and splint are now removed, followed by test distraction on both sides and wound closure. The concluding distraction results in a class I occlusion (**Figs. 35.18, 35.19**).

Maxillary Retrognathia

Indication

Up to now the retrognathic maxilla was usually distracted extraorally. This was performed with a halo frame fixed with spikes onto the skull, which due to its size and visibility naturally limited the length of the retention period. This resulted in relapses with a reduction in distraction distance of between 20 and 25 %. The development and use of transantral distractors is new and allows an unlimited retention period and consequently a minimal relapse distance (**Fig. 35.20**).

Prerequisites for exclusive maxilla distraction to correct a malpositioned maxilla are orthodontic treatment with formation of congruent dental arches, completed skeletal growth, and normal position of the mandible.

In cases of extreme congenital maxillary retrognathia an earlier maxillary distraction may be indicated, usually for psychological reasons. In this case the maxillary space must at least be so far developed that the Le Fort I osteotomy can avoid damaging the high-lying canine tooth germs. A CT-scan is indicated. Experience shows that distraction can begin at around 10 years of age.

Surgical Technique

Under transnasal intubation anesthesia, the maxilla is exposed through a standard LeFort I incision at the height of the buccal vestibule from the region of the upper first molar to the contralateral first molar. After subperiostal dissection of the complete maxilla and the lower nasal passages, the Le Fort I osteotomy is performed without mobilizing the pterygoid process. This is followed by a down fracture with complete mobilization of the maxilla (**Fig. 35.21**). Both transantral distractors are fixed in the area of the piriform aperture with each of the straight, three-holed miniplates (**Fig. 35.22**). The distractor length is adjusted to fit the size of the maxillary space. This is done by using a screwdriver to insert the spike at the posterior end of the distractor into the front of the processus pterygoideus cranial to the osteotomy line

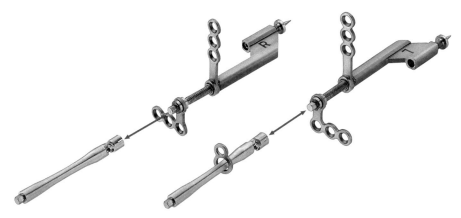

Fig. 35.20 Bilateral transantral distraction devices for maxillary advancement: left and right device in the distracted position. The distraction screw-tap is to be seen left and right. The size of the device can be changed with a screwdriver by extending the blunt spike, which will be stuck into the bony rear wall of the sinus. The straight, three-hole miniplate fixed onto the front border of the distraction cylinder is fixating the device onto the piriform aperture. The angled miniplate is fixed on the canine fossa of the mobile maxilla to push it forward. Intraoperative distraction will be performed by anticlockwise rotation of the distraction screw (upper end of red arrow). The angled extension piece (lower end of red arrow) causes transmucosal activation in the maxillary floor of the mouth and may be removed after distraction is complete. For security reasons, a fixation ring around the extension piece (drawn only in the left device) can be stitched in the maxillary vestibule.

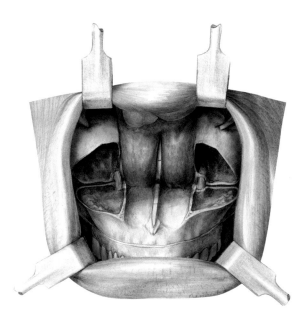

Fig. 35.21 Le Fort I osteotomy with down fracture. The greater palatine neurovascular bundle is dissected. Damage to the posterior wall of the maxillary sinus must be avoided, as it serves as a distal support for the distractors.

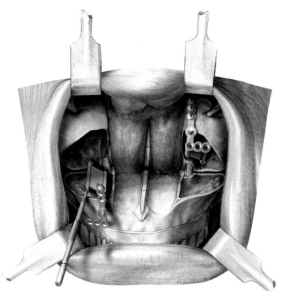

Fig. 35.22 Fitting the transantral distractor.

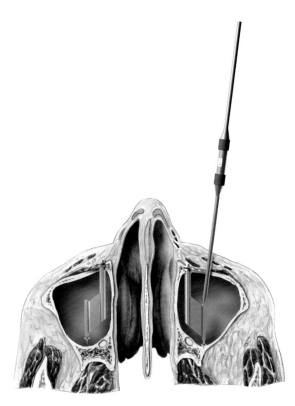

Fig. 35.23 The rear spike of the distractor is extended with the screwdriver in accordance with the depth of the maxilla and inserted into the bony rear wall of the maxillary sinus lateral to the neurovascular bundle.

(**Fig. 35.23**). Care should be taken to ensure that the distractors are in a parallel position (**Fig. 35.24**). The mobilized maxilla is now folded back and the osteotomy border and the angled miniplates are screwed into the area of the canine fossa (**Fig. 35.25**). The extension pieces of the distraction axis are put into place and guided through the mucous membrane into the maxillary vestibule as the wound is sutured (**Figs. 35.26, 35.27**). Daily distraction in the maxillary vestibule is problem-free. Finally, the extension pieces are removed so that the end of the distractor disappears under the mucous membrane (**Fig. 35.28**). Open bites can also be closed if the distraction direction in the area of the piriform aperture is lowered (Kretschmer and Wangerin, 2006) (**Fig. 35.29**).

Transversal Mandibular Deficiency

Indication

Transversal dental arch discrepancies caused by too small mandibular dental arches (**Fig. 35.30**) can be treated successfully with transversal median mandibular distraction. Indications might include facial types with a narrow mandible, crowding of the lower frontal dental segment, when a bilateral premolar extraction with a gain of 14 mm space is considered too large and a front tooth extraction with a gain of 5 mm space is too small. An exact treatment plan and an orthodontic space analysis are prerequisites, taking into consideration the anterior–posterior position of the frontal teeth.

Follow-up examinations of our patients up to now have shown that transversal mandibular distraction not only

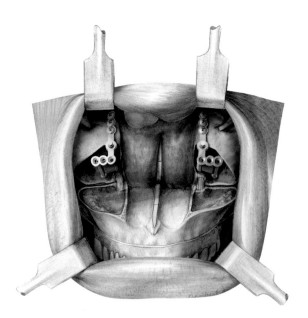

Fig. 35.24 The parallel position is achieved by fixation of the distractor to the piriform aperture.

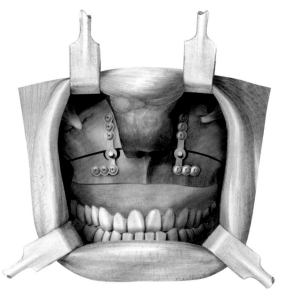

Fig. 35.25 The mobile maxilla is now folded up and with the aid of the angled miniplates is fixed on the lateral upper border of the osteotomy near the canine fossa.

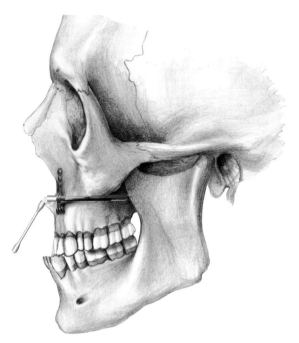

Fig. 35.26 The extension segment is placed onto the distraction rod and a joint is used to guide it through the mucous membrane into the maxillary vestibule, enabling a problem-free distraction to bring forward the retrognathic maxilla.

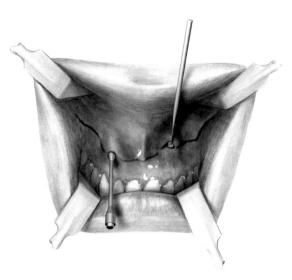

Fig. 35.27 The extension pieces of the distraction axis are put into place and guided through the mucous membrane into the maxillary vestibule as the wound is sutured.

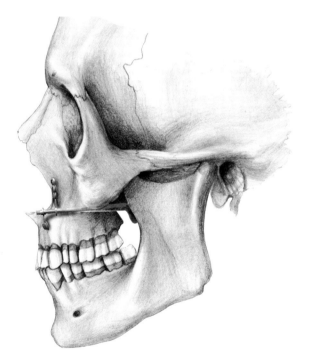

Fig. 35.28 After distraction is completed the extension segment is pulled out through the mucous membrane, the distractor thus remaining completely covered by tissue. The duration of the subsequent retention period is unlimited.

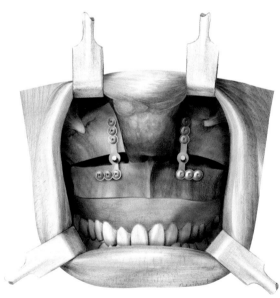

Fig. 35.29 The direction of distraction can be varied, but it is essential to plan it well before surgery. Vertical rearrangement of miniplate fixation can also be used to close an open bite.

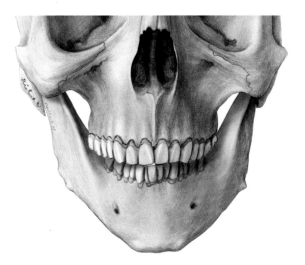

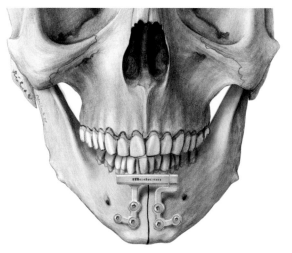

Fig. 35.30 Indication for transversal mandibular distraction. A narrow mandible with frontal crowding.

Fig. 35.31 A mucosal incision is made in the mandibular vestibule under local anesthesia, the mentalis muscle is dissected, and the distractor temporarily screwed in. After complete median osteotomy, the distractor is replaced with closure of the mucous membrane.

promotes bone growth with formation of a strong mandible, but also serves to increase the distance between the canine teeth, enabling the use of alternative orthodontic treatment methods. Up to now orthodontic therapy was built up around a constant distance between the lower canine teeth that could not be influenced by therapy.

Surgical Technique

Following local analgesia, an anterior labial vestibular mandibular incision is made beyond the reflection of the mucogingival junction, well into mobile mucosa. The mentalis muscle is dissected bilaterally, the median osteotomy lines are marked, and both the angulated distractor miniplates are pre-bent. They are then temporarily fixed on both sides with a 7 mm long miniscrew. The distraction cylinder should be lying horizontally at the level of the height of gingival margin of the incisors. Then all the remaining holes are drilled and the distractor is once again removed. The mandibular symphysis is sectioned with a saw and levered apart with a chisel so that it is completely fractured and no inter-radicular manipulation is necessary. In case of crowding this could lead to tooth root damage. The distractor is reinserted and completely fixated with monocortical screws (**Fig. 35.31**). A test distraction is performed and the wound closed. After healing, distraction can be performed according to plan (**Fig. 35.32**). The tooth movement into the diastema should be performed in close cooperation with the orthodontist, who can at the same time begin to form the upper dental arch (**Figs. 35.33, 35.34**).

Transversal Maxillary Deficiency

Indication

A narrow maxilla can be corrected orthodontically as well as surgically. Rapid maxillary expansion is a therapeutic measure which is performed during the skeletal growth period by the orthodontist alone. The median maxillary suture can be broken by activating a transversal extension apparatus which is fixed to the teeth, enabling transversal widening of the maxilla as required. After skeletal growth is complete, however, this method is relatively unreliable and needs operative assistance. It is possible to perform a purely transversal parallel expansion of the maxilla, resulting in a diastema and expansion of the lateral dental arch segments.

A therapeutic variation is the use of the fanlike expansion screw, which becomes necessary when the maxillary tooth bow is underdeveloped in the front and needs to be expanded obliquely. At the rear of the maxilla expansion is hardly ever achieved (**Figs. 35.35, 35.36**). Also, boneborne devices are used in cases of periodontitis or partial edentulism; however, the directional control over the movement of the maxillary segments is largely unpredictable, due to poor fixation of the deliberately small-sized fixation part of the device.

Surgical Technique

After the premolars and molars have been separated and the distractor has been worn temporarily, under transnasal intubation anesthesia an incision is made in the midline of the hard palate and in the maxillary buccal vestibule from the region of the second premolar to the contralateral second premolar. After exposure of the me-

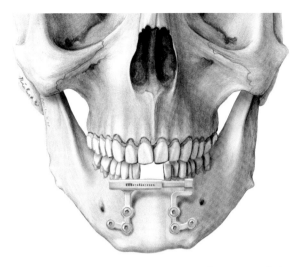

Fig. 35.32 To ensure that the inicisors in the vicinity of the osteotomy do not loosen or wander into the distraction gap too soon, they are fixated orthodontically so that a wide diastema ensues.

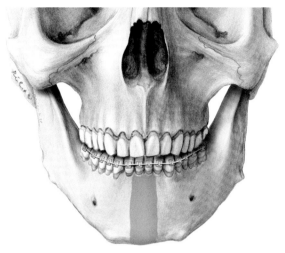

Fig. 35.33 After about 2 months the teeth are orthodontically moved into the new bone-filled gap, until the dental arch is accurately aligned.

dian hard palate and the maxilla, including the lower nasal passages, a bilateral Le Fort I osteotomy is performed, followed by a paramedian bilateral sagittal palatal osteotomy via the approach on the hard palate. The two osteotomy lines meet in the midline in the area of the premaxilla, so that both maxillary segments can be mobilized between the two central incisors after osteotomy of the anterior nasal spine and anterior median osteotomy. In the Le Fort I plane also both maxillary segments are mobilized without performing a down fracture. To avoid tipping during transversal distraction, wedge-shaped bone pieces are removed at the region of zygomatic buttresses on both sides. The final step is wound closure and cementing of the distractor onto the teeth.

Combinations

Of course it is possible to perform distraction of the maxilla and mandible at the same time. This indication is seen in occasional cases of a narrow jaw with frontal crowding. Combined orthodontic rapid palatal expansion with transverse mandibular distraction may certainly in some cases be justified during puberty.

Conclusion

In its early days distraction therapy gave rise to a certain euphoria, as the indications and equipment development appeared to be inexhaustible. Many wrong paths were taken. Thankfully, complications caused by inefficient dis-

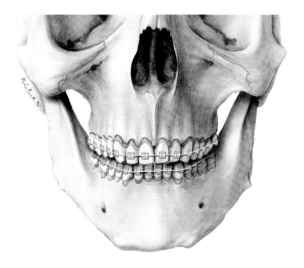

Fig. 35.34 The upper dental arch must be aligned accurately to obtain a class I occlusion by the end of treatment.

tractors and faulty operation techniques are now a thing of the past.

Enoral distraction techniques have replaced extraoral methods. Although Ilizarov (1988) recommended beginning distraction 1 week postoperatively, we have learned that it is advisable to begin distraction in children as early as the third, and in adults the fourth, postoperative day. Distraction speed of 1 mm per day, as described in the literature, is also variable. In children we distract 0.8–1.0 mm mornings and evenings (1.6–2.0 mm per day), to prevent premature ossification, and in older pa-

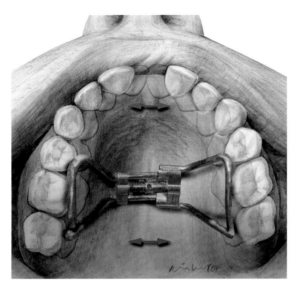

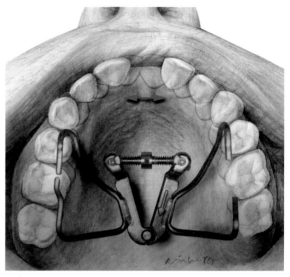

Fig. 35.35 Transversal maxillary distraction with a transversal tooth-fixated extension screw, to evenly expand the whole dental arch transversally in the front and in the canine area.

Fig. 35.36 Fanlike maxillary distraction for anterior widening, producing a wide diastema. Even the opposite transversal distraction is possible by turning the device round 180° to widen the posterior parts of the maxilla.

tients we suggest only 0.4–0.5 mm mornings and evenings (0.8–1.0 mm per day) to avoid infections and osteomyelitis.

It is now possible to improve severe facial deformities with simple procedures to normalize the functions. A therapy method formerly reserved for adults has been extended for use in children. We now know that distracted bone also continues growing, although later it always lags behind the growth of normally formed bony structures.

It is possible to repeat distraction without hesitation after a year. In severe syndromes distraction may be com-

bined with all other operative treatment methods (Wangerin, 2006; Wangerin et al., 2006).

Experience over the past 12 years has shown that distraction has become an indispensable part of therapy of congenital malformations and acquired bony defects in the craniomaxillofacial area.

The concept of enoral distraction describes standardized and systematic ways to safely and satisfactorily treat malformations during and after the skeletal skull growth period. In severe cases this enables a therapy plan covering several time periods, resulting in ultimate success.

36 Microsurgical Anastomosis of the Fibula Bone

Friedrich W. Neukam, Rainer Schmelzeisen, and Emeka Nkenke

Introduction

Reconstruction of mandibular and maxillary defects represents a challenge to the oral and maxillofacial surgeon. The restoration of form and function is paramount for rehabilitation of the affected patient. As a consequence, the shape and size of the graft should correspond with the bone segment that has to be replaced. The vascular pedicle should be long, constant, and offer the possibility of concomitant transfer of soft tissue for replacement of mucosal and cutaneous defects.

To facilitate masticatory rehabilitation by the placement of dental implants, the grafts should consist of a thick cortical plate surrounding cancellous components of high density. Vertical bone height of 7–10 mm and a bone width of 6 mm are required as a minimal volume.

To date, the fibula flap is one of the most popular options for bony reconstruction in oral and maxillofacial surgery. It is the workhorse of modern-day mandibular reconstruction. Free vascularized osseous or osteocutaneous flaps can be adopted for the reconstruction of extensive bony and soft-tissue defects. The fibula allows division into segments using a wedge osteotomy technique to precisely recreate the shape of the resected bone.

In contrast to the homogenous structure of the alveolus, the fibula is the best flap to be harvested in obese patients. There is only limited donor site morbidity. It offers a reliable donor site. However, variations in vascularization of the fibula are possible, and thus preoperative angiography or color Doppler ultrasonography is recommended.

The fibula is composed of heterogeneous portions consisting of a dense cortical margin and a small cancellous core. The placement of implants into dense fibular free flaps results in a high primary stability. Sometimes primary stability is high enough to permit immediate functional loading of these implants (Chen, Chen, and Hahn, 1994; Hidalgo, 1989, 1991, 1994; Hidalgo and Pusic, 2002; Hidalgo and Rekow, 1995; Hausamen and Neukam, 1994; Neukam and Hausamen, 1996; Neukam, Schmelzeisen, and Schliephake, 1994; Schmelzeisen et al., 1996; Peled et al., 2005).

Anatomical Considerations

The fibula is a straight bone that is up to 40 cm long. To maintain the integrity of the knee and ankle joints, 7 cm of bone proximally to the neck of the fibula and distally to the lateral malleous have to be preserved. Segments of fibular bone up to 26 cm in length can be harvested. Segmentalization of the fibula to restore symphyseal contour and jaw relationship with a view to future implant rehabilitation is a demanding aspect of the reconstruction because of the inherent risks of devascularization, instability, and malposition of the segments (Baehr et al., 1998). However, wedge excision osteotomy is a reliable technique to achieve the required shape of the graft.

One disadvantage of the fibula graft is its limited vertical height that may cause problems during prosthetic reconstruction (Klespers et al., 2000). If placed at the caudal border of the mandible, the distance between implant shoulder and the occlusal plane is large, leading to unfavorable crown-to-implant ratios. Doubling of the fibula helps to mitigate this problem (Baehr et al., 1998). An alternative method is vertical distraction osteogenesis of the graft (Chiapasco et al., 2000).

The peroneal artery provides the blood supply of the fibula by an endosteal nutrient medullary artery as well as periosteal circulation (**Fig. 36.1**). The graft can be raised as a free osseous or a free osteocutaneous flap with a thin pliable paddle of skin. The venous drainage is secured by two venae comitantes. The vascular pedicle is short but consistent in location. Usually, the pedicle is approximately 5 cm long and the diameter of the artery is 2–3 mm. Possible variations of vascularization prompt preoperative angiography (Whitley et al., 2004). If any of the three tibial arteries is missing, or only weakly developed, harvesting of a fibular flap should be avoided to prevent ischemic complications.

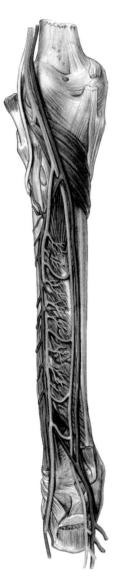

Fig. 36.1 Posterior view of the vascular supply of the left fibula.
A nutrient artery enters the bone 13 cm below the head of the
fibula. In addition to the endosteal vascular supply to the fibula by
the nutrient medullary artery, the peroneal artery provides vascular
supply through numerous periosteal feeders. The common peroneal
nerve passes 1–2 cm below the fibula head.

Preoperative Diagnostics for Graft Shaping

The fibula is one of the most popular grafts for mandibular
reconstruction. It is superior in terms of bone characteristics compared with other vascularized bone grafts (Klespers et al., 2000). There is enough bone available to reconstruct any length of mandibular defect. The nature of
the fibular blood supply allows a precise graft-shaping by
multiple osteotomies.

Preoperative evaluation of the lower extremity vessels
is recommended to assess vascular disease that may preclude transfer. Sometimes variations of vascularization
can be encountered. Therefore, to exclude variations in
vascularization of the fibula, preoperative angiography or
color Doppler ultrasonography is performed. Today, magnetic resonance angiography has replaced traditional angiography as the technique of choice.

The correct anatomical relation of the outer contour of
the reconstructed mandible to the maxilla (maxillomandibular relation) is important to gain satisfactory aesthetic
results (Metha and Deschler, 2004).

To facilitate reconstruction, three-dimensional models
of mandible or maxilla and the fibula can be obtained
from computed tomography (CT) scan data. The length
of the fibula to be harvested is predetermined by measurement of the simulated or existing defect on the jaw
stereomodel. A reconstruction plate or miniplates can be
pre-bent and shaped to fit the jaw contour. The stereomodel fibula is divided into multiple segments and the
segments are placed on the jaw stereomodel in the ideal
position against the opposing dentition. Even the angular
contour of the mandible can be reconstructed for best
comesis. The predetermined bony segments are measured
and the system is transferred to the patient in the operation room using acrylic locating splints (Yeung et al.,
2007).

Technique

A lateral approach gives easy access to the donor site
(Gilbert, 1979). Because of the location of the fibula, a
two-team approach allows simultaneous harvesting of
the graft while head and neck surgery is going on (Cordeiro et al., 1999). Flap harvesting in anemia should be
preferred using a tourniquet. After palpation of the fibula,
the bone is outlined on the skin. The peroneal nerve
passes 1–2 cm below the fibular neck. The skin incision
is placed on a straight line between the fibular head and
the epicondyle of the ankle (**Fig. 36.2**). If a skin flap is to be
removed in addition, its axis is marked over the posterior
cural septum at the boundary from the middle to the
distal section of the fibula. The skin paddle is designed

in a fusiform shape over the posterolateral aspect of the fibula and centered near its midpoint.

After incision of the skin, subcutaneous tissue, and the fascia overlying the peroneous longus and brevis muscle, the anterior skin margin is reflected to expose the intermuscular septum.

If septocutaneous vessels are not identified, musculo-cutaneous vessels derived from the peroneal artery and perforating the soleus muscle must be included when raising the posterior part of the flap. Access to the fibula is gained along the intermuscular fascia. During this approach, septocutaneous perforators must not be harmed. Dissection is continued along the anterior aspect of the fibula. A cuff of muscle of a few millimeters in thickness is retained on the fibular bone to protect the periosteal blood supply. After retraction of the peroneus longus, peroneus brevis, and extensor hallucis longus muscles, the anterior tibial artery and vein can be identified in the anterior compartment. Further dissection along the medial aspect of the fibula allows exposure of the interosseous membrane, which is incised. For posterior dissection, the posterior incision around the skin flap is made to expose the fascia of the soleus muscle and to identify the septocutaneous perforators. Preserving the posterior intermuscular septum, the soleus and flexor hallucis muscle are retracted. After reflecting the periosteum, the fibula is sectioned proximally and distally, using an oscillating saw. The osteotomized fibula is retracted laterally; the peroneal artery and vein are identified and ligated distally. The vascular pedicle is dissected, up to the bifurcation with the posterior tibial artery and vein, by transecting the flexor hallucis longus muscle, leaving a small cuff of muscle on the fibula bone. After reflecting the periosteum from the outer and inner cortex, the straight fibula bone graft can be contoured by wedge osteotomies, using an oscillating saw and rotating burrs (Schmelzeisen et al., 1996).

Graft Fixation

The two most popular options for the fixation of vascularized fibular bone grafts are a single large plate or several miniplates. Both techniques allow for rigid internal fixation that spans all osteotomy sites.

A large plate safely connects the remaining segments of the mandible. Even fibular grafts that have been repeatedly osteotomized can be rigidly fixed to the plate. However, graft shaping is limited because the large plate predetermines the bony contour. Moreover, a large plate adds bulk to the external contour of the graft.

Miniplates have been used in the treatment of facial fractures and provide adequate fixation without the need for additional measures such as maxillomandibular fixation (Champy et al., 1977; Gerlach et al., 1982). Different shapes of the plates are available (straight, L-shaped, Y-

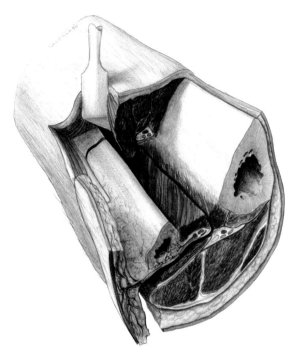

Fig. 36.2 Schematic drawing of the elevation of a combined osteocutaneous fibula flap. The septocutaneous perforators may run through the septum or as musculocutaneous perforators through the flexor hallucis longus and soleus muscle.

shaped, H-shaped, etc.). Two to three plates are placed on the outer surface and the lower border of the graft and jaw segments without stripping the periosteum at the osteotomy sites (**Figs. 36.3, 36.4**). Self-tapping, monocortical screws allow rapid placement and do not compromise the free graft to a critical degree (Hidalgo, 1989).

Miniplates provide sufficient stability and safely prevent torsional instability. They are easily contoured for each osteotomy site. Therefore, miniplates offer an excellent option for fixation and preservation of symmetric contours of the reconstructed midface or mandible (**Figs. 36.5–36.7**).

The risk of compromising the vascularization of the fibular graft by miniplates is minimal, because most of the periosteum and muscular attachment are left intact and screws are only fixed monocortically.

Miniplates provide sufficient stability for early functional loading of the graft. The required contour of the bone is safely maintained.

About 3–4 months after bone grafting, the plates can be removed if necessary, and endosseous implants can be inserted for later oral rehabilitation. However, there is no real need for miniplate removal, because the monocortical screws do not interfere with dental implants in most cases.

Simultaneous implant installation into the fibular graft during maxillary or mandibular reconstruction is possible

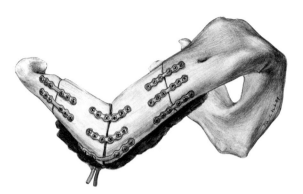

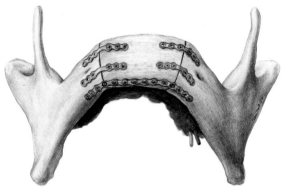

Fig. 36.3 Graft shaping and stabilizing in the lateral view. The fibula graft is shaped by several osteotomies in the subperiosteal plane to precisely duplicate the contour of the inferior border of the mandible. The cuts are planned in such a way that the pedicle is later located lingually of the mandible graft. Miniplates in two planes are typically placed on the facial aspect of the mandible graft

Fig. 36.4 Graft shaping and stabilizing in the frontal view of the mandible.

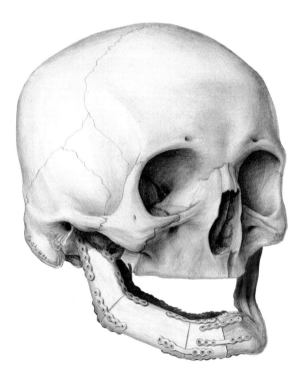

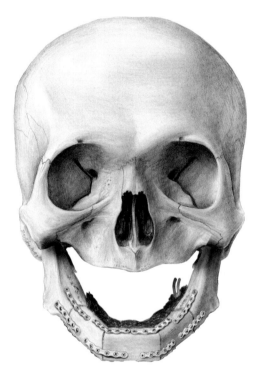

Fig. 36.5 Lateral grafts. One osteotomy is performed to form the angle of the mandible. In most cases the body of the graft requires one more osteotomy to duplicate the horizontal ramus of the mandible. The segments are fixed by miniplates in two planes.

Fig. 36.6 Anterior grafts. These consist of a central segment and two lateral segments, which may need a further osteotomy on both sides during the graft-shaping process if the mandibular defect extends to the angle of the mandible. The graft is fixed to the mandibular stumps and the osteotomies are stabilized by miniplates in two planes. Microvascular anastomoses are performed after shaping and fixation of the graft is complete.

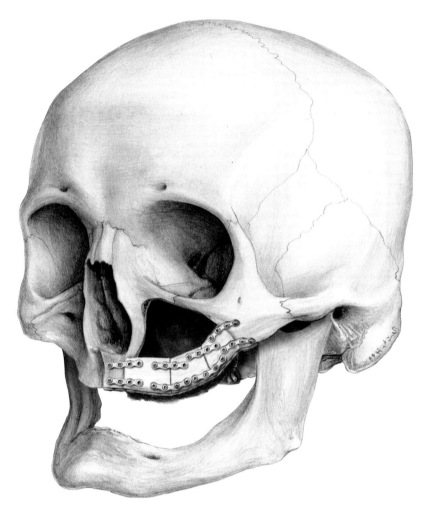

Fig. 36.7 The fibula is shaped by several osteotomies in the subperiosteal plane to duplicate the alveolar process of the maxilla. The cuts are planned so that the pedicle is later located laterally to the maxillary graft. Miniplates in two planes are fixed by monocortical screws to the maxillary graft.

without harming the blood supply of the graft. However, implant placement after a healing period of 3 months allows for optimal positioning of the dental implants, which makes the prosthodontic treatment easier and secures long-term success of implants and superstructure (Gbara et al., 2007).

37 Microsurgical Anastomosis of the Scapula Bone

Rainer Schmelzeisen and Friedrich W. Neukam

Introduction

The scapula region offers the unique possibility of allowing the harvest of one or two soft-tissue flaps in combination with a vascularized bone graft (Sieverberg, Banis, and Acland, 1985; Swartz et al., 1986). Different aspects of the flap can be mobilized independently from each other, yet vascularized via one pedicle. Since the medial aspect of the scapula is rather thin and often has to be placed at the upper border of the mandible, the bone graft is frequently not suitable for insertion of dental implants (Schultes, Gaggl, and Karcher, 2002). The skin of the scapula offers a good color match with that of the head and neck area, and has the added advantage of being thin and pliable (Smith et al., 2007).

Anatomical Considerations

The vascular supply of the scapula region is derived from the subscapular artery, which divides into thoracodorsal and circumflex scapular artery 1–2 cm below the axillary artery. The circumflex scapular artery passes through the triangular space bordered by the teres major and minor muscles and by the long head of the triceps muscle. The artery supplies the infraspinatus muscle and the lateral border of the scapula at the proximal aspect of the bone. The inferior third of the lateral border of the scapula is vascularized by the angular branch of the thoracodorsal artery (**Fig. 37.1**).

After it has passed through the muscular triangle, the circumflex scapular artery divides into a descending cutaneous branch (the parascapular flap), and a transverse cutaneous branch (the scapula flap) (**Fig. 37.2**).

Harvesting

For harvesting a combined osteocutaneous flap, the parascapular orientation of the soft-tissue pedicle offers a safe vascular supply.

For harvesting the bone, the teres major muscle must be cut at the scapula tip. However, some muscular attachment has to be left on the bone to avoid interference with the periosteal blood supply. In general, it is sufficient to harvest 2–2.5 cm from the lateral border to match the height of the mandible. The inferior third of the scapula is nourished by the angular branch of the thoracodorsal artery. This autonomous vascularization does not allow an osteotomy, if it is necessary to bend the bone graft (**Fig. 37.3**). The disadvantage of the soft-tissue pedicles of the scapula region, in common with most free flaps, is that there is no sensory supply.

Indications

The scapula region offers unique opportunities for reconstruction of skin, bone, subcutaneous tissue, and, especially, combinations of bone and soft tissues. Among all flaps derived from the head and neck area, the texture and color of the skin at the scapula region almost perfectly match the texture and color of the facial skin. Although the skin is relatively thick, it is not as bulky as that of myocutaneous grafts, or free flaps from the iliac crest. In general, scapula grafts should always be considered for complex soft-tissue defects, or combined bone and soft-tissue defects, as long as neither massive volume augmentation nor large bone volume are required (Fairbanks and Hallock, 2002).

Isolated de-epithelized scapula soft-tissue grafts may also be used and are ideal for tissue augmentation, for example, in patients with hemifacial microsomia.

Combined osteocutaneous flaps are suitable for reconstruction of the posterior aspect of the mandible and the ascending ramus, when implant insertion is not a requirement. The soft-tissue pedicle may be used for reconstruction of the floor of the mouth or for extraoral lining. As the scapular and parascapular skin and the bone can be mobilized independently from each other, the flaps are ideal for reconstruction of combined oral and extraoral defects (Coleman et al., 2000). Only rarely will there be a need to harvest bone grafts alone.

As bone of the medial extension of the scapula is thin, it is often used for reconstruction of the maxilla. The soft-tissue pedicle then allows a separation into different functional units, such as the nasal and oral cavity and the maxillary sinus (Barnouti and Caminer, 2006).

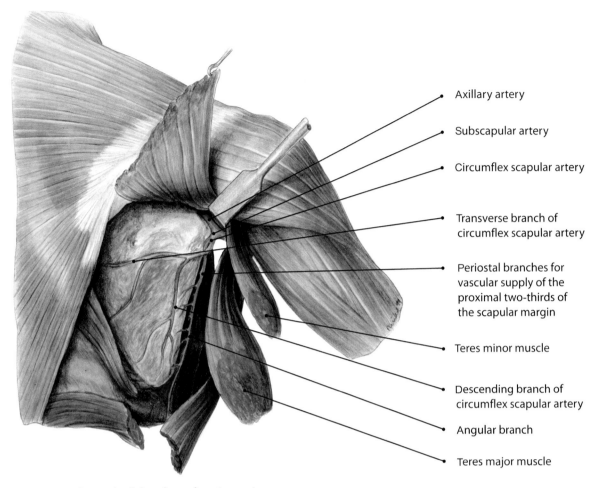

Axillary artery

Subscapular artery

Circumflex scapular artery

Transverse branch of circumflex scapular artery

Periostal branches for vascular supply of the proximal two-thirds of the scapular margin

Teres minor muscle

Descending branch of circumflex scapular artery

Angular branch

Teres major muscle

Fig. 37.1 Vascular supply of the subscapular artery system.

Mandibular Reconstruction

In every microsurgical reconstruction, preparation of suitable vessels at the recipient site in the neck has to be performed before flap harvesting is begun. The facial vessels of the ipsilateral side are often suitable. In defects with suitable ipsilateral recipient vessels the osteocutaneous scapula graft is harvested from the contralateral side (**Fig. 37.4**). The residual stump of the mandible first has to be returned to its original position. In situations where the ascending ramus is still present, it has to be prepared, mobilized and moved inferiorly and laterally, after resection of any residual scarring. The mandibular borders have to be prepared with an oscillating saw or a rotating burr until bleeding bone is seen. The bony edges may be osteotomized in an oblique manner to create a large contact surface for the graft, which improves healing between the residual mandibular stumps and the bone graft.

If suitable ipsilateral vessels are not available, contralateral vessels must be identified (**Fig. 37.5**). To allow sufficient mobilization of the recipient arteries, the external carotid artery may be ligated cranially. Then, for example, the facial artery can be mobilized almost to the midline of the neck.

As the vascular pedicle in general must be oriented toward vessels in the angle of the mandible, the thicker lateral aspect of the scapula often becomes the inferior border of the new mandible. In patients with an intraoral soft-tissue deficit the soft-tissue pedicle is located medially and inferior to the scapula bone, and therefore has to be elevated and trimmed. It is sutured into the defect with minimal tension. Then the bone is fixed into position with miniplates and monocortical screws. When the residual segments are osteotomized obliquely to enhance the bony contact area, the screws may pass through the thin scapula bone graft and the residual stump of the mandible and act as lag screws.

In general, two miniplates are placed with a minimum of two screws per segment. It is not necessary to remove

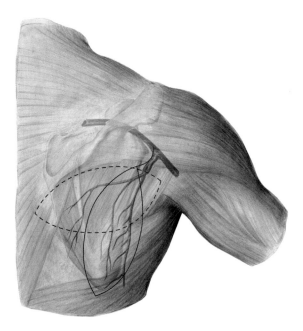

Fig. 37.2 Schematic drawing showing the relationship of the scapula and parascapular flap below the transverse branch, and the access of the descending branch.

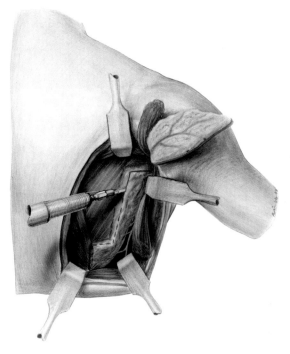

Fig. 37.3 Elevation of a combined osteocutaneous parascapular flap. After preparation of the muscular triangle, the vessels to the bone are identified and a muscular cuff must remain at the lateral border of the scapula. The teres major muscle is dissected and the lateral border of the scapula is osteotomized.

the periosteum before fixation of the miniplates. Lag screws alone do not provide sufficient stability for bone graft fixation.

In predominantly extraoral soft-tissue defects the bone is inserted first, and then the cranial margin of the soft tissue flap is inserted. Final fixation of the flap is performed after vascular anastomoses are completed. Then the extraoral flap is sutured tightly into position.

If the ascending ramus including the condyle has to be reconstructed, the tip of the contralateral scapula can be shaped to act as a new condylar head. The vascular pedicle is then at the inner aspect of the bone graft, pointing toward the vessels in the mandibular angle.

Reconstruction of the Maxilla and Midface

Flaps from the scapula region are ideally suited for reconstructing soft tissue and bone areas in the midface.

In simple maxillary defects it may be possible to reconstruct aspects of the nasal mucosa to create a layer toward the nasal cavity and the maxillary sinus. Then the flat scapula bone is fixed securely to residual aspects of the zygoma. The bony contact between the residual maxillary bone and the bone graft should be as extensive as possible, to allow good bone healing in that area. The soft tissue then can be used to create the oral lining. In later surgical procedures, an additional bone graft can be fixed to the scapula bone to form a new alveolar process suitable for the insertion of dental implants (**Fig. 37.6**).

It is not always possible to position the thicker lateral border of the scapula to form the alveolar process in the maxilla, because care must be taken for a tensionless vascular anastomosis to submandibular recipient vessels. For that purpose the marginal branch of the facial nerve is identified and protected using a paramandibular incision or subfacial preparation in the typical manner. Preparation is continued on the lateral surface of the masseter muscle and a tunnel is created toward the maxilla. Care has to be taken to enlarge the tunnel to avoid compression of the vascular pedicle in the postoperative period.

The superficial temporal vessel has proven not to be very useful for vascular anastomosis, because of the thin and fragile superficial temporal vein.

Postoperatively, the subcutaneous volume of the scapula skin graft may have to be thinned.

For lateral aspects of the midface, combined scapula grafts are useful. The thin scapula bone can be used for reconstruction of the infraorbital rim, whereas partially de-epithelized aspects of the parascapular skin pedicle are used for augmentation of the skin (**Fig. 37.7**). Another aspect of the parascapular flap, or an additionally harvested scapula flap, can then be positioned caudally, to form the oral lining of the alveolar process of the maxilla.

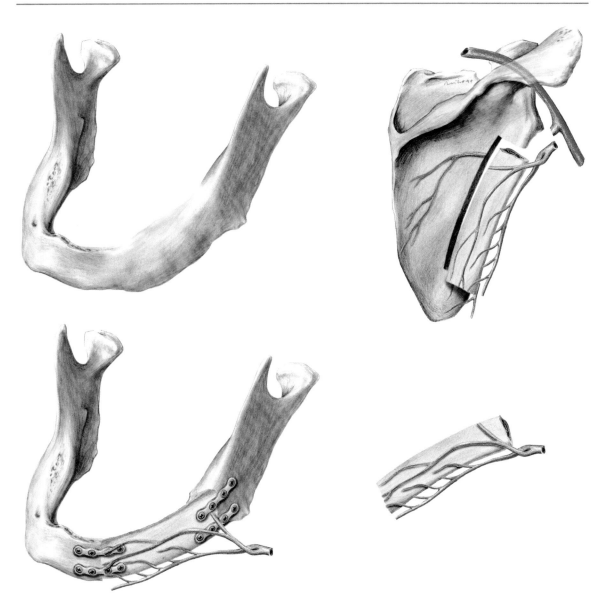

Fig. 37.4 If the mandibular defect and the recipient vessels are on the same side, the scapula is harvested from the contralateral shoulder. This allows the vascular pedicle to be located in the angle of the mandible.

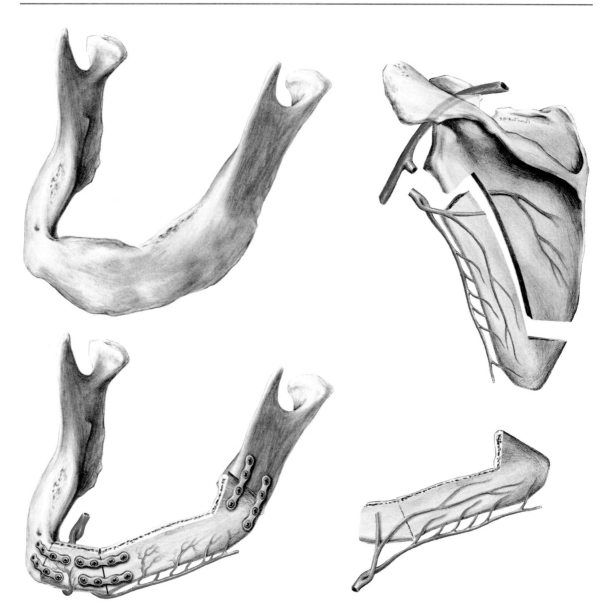

Fig. 37.5 If the vessels are located on the side contralateral to the mandibular defect, the ipsilateral scapula may be more suitable for vascular anastomosis to the opposite neck.

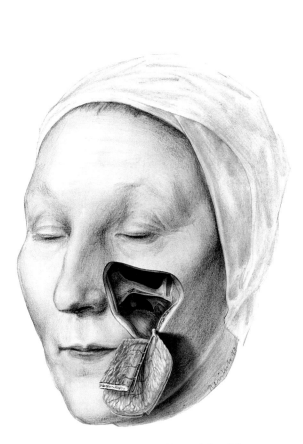

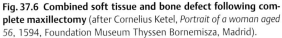

Fig. 37.6 Combined soft tissue and bone defect following complete maxillectomy (after Cornelius Ketel, *Portrait of a woman aged 56*, 1594, Foundation Museum Thyssen Bornemisza, Madrid).

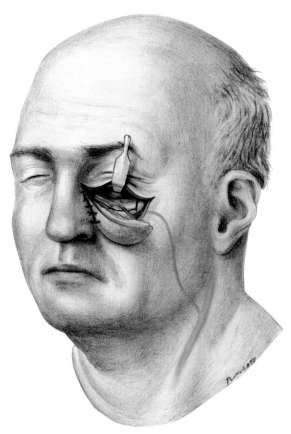

Fig. 37.7 Soft tissue and bone defect following resection of a maxillary carcinoma (after Jan Polack, *Portrait of a Benedictine abbot*, 1484, Foundation Museum Thyssen Bornemisza, Madrid).

Volume augmentation in the lateral midface with a de-epithelized parascapular flap can also be combined with a scapula bone graft used for reconstruction of parts of the zygoma, as for example the zygomatic arch. Therefore, hemifacial microsomia patients may be suitable candidates for soft tissue and bone reconstruction with scapula grafts (Warren et al., 2007).

Conclusion

Indications for the use of scapula grafts are isolated soft-tissue defects or combined defects with a predominant soft-tissue problem. The grafts can be used for reconstruction of posterior aspects of the mandible and the ascending ramus with additional intraoral or extraoral soft-tissue defects. Scapula grafts are the grafts of choice for reconstructing combined defects in the maxilla or midface.

38 Titanium Plate Removal: Yes or No?

Hendrik Terheyden and Maxime Champy

Introduction

The early plating systems were made of stainless steel (Spiessl, 1969; Becker and Machtens, 1973; Champy, Wilk, and Schnebelen, 1975) or of Vitallium (Luhr, 1968). Removal of the hardware, once the fracture had consolidated and the plate had ceased to function, was advocated as part of the total treatment (Champy et al., 1976; Alpert and Seligson, 1996). Subsequently, the evolution of plating systems was characterized by smaller implants, often placed in inaccessible areas, improved surgical techniques, and the use of titanium (Weber et al., 1990; Oikarinen, Ignatius, and Silvennoinen, 1993). Titanium is the preferred metal for bone appliances (Zitter and Plenk, 1987). The seminal discovery that titanium develops a direct bony anchorage has had a decisive impact on dental implantology (Brånemark, 1983). Titanium is one of the most biocompatible and corrosion-resistant metals (Rae, 1986; Alpert and Seligson, 1996). Titanium has an elastic modulus closer to that of bone than other metals used in bone surgery (Katou et al., 1996; Haug, 1996). Thus, retention of titanium hardware seemed possible and controversy about elective removal of asymptomatic plates has developed as a consequence (Hildebrand and Champy, 1987; Haug, 1996).

Removal of *symptomatic* plates is not controversial. Symptomatic plates are those involved in infection, dehiscence, or extrusion (MacLeod and Bainton, 1992), and loose, fractured, or migrating plates. Similarly, there is no controversy about the removal of plates that cause pain, temperature sensitivity, and foreign body reactions (Alpert and Seligson, 1996). Elective removal of *asymptomatic* plates is more difficult to agree with, but may be necessary in a few indications. Material at the alveolar process can interfere with dentures and is subject to extrusion after tooth loss and subsequent atrophy of the ridge. In the growing craniofacial skeleton, plates can become buried or dislocated into the brain (Hönig, Merten, and Luhr, 1995; Yaremchuk and Posnick, 1995) or cause growth restriction (Yaremchuk et al., 1994).

Corrosion and Metal Release from Titanium Plates

According to Semlitsch (1987), titanium in plates is usually alloyed as Ti–6Al–4V (6% aluminum and 4% vanadium) or Ti–6Al–7Nb (6% aluminum and 7% niobium). Commercially pure titanium (cpTi) is 99.99% pure. However, the remaining 0.01% is unspecified (Moberg, Nordenram, and Kjellmaru, 1989). Unlike stainless steel (Fe–Cr–Ni alloy) or Vitallium (Co–Cr alloy), titanium is virtually free from pitting and crevice corrosion (Gerstorfer and Weber, 1988; Haug, 1996). Titanium spontaneously forms a film of oxides approximately 10 µm thick, which protects against acids under body conditions (Scales, 1991). Although cpTi and alloys are different metals with different electrochemical potentials, their combined use appears not to produce a galvanic effect (Haug, 1996). Despite these properties, however, metal release occurs in maxillofacial applications from bending of the plates and from movement of the screws against them (Solar, Pollak, and Korostoff, 1979) or against the bone (Muster et al., 1987; Galante et al., 1991). Titanium is one of the least wear-resistant metals currently in use as biomaterial (Rae, 1979) and is susceptible to fretting corrosion (Agins et al., 1988). Fretting corrosion is considerably enhanced in the presence of hydrogen peroxide (H_2O_2). Activated macrophages are a possible source of H_2O_2 (Tengvall et al., 1990; Montague et al., 1996).

Toxicity and Accumulation in the Body

Titanium in ionic form is cleared through the kidneys (Jacobs et al., 1991). Titanium ions exhibit lower toxicity to osteoblasts than aluminum, vanadium, and chromium (Maurer, Merritt, and Brown, 1994; McKay et al., 1996; Thompson and Puleo, 1996; Ito et al., 1995). Elevated titanium in blood (Jacobs et al., 1991) and in hair (Trinchi, Nobis, and Cecchele, 1992) was measured in patients with loose joint replacements. Concentrations of 0.1–100 ng/mL of Ti ions in joint fluid after hip replacements have been reported (Jacobs et al., 1991).

Vanadium is rapidly released from Ti–Al–V alloy particles in ionic form (Lalor et al., 1991). Vanadium salt is a source of this essential trace element, but in elevated concentrations it is frankly toxic to many tissues (Dafnis and Sabatini, 1994), its effects including reproductive and developmental toxicity (Sakurai, 1994; Domingo, 1996).

Aluminum ions are cleared through the kidneys (Merritt, Margevicius, and Brown, 1992) but can accumulate in renal insufficiency (Exley et al., 1996). Aluminum ions are toxic to the central nervous system (Julka and Gill, 1996) and have been associated with Alzheimer dementia (Morris et al., 1994). Reproductive and developmental toxicity has been reported (Domingo, 1995). After Ti–Al–V hip replacement, elevated concentrations of aluminum in blood (Dittert, Warnecke and Willert, 1995) and hair (Trinchi, Nobis, and Cecchele, 1992) were observed.

Titanium, in particular, has a low toxicity in vitro and in vivo (Edel, Marafante, and Sabbioni, 1985; Rae, 1986) compared with Co–Cr particles (Haynes et al., 1993). The main corrosion product, the dioxide rutile, is almost insoluble in body fluids. Thus, it accumulates in lymph nodes, liver, spleen, bone marrow, and brain (Case et al., 1994). Titanium debris appears as gray discoloration at the implantation site (Lalor et al., 1991; Scales, 1991) and may be entrapped by collagen fibers after unsuccessful degradation by macrophages (Schliephake et al., 1993, Nakamura, Takenoshita, and Masuichiro, 1994). However, titanium particles are also transported from the site of origin by the blood (Hillmann and Donath, 1991) and the lymphatic route (Onodera, Ooya, and Kawamura, 1993; Weingart, Steinemann, and Schilli, 1994). Titanium debris is not inert (Case et al., 1994). In the lymph nodes, sinus histiocytosis (Albores-Saavedra et al., 1994), necrosis and fibrosis (Case et al., 1994) and a symptomatic granulomatous reaction in liver and spleen have been demonstrated (Peoc'h et al., 1996).

Toxicity of the alloyed metals may be a reason for plate removal. However, toxicity depends on dosage, and the systemic doses of aluminum and vanadium resulting from facial plates are supposed to be low. However, toxic effects are cumulative. In renal insufficiency especially, removal should be mandatory.

Inflammatory Response

Inflammatory complications like peri-implantitis, aseptic loosening of hip replacement, or persistent inflammation of skin-penetrating implants occur in various fields of titanium application (Jacobson et al., 1987). The primary cell type to react against titanium is the macrophage (Anderson and Miller, 1984). Macrophages have been shown to react to titanium particles in phagocytable sizes, with activation of lysosomal enzymes and a partial degradation of titanium (Elagi, Vérnon, and Hildebrand, 1995; Wooley, Nasser, and Fitzgerald, 1996). Activated macrophages release inflammatory mediators. Bone-resorbing cytokines, interleukin (IL)-1δ, IL-6 and tumor necrosis factor-α, were demonstrated after stimulation of macro-

phages with particles, and Ti–AL–V was more potent than cpTi (Shanbhag et al., 1995). Titanium ions also enhanced the release of bone-resorbing cytokines and inhibited bone-protecting cytokines (Wang et al., 1996a). Co–Cr particles result in early cell death after phagocytosis, whereas the less toxic Ti–Al–V particles lead to an inflammatory response (Haynes et al., 1993). Thus, titanium particles may exhibit inflammatory effects because they are nontoxic and insoluble. Clinically, in the maxillofacial region a chronic inflammatory response was demonstrated immunohistochemically in retrieved tissue (Katou et al., 1996). Granulation tissue, bone resorption, or loose hardware was found in 50% of maxillofacial patients (Kim, Yeo, and Lim, 1997). Thus the argument of macrophage activation and inflammatory response supports elective plate removal.

Sensitivity to Titanium

Titanium is used extensively as an ingredient in house paints, in paper, as a food additive, in cosmetic articles (Moran et al., 1991), in ointments or topical dental fluorides (Lalor et al., 1991; Charvat et al., 1995). Sensitivity to titanium is not common, in contrast to nickel and chromium (Rudner, Clendenning and Epstein, 1975; Goh, 1986; Haug, 1996). However, titanium from corrosion products does bind to cells and proteins and can stimulate immunological responses (Maurer, Merritt and Brown, 1994; Ikarashi et al., 1996). Titanium pacemaker rejection (Peters et al., 1984; Verbov, 1985; Abdallah, Balsara and O'Riordan, 1994), sensitivity to titanium joints (Black et al., 1990, Lalor et al., 1990, Merritt and Rodrigo, 1996), asthma (Breton, Louis and Garnier, 1992), and reactions to skin-penetrating titanium implants (Holgers et al., 1992) are reported. Titanium sensitivity was correlated to aseptic loosening of joint replacement (Lalor et al., 1991; Merritt and Rodrigo, 1996). T-lymphocyte activation adjacent to maxillofacial titanium plates has been observed (Torgensen et al., 1995; Katou et al., 1996).

Contact sensitivity to aluminum (Dwyer and Kerr, 1993; Lopez et al., 1994) and vanadium (Motolese et al., 1993) has occasionally been reported in the literature. Vanadium sensitization was reported in a group of patients with hip replacement (Cancilleri et al., 1992).

Contact sensitization is a slow type IV reaction and takes several months to develop. Studies monitoring contact sensitivity to metal appliances showed no sensitization before 6–12 months, by which time the device has usually fulfilled its function (Merritt and Rodrigo, 1996). Contact sensitization may be an argument for elective plate removal, since the prevalence of sensitivity depends on the number of exposed individuals and the duration of exposure (Merritt and Rodrigo, 1996).

Carcinogenity

Associations of soft-tissue malignancy (Goodfellow, 1992) or hepatopoietic malignancy (Gillespie et al., 1991; Visuri and Koskenvuo, 1991) with metallic implants have been reported. However, cases are rare compared with the number of incorporated metallic implants (Haug, 1996). Experimentally, nickel alloys evoked sarcomas in rodents (Takamura et al., 1994). It is advocated that nickel-containing alloys (stainless steel) should be removed (Haug, 1996). Tumors in the vicinity of titanium implants are comparatively rare (Fraedrich et al., 1984, Friedman and Vernon, 1983) and have not been induced experimentally. Carcinogenity does not appear to be an argument for plate removal in the maxillofacial region (Haug, 1996).

Infection

Metal hardware may serve as a foreign body, prone to infection through blood-borne bacteria, and may act as a focus for immunological disorders in young patients (Dobbins, Seligson, and Raff, 1988). One reason for infection around titanium plates may be the inhibition of T and B cell proliferation by titanium, cobalt, and chromium mediated by IL-2 and IL-6 (Wang et al., 1996b). Titanium-induced dysfunction of alveolar macrophages to kill *Staphylococcus epidermidis* may be another reason (Giridhar, Myrvik, and Gristina, 1995). Plates have to be removed once an infection is clinically evident. In contrast to orthopedic surgery, delayed infection and septic loosening of implants is not an important clinical issue in maxillofacial surgery.

Diagnostic and Therapeutic Radiation Scattering

Magnetic resonance imaging and computed tomographic imaging artifacts of titanium plates are significantly reduced compared with Vitallium and stainless steel plates (Eppley et al., 1993; Fiala, Novelline and Yaremchuk, 1993; Fiala et al., 1994). Scattering of diagnostic radiation by titanium implants does not apepar to be harmful (Rosengren et al., 1993). Back-scattering of therapeutic radiation has been a problem. Radiotherapists, however, have managed this problem and found solutions (Gullane, 1991; Castillo et al., 1988).

Stress Shielding

Stress shielding by plates, leading to localized osteoporosis and risk of refracture after plate removal, is a problem in orthopedic surgery (Frankel and Burstein, 1968; Uthoff, Boisvert, and Finnegan, 1994) and has been demonstrated experimentally in maxillofacial surgery (Kennady et al., 1989). Based on the absence of clinical reports, refracture due to stress shielding does not appear to be an issue in facial fractures (Haug, 1996).

Conclusion and Ethical Considerations

Toxic effects of aluminum and vanadium, sensitization to metals, a proliferative and inflammatory stimulus, and widespread dissemination of titanium debris in the body are the main arguments for elective plate removal, especially in young individuals. Corrosion of titanium may be enhanced considerably by hydrogen peroxide released from activated macrophages.

However, under certain conditions, characteristics of biocompatibility may manifest differently (Katou et al., 1996). In dental implantology, titanium is encapsulated by bone. Thus, interaction of titanium and the organism is reduced. In orthopedic devices the quantities of metal and production of wear particles usually differ from maxillofacial plates. Thus, results from dental implantology and orthopedic surgery do not easily transfer to maxillofacial plating.

The following statement was issued during the 1991 Strasbourg Osteosynthesis Research Group meeting:

A titanium plate which is intended to assist the healing of bone becomes a nonfunctional implant once this role is complete. It may then be regarded as a foreign body. While there is no clear evidence to date that a titanium plate causes any actual harm, our knowledge still remains incomplete. It is therefore not possible to state with certainty that an otherwise symptomless titanium plate left in situ in the long term is harmless. The removal of a nonfunctioning titanium plate is desirable provided that the procedure to remove the plate does not cause any undue risk to the patient (Black, 1988; Bos, 1993).

In many countries, the need for a general anesthetic to remove these plates or the need to open old incisions constitutes just such an "undue risk to the patient."

39 Complications: Causes and Management

Klaus Louis Gerlach, Hans-Dieter Pape, and Maxime Champy

Introduction

Complications connected with miniplate osteosynthesis are more frequently observed after treatment of mandibular fractures than in other situations. The most important complications include wound healing; for example, suture dehiscences, abscesses, osteomyelitis, and pseudarthrosis. The main factors predisposing to these are delayed treatment, missing perioperative antibiotic treatment, and insufficient fracture stability. Long-term follow-up studies indicated that some errors in technique and management led to certain complications, which were seldom seen by experienced surgeons (Champy et al., 1976b; Gerlach et al., 1985; Champy and Blez, 1992).

Suture Dehiscences

A breakdown in the intraoral closure commonly occurs between the fourth and eighth postoperative day after treatment of mandibular fractures. This complication is encountered mainly in the posterior region where the plate was located close to the external oblique ridge. In unselected series the incidence of this complication was reported to be between 2.7% and 12% after osteosyntheses (Champy et al., 1976b; Champy et al., 1978a; Cawood, 1985; Gerlach et al., 1985; Champy et al., 1986b; Champy and Blez, 1992).

Suture dehiscences were more frequently found if there had been an undue delay between the time of trauma and the time of operation; they can also occur following an inappropriate incision within the region of the attached gingiva. The incision line should be placed 5 mm below the attached gingiva or on the marginal rim. Pre-existing mucosal tears and poor oral hygiene were other possible factors contributing to wound dehiscence. In such cases, after removal of the sutures and wound cleaning with 1.5% hydrogen peroxide, the wound is dressed with an iodoform Vaseline pack. A secondary suture is not necessary. An unimpaired bony union is ensured by normal, open-wound treatment.

Infection

Postoperative infections with abscess formations are also commonly observed in those patients whose treatment had been delayed for some days following trauma and who received no antibiotic prophylaxis (Champy et al., 1976b). This became obvious when, with the decrease of the preoperative time interval, the frequency of abscess formation also diminished from 6.6% to 3.4% (Gerlach et al., 1985; Champy and Blez, 1992). In larger series, the quota of postoperative infections was reported between 1% and 6% (Cawood, 1985; Champy, 1986b; Nakamura, Takenoshita, and Masuichiro, 1994; Tuovinen et al., 1994; Reinhart et al., 1996; Kakoschke, Mohr, and Schettler, 1996; Pape et al., 1996).

As well as the early treatment of fractures, a perioperative antibiotic treatment is recommended to avoid infections. In a randomized prospective study 200 patients with differing therapeutic regimes were compared (Gerlach and Pape, 1988). Patients received antibiotics prophylactically for different periods: 50 patients for 1 day, 49 patients for 3 days, 50 patients a one-shot prophylaxis, and 51 patients had no antibiotics. The first administration of a combination of mezlocillin and oxacillin was given in all cases 30 minutes before the operation. Infections were found in 23 of 200 patients. The analysis of the examined groups indicated 15 infections in the control group and one, three, and four infections, respectively, in the different prophylaxis groups. A 1-day perioperative antibiotic treatment is recommended.

If an abscess develops, incision and drainage generally lead to normal bone healing. Usually the plates can be retained in situ. Only in cases of delayed infections after 1 or 2 months postoperatively, should the osteosynthesis material be removed if it does not assure immobilization. This is usually caused by poor reduction or poor stabilization from badly placed plates. If bony union is insufficient, intermaxillary fixation becomes necessary.

Osteomyelitis

Osteomyelitis of the fracture site is the most serious form of infection, but this complication seldom occurs. All series reported incidences between 0.2% and 1% only (Champy and Blez, 1992).

In those cases, inadequate immobilization of the fragments was the cause. For example, the use of only one miniplate in the region anterior to the canines, fracture fixation with only a single screw in one of the fragments, and application of plates outside the correct osteosynthesis tension line. Furthermore, these patients often failed to keep outpatient appointments. In case of osteomyelitis, removal of the plate and a period of intermaxillary fixation following incision and drainage of the infected fracture line are necessary. Bone healing usually follows this treatment.

Delayed Union (Pseudarthrosis, Fibrous Union)

Delayed union, or even pseudarthrosis, is a very rare complication. Champy and Blez (1992) quoted an incidence of 0.5% after a follow-up of 2600 osteosyntheses. This complication generally occurred after an incorrect fracture reduction or plate fixation, inadequately treated infection, and malocclusions. In the early postoperative period, reoperation with removal of the plates, proper reduction of the fragments, and repeat osteosynthesis with longer plates is recommended. In cases of pseudarthrosis, after removal of the plates, the bone ends should be exposed and the eburnated bone removed with burrs. The bone defect has to be filled with cancellous bone or iliac bone grafts. It is preferable to bridge the defect with two parallel running miniplates (see Chapter 34).

The following recommendations are made in the interest of preventing breakdown of the suture line and impaired wound healing:

- If possible, the osteosynthesis should be performed within the first 24 hours after trauma.
- When fracture treatment can be performed only at a later time, temporary immobilization with intermaxillary fixation is helpful.
- Careful preoperative and postoperative oral hygiene must be observed.
- Perioperative antibiotic treatment is recommended.
- The line of the incision should lie 4–5 mm below the level of the attached gingiva or it should be made as a marginal rim incision.
- The wound edges should be protected during surgery. Wider exposure provides greater visibility and prevents mucosal tears.
- Hematomas can be avoided by suction drainage, by rubber drainage in the incision line for 24 hours, or by extraoral elastic bandages.

Malocclusion

Postoperative disturbances to the occlusion and displacement of fragments result from incorrect reduction and inadequate occlusal fixation of the fragments during osteosynthesis. Large errors of occlusion necessitate a new osteosynthesis. If the error is minimal it can be compensated by selective occlusal grinding after bony union is completed. These complications can be avoided by a precise occlusal fixation during surgery. Only an experienced operating team will be able to establish the occlusion manually during the osteosynthesis. However, securing the occlusion during surgery by intermaxillary fixation or by fixation of the fracture with a towel-clip type bone-holding forceps is recommended, as a safer method.

Special evaluations indicated that the restoration of form and function with regard to the occlusion was satisfactory. The occlusion and articulation of 180 patients were checked by clinical tests and function analysis. Among the fully dentate patients there were eight major and 14 slight occlusional discrepancies. Grinding and, in some cases, use of functional appliances led to a normal occlusion in all patients (Gerlach, Pape, and Tuncer, 1982). In other reports, malocclusion was reported in 3.6% to 8% of cases (Champy and Lodde, 1976; Cawood, 1985; Nakamura, Takenoshita, and Masuichiro, 1994; Tuovinen et al., 1994).

Damage to Dental Roots

Injuries to the dental apices may result from application of the osteosynthesis plate at a too high a level. This complication was seen significantly more often in the posterolateral regions, where the positions of the root apices are not so easily located through the cortical bone, and the space between the apex and the cortical bone is minimal. Injury to the root tips is not likely to occur if the drill holes are made below the alveolar crest at a distance of approximately twice the height of the crown of the tooth (Gastelo, 1978). In 787 fractures treated by miniplates, Gerlach et al. (1985) found root-tip injuries in 30 teeth; only four cases showed a negative pulp vitality and apicectomy and root filling had to be performed.

Damage to the Inferior Alveolar Nerve

Sensory disturbance of the inferior alveolar nerve may occur. In the literature either this complication was not noted or sensory disturbances persisting 12 months postoperatively were described as a result of the injury and prior to osteosynthesis (Tuovinen et al., 1994). In 1985, Cawood noted iatrogenic damage of the inferior alveolar nerve in 8 % of cases. This was associated with a fracture in the vicinity of the mental foramen. Careful protection of the mental nerve with an elevator is recommended while inserting the plate, especially in this region.

Angle Fractures: One or Two Plates?

Despite encouraging results with a low rate of complications, some authors have raised doubts about the functional stability of Champy miniplates, especially for angle fractures. Based on the biomechanical studies of Kroon et al. (1991), Levy et al. (1991) compared the use of one miniplate versus two miniplates in 63 angle fractures and found one complication in 44 patients treated with two miniplates but five in the control group with one miniplate. Ellis and Walker (1994) reported an unacceptable rate of complications (28 %) after treatment of 69 fractures of the angle using two miniplates. In contrast to these observations, Kakoschke et al. (1996) discovered 19 cases of infection, two pseudoarthroses and five malocclusions after treatment of 517 angle fractures with one plate. Pape et al. (1996) observed 433 fractures followed by infection (4 %) and seven cases of malocclusion. Finally, Ellis and Walker (1996), after treatment of 81 angle fractures according to the recommendations of Champy, found only three cases with slight malocclusion and two patients requiring treatment for abscess: one of these developed a pseudoarthrosis. They concluded that the use of a miniplate for fractures of the angle is a simple, reliable technique with a low number of major complications. In conclusion, the results of all these studies confirm Champys recommendation to use miniplate osteosynthesis for treatment of all kinds of mandibular fractures, in dentate as well as edentulous patients.

References

Abdallah HI, Balsara RK, O'Riordan AC. Pacemaker contact sensitivity: clinical recognition and management. *Ann Thorac Surg* 1994;57:1017–1018

Agins HJ, Alcock NW, Bansal N, et al. Metallic wear in failed titanium alloy total hip replacements: a histological and quantitative analysis. *J Bone Joint Surg Am* 1988;70:347–356

Al-Kayat A, Bramley P. A modified pre-auricular approach to the temporomandibular joint and malar arch. *Br J Oral Surg* 1979;17:91–103

Albores-Saavedra J, Vuitch F, Delgado R, et al. Sinus histiocytosis of pelvic lymph nodes after hip replacement. A histiocytic proliferation induced by cobalt-chromium and titanium. *Am J Surg Pathol* 1994;18:83–90

Alpert B, Seligson D. Removal of asymtpomatic bone plates used for orthognathic surgery and facial fractures. *J Oral Maxillofac Surg* 1996;54:618–621

Amir LR, Becking AG, Jovanovic A, et al. Vertical distraction osteogenesis in the human mandible: a prospective morphometric study. *Clin Oral Implants Res* 2006;17: 417–425

Anastassov GE, Rodriguez ED, Schwimmer AM, Adamo AK. Facial rhytidectomy approach for treatment of posterior mandibular fractures. *J Craniomaxillofac Surg* 1997;25:9–14

Anderson JM, Miller KM. Biomaterials biocompatibility and the macrophage. *Biomaterials* 1984;5: 5–10

Arthur G, Berardo N. Simplified technique of maxillomandibular fixation. *J Oral Maxillofac Surg* 1989;47: 1234–1235

Asprino L, Consani S, de Moraes M. A comparative biomechanical evaluation of mandibular condyle fracture plating techniques. *J Oral Maxillofac Surg* 2006;64: 452–456

Atwood DA. Postextraction changes in the adult mandible as illustrated by microradiographs of midsagittal sections and serial cephalometric roentgenograms. *J Prosthet Dent* 1963;13:810–824

Axhausen G. Die operative Freilegung des Kiefergelenks. *Chirurg* 1931;31:713–719

Bähr W, Stoll P, Wächter R. Use of the "double barrel" free vascularized fibula in the mandibular reconstruction. *J Oral Maxillofac Surg* 1998;56:38–44

Baker DL, Stoelinga PJW, Blijdorp PA, Brouns JJA. Longterm stability after inferior maxillary repositioning by miniplate fixation. *Int J Oral Maxillofac Surg* 1992;21:320–326

Bähr W, Bagambisa FB, Schlegel G, Schilli W. Comparison of transcutaneous incisions used for exposure of the infraorbital rim and orbital floor. A Retrospective Study. *Plast Reconstr Surg* 1992;90:585–591

Barnouti L, Caminer D. Maxillary tumours and bilateral reconstruction of the maxilla. *ANZ J Surg* 2006;76:267–269

Becker R, Machtens E. Druckplattenosteosynthese zur Frakturbehandlung und bei orthopädisch chirurgischen Maßnahmen am Gesichtsschädel. *Osteo News (Schweiz)* 1973;19:2–6

Bell WH. Le Fort I osteotomy for correction of maxillary deformities. *J Oral Surg* 1975;33:412–426

Bell WH, Epker BN. Surgical-orthodontic expansion of the maxilla. *Am J Orthod* 1976;70:517–528

Berg St, Pape H-D. Teeth in the fracture line. *Int J Oral Maxillofac Surg* 1992;21:145–146

Bernauer E. Studie über die Aa. interalveolares (Tsusaki-Vessels) und ihre Eintritte in den Knochen an 1600 mazerierten Mandibeln [Dissertation]. Innsbruck, 2004

Bessho K, Fujimura K, Iizuka T. Experimental long-term study of titanium ions eluted from pure titanium miniplates. *J Biomed Mater Res* 1995;29:901–904

Betts NJ, Vanarsdall RL, Barber HD, et al. Diagnosis and treatment of transverse maxillary deficiency. *Int J Adult Orthodon Orthognath Surg* 1995;10:75–96

Binger T, Landau H, Binger A, Spitzer W. Analyse pathologischer Unterkieferfrakturen nach enossaler Implantation: zwei Fallberichte. *Stomatologie* 1999;96:209–212

Black J. Does corrosion matter? *J Bone Joint Surg Br* 1988;70(4): 517–520

Black J, Sherk H, Bonini J, et al. Metallosis associated with a stable titanium alloy femoral component in total hip replacement: a case report. *J Bone Joint Surg Am* 1990;72:126–130

Block MS, Chang A, Crawford D. Mandibular alveolar ridge augmentation in the dog using distraction osteogenesis. *J Oral Maxillofac Surg* 1996;54:309–314

Bockenheimer P. Eine neue Methode zur Freilegung der Kiefergelenke ohne sichtbare Narben und ohne Verletzung des Nervus facialis. *Zentralbl Chir* 1920;47:1560–1579

Boffetta P. Carcinogenicity of trace elements with reference to evaluations made by the International Agency for Research on Cancer. *Scand J Work Environ Health* 1993;19(Suppl 1): 67–70

Borges AF, Alexander JE. Relaxed skin tension lines, Z-plasties on scars and fusiform excision of lesions. *Br J Plast Surg* 1962;15:242–254

Borges AF, Alexander JE, Block LL. Z-plasty treatment of unesthetic scars. *Eye Ear Nose Throat Mon.* 1965;44:39–44

Borges AF. Elective incision and scar revision. Boston: Little Brown; 1973:1–14

Borstlap WA, Stoelinga PJW, Hoppenreijs ThJM, et al. Stabilisation of sagittal split advancement osteotomies with miniplates: a prospective, multicentre study with two-year follow-up. Part I Clinical parameters, part II Radiographic parameters. *Int J Oral Maxillofac Surg* 2004; 33: 433-441, 535–542

Borstlap WA, Stoelinga PJ, Hoppenreijs TJ, van't Hof MA. Stabilisation of sagittal split set-back osteotomies with miniplates: a prospective, multicentre study with two-year follow-up (Clinical and Radiographic parameters). *Int J Oral Maxillofac Surg* 2005;34:487–494

Bos RM. Implant removal. In: Prein J, ed. AO-ASIF Maxillofacial course. Rigid fixation with plates and screws in cranio-maxillofacial trauma. Davos: Syllabus; 1993:17

Boutault F, Fabie M, Cadenat H, Baro JP. Ostéosynthèse trans-jugale par mini-vis à compression dans les ostéotomies sagittales des branches montantes. *Rev Stomatol Chir Maxillofac* 1987;88:257–265

Boutault F, Cadenat H, Poirot A, Bodin H. Intérêt des mini-vis à compression en chirurgie maxillo-faciale. *Ann Chir Plast Esthet* 1989;34:51–57

Boyne PJ. Restoration of osseous defects in maxillofacial casualites. *J Am Dent Assoc* 1969;78:767–776

Boyne PJ. Free grafting of traumatically displaced or resected mandibular condyles. *J Oral Maxillofac Surg* 1989;47: 228–232

Boyoud A, Paty Y. Etude biomécanique des osteosynthèses mandibulaires par plaques vissées. Strasbourg: GEBOAS Faculté de Médecine; 1975

Bradley JC. A radiological investigation into the age changes of the inferior dental artery. *Br J Oral Surg* 1975;13:82–87

Branemark PI. Osseointegration and its experimental background. *J Prosthet Dent* 1983;50:399–410

Breton JL, Louis JM, Garnier G. Asthme aux metaux durs: responsabilite du titane. *Presse Med* 1992;21:997

Brown JS, Trotter M, Cliffe J, et al. The fate of miniplates in facial trauma and orthognathic surgery: a retrospective study. *Br J Oral Maxillofac Surg* 1989;27:306–312

Brown JS. Deep circumflex iliac artery free flap with internal oblique muscle as a new method of immediate reconstruction of maxillectomy defect. *Head Neck* 1996;18:412–421

Buijs GJ, Stegenga B, Bos RR. Efficacy and safety of biodegradable osteofixation devices in oral and maxillofacial surgery: a systematic review. *J Dent Res* 2006;85:980–989

Busch RF, Prunes F. Intermaxillary fixation with intraoral cortical bone screws. *Laryngoscope* 1991;101:1336–1338

Busch RF. Maxillomandibular fixation with intraoral cortical bone screws: a 2-year experience. *Laryngoscope* 1994;104: 1048–1050

Cadenat E, Cadenat H. Utilisation des broches de Kirschner dans les fractures des machoires et de la face. *Rev Stomatol Paris* 1956;57:230–269

Cancilleri F, de Giorgis P, Verdoia C, et al. Allergy to components of total hip arthroplasty before and after surgery. *Ital J Orthop Traumatol* 1992;18:407–410

Car M, Tic A, Sambunjak T, et al. Nasa iskustva u lijecenju prijeloma kostiju lica s posebnim osvrtom na metodu intermaksilarne imobilizacije metalnim kukicama. *Chir Maxillofac Plast* 1986; 16:9–16

Case CP, Langkamer VG, James C, et al. Widespread dissemination of metal debris from implants. *J Bone Joint Surg Br* 1994; 76:687–691, 701–712

Castillo MH, Button TM, Homs MI, et al. Effects of radiation therapy on mandibular reconstruction plates. In: Transactions of the forty-first annual cancer symposium. New Orleans: Society of Surgical Oncology; 1988:114

Cawood JI. Small plate osteosynthesis of mandibular fractures. *Br J Oral Maxillofac Surg* 1985;23:77–91

Cawood JI, Howell RA. A classification of the edentulous jaws. *Int J Oral Maxillofac Surg* 1988;17:232–236

Cawood JI, Howell RA. Reconstructive preprosthetic surgery–anatomical considerations. *Int J Oral Maxillofac Surg* 1991;20: 75–82

Cawood JI, Stoelinga PJW. Reconstruction of the severely resorbed Class VI maxilla. *Int J Oral Maxillofac Surg* 1994;23: 219–225

Cawood JI, Stoelinga PJW. Report of the International Research Group on Reconstructive Preprosthetic Surgery. *Int J Oral Maxillofac Surg* 1996;25:81–84

Cawood JI, Stoelinga PJW. International Academy for Oral and Facial Rehabilitation. Consensus Report. *Int J Oral Maxillofac Surg* 2006;35:195–198

Cawood JI, Stoelinga PJW, Blackburn TK. The evolution of preimplant surgery from preprosthetic surgery. *Int J Oral Maxillofac Surg* 2007;36:377–385

Champy M, Wilk A, Schnebelen JM. Die Behandlung der Mandibularfrakturen mittels Osteosynthese ohne intermaxilläre Ruhigstellung nach der Technik von F.X. Michelet. *Dtsch Zahn-Mund- u. Kieferheilk.* 1975;63:339–341

Champy M, Lodde JP, Wilk A. A propos des osteosyntheses frontomalaires par plaques vissees. *Rev Stomatol.* 1975;76:483–488

Champy M, Lodde JP, Jaeger JH, Wilk A. Osteosynthèses mandibulaires selon la technique de Michelet. I-Bases biomécaniques. *Rev Stomatol.* 1976a;77:569–576

Champy M, Lodde JP, Jaeger JH, et al. Ostéosynthéses mandibulaires selon la technique de Michelet. II Presentation d'un nouveau materiel. Resultats. *Rev Stomatol.* 1976b;77:577–582

Champy M, Lodde JP. Synthèses mandibulaires. Localisation des synthèses en fonction des contraintes mandibulaires. *Rev Stomatol.* 1976;77:971–979

Champy M, Lodde JP. Etude des contraintes dans la mandibule fracturée chez l'homme. Mesures théoriques et vérification par jauges extensométriques in situ. *Rev Stomatol.* 1977; 78:545–556

Champy M, Lodde JP, Grasset D, et al Les osteosyntheses par plaques miniaturisées vissées en chirurgie faciale et cranienne. A propos de 400 cas. *Ann Chir Plast.* 1977;22:165–167

Champy M, Lodde JP, Schmitt R, Jaeger JH, Muster D. Mandibular osteosynthesis by miniature screwed plates via a buccal approach. *J Oral Maxillofac Surg* 1978a;6:14–21

Champy M, Lodde JP, Wilk A, Grasset D. Plattenosteosynthesen bei Mittelgesichtsfrakturen und Osteotomien. *Dtsch Z Mund Kiefer Gesichtschir* 1978b;2:26–36

Champy M, Lodde JP, Wilk A, et al. Probleme und Resultate bei der Verwendung von Dehnungsmeßstreifen am präparierten Unterkiefer und bei Patienten mit Unterkieferfrakturen. *Dtsch Z Mund Kiefer Gesichtschir* 1978c;2:41–43

Champy M. Surgical treatment of midface deformities. *Head Neck Surg* 1980;2:451–454

Champy M. Biomechanische Grundlagen der Straßburger Miniplattenosteosynthese. *Dtsch Zahnarztl Z* 1983;38:358–360

Champy M, Lodde JP, Kahn JL, Kielwasser P. Attempt at systematization in the treatment of isolated fractures of the zygomatic bone: techniques and results. *J Otolaryngol* 1986a; 15:39–43

Champy M, Pape HD, Gerlach KL, Lodde JP. The Strasbourg miniplate osteosynthesis. In: Krueger E, Schilli W, Worthington P, eds. Oral and maxillofacial traumatology Vol. II. Chicago: Quintessence; 1986b:19–43

Champy M, Blez P. Results of small plate osteosynthesis in fractures of the mandible in the departments of maxillo-facial surgery of Cologne and Strasbourg. In: Shimuzu M, Yanagisawa S, eds. Oral and maxillofacial surgery: Proceedings of the 16th Congress of IAMFS. Masama Saika Insatzu 1992:49–52

Champy M. Small plate osteosynthesis in facial and cranial surgery. Cours sur l'ostéosynthèse faciale et cranienne par plaques miniaturisées, 23 sept. 1978, Strasbourg. Strasbourg Service de Stomatologie et Chirurgie Maxillofaciale, Hospices Civils de Strasbourg.

Champy M, Blez P, Kahn JL, Muster D. Utilisation de plaques résorbables dans l'ostéosynthèse du tiers moyen de la face. *Acta Biomater* 1993;2:47–54

Charvat J, Soremark R, Li J, Vacek J. Titaniumtetrafluoride for treatment of hypersensitive dentine. *Swed Dent J* 1995;19: 41–46

Chen CT, Lai JP, Tung TC, Chen YR. Endoscopically assisted mandibular subcondylar fracture repair. *Plast Reconstr Surg* 1999;103:60–65

Chen YB, Chen HC, Hahn LH. Major mandibular reconstruction with vascularized bone grafts: Indications and selection of donor tissues. *Microsurgery* 1994;15:227–237

Chiapasco M, Brusati R, Galioto S. Distraction osteogenesis of a fibula revascularized flap for improvement of oral implant repositioning in a tumour patient: a case report. *J Oral Maxillofac Surg* 2000;58:1434–1440

Chiapasco M, Zaniboni M, Rimondini L. Autogenous onlay bone grafts vs. alveolar distraction osteogenesis for the correction of vertically deficient edentulous ridges: a 2–4-year prospective study on humans. *Clin Oral Implants Res* 2007;18: 432–440

Chin M, Toth BA. Distraction osteotogenesis in maxillofacial surgery using internal devices—review of five cases. *J Oral Maxillofac Surg* 1996;54:45–53

Chin M. Transoral or coronal Le Fort III advancement: internal, self-retaining distractors. Book of Abstracts: International Congress on Cranial and Facial Bone Distraction Processes, Paris 1999

Choi BH, Huh JY, Yoo JH. Computed tomographic findings of the fractured mandibular condyle after open reduction. *Int J Oral Maxillofac Surg* 2003;32:469–473

Choi BH, Yi CK, Yoo JH. Clinical evaluation of 3 types of plate osteosynthesis for fixation of condylar neck fractures. *J Oral Maxillofac Surg* 2001;59:734

Choi BH, Kim KN, Kim HJ, et al. Evaluation of condylar neck fracture plating techniques. *J Craniomaxillofac Surg* 1999;27: 109

Chotkowski GC. Symphysis and parasymphysis fractures. *Atlas Oral Maxillofac Clin North Am* 1997;5(1):27–59

Chuong R, Piper MA. Open reduction of condylar fractures of the mandible in conjunction with repair of disc injury: a preliminary report. *J Oral Maxillofac Surg* 1988;46:257–263

Clavero J, Lundgren S. Ramus or chin grafts for maxillary sinus inlay and local onlay augmentation: comparison of donor site morbidity and complications. *Clin Implant Dent Relat Res* 2003;5:154–160

Cohen L. Further studies into the vascular architecture of the mandible. *J Dent Res* 1960;39:936–943

Cohen SR, Rutrick RE, Burstein FD. Distraction osteogenesis of the human craniofacial skeleton: initial experience with a new distraction system. *J Craniofac Surg* 1995;6:368–374

Coleman SC, Burkey BB, Day TA, et al. Increasing use of the scapula osteocutaneous free flap. *Laryngoscope* 2000;110: 1419–1424

Coleman F. Some points in connexion with fractures of the jaw. *St Bartholomews Hosp J* 1910;17:134–138

Coleman F. An important sign in the diagnosis of fracture of the jaw. *Proc R Soc Med* 1912;5:13–15

Cordeiro PG, Disa JJ, Hidalgo DA, Hu QY. Reconstruction of the mandible with osseous free flaps: a 10-year experience with 10 consecutive patients. *Plast Reconstr Surg* 1999;104: 1314–1320

Cornell CN, Lane JM. Newest factors in fracture healing. *Clin Orthop Relat Res* 1992;277:297–311

Dafnis E, Sabatini S. Biochemistry and pathophysiology of vanadium. [editorial] *Nephron* 1994;67:133–143

Dal Pont G. Retromolar osteotomy for the correction of prognathism. *J Oral Surg* 1961;19:42–47

Dal Pont G. Sull'impiego di ganci metallici iuxtaossei nel bloccagio intermascellare in sogetti presentanti fratture die mascellari. *Riv Ital Stomatol* 1965;20:791–797

Dal Santo P, Mille P, Cornet A, Champy M. Reconstitution mandibulaire par plaques miniaturisés vissées. AUM, ed. Acta du 12ème Congrès de Mécanique, Strasbourg, Vol. 1 1995:13–16

Daniels AU, Chang MKO, Andriano KP. Mechanical properties of biodegradable polymers and composites proposed for internal fixation of bone. *J Appl Biomater* 1990;1:57–78

Danis R. Théorie et pratique de l'ostéosynthèse. Paris: Masson; 1949

de Brul EL. The Skull. In: de Brul EL, ed. Sicher's oral anatomy. St. Louis: Mosby; 1970:85–93

Desault PJ. Mémoires sur la fracture des condyles de la machoire inférieure. Oeuvres chirurgicales ou exposé de la doctrine et de la pratique de P.J. Desault par son élève Xavier Bichat. 1e Edition, tome I. Paris: Méquignon l'Aine; 1798

Diner PA, Kollar EM, Martinez H, Vazquez MP. Intraoral distraction for mandibular lengthening: a technical innovation. *J Craniomaxillofac Surg* 1996;24:92–95

Dittert DD, Warnecke G, Willert HG. Aluminum levels and stores in patients with total hip endoprostheses from TiAlV or TiAlNb alloys. *Arch Orthop Trauma Surg* 1995;114:133–136

Dobbins JJ, Seligson D, Raff MJ. Bacterial colonization of orthopedic fixation devices in the absence of clinical infection. *J Infect Dis* 1988;158:203–207

Domingo JL. Reproductive and developmental toxicity of aluminum: a review. *Neurotoxicol Teratol* 1995;17:515–521

Domingo JL. Vanadium: a review of the reproductive and developmental toxicity. *Reprod Toxicol* 1996;10:175–182

Ducheyne P, Bianco PD, Kim C. Bone tissue growth enhancement by calcium phosphate coatings on porous titanium alloys: the effect of shielding metal dissolution product. [published erratum appears in Biomaterials. 1992;**13**:800] *Biomaterials* 1992;13: 617–624

Dumbach J, Steinhäuser EW. Resektion und Rekonstruktion des Unterkiefers mit dem Titangitter bei osteomyelitischen Pseudoarthrosen. *Dtsch Zahnärztl Z* 1983;38:423–425

Dumbach J. Mandibular reconstruction after infected posttraumatic defects In: Hjrrting-Hansen E, ed. Oral and maxillofacial surgery. Chicago: Quintessence; 1985:527–530

Dumbach J. Unterkieferrekonstruktion mit Titangitter, autogener Spongiosa und Hydroxyl-apatit. Biomechanische, tierexperimentell-histologische und klinische Untersuchungen. Munich: Hanser; 1987

Dumbach J, Rodemer H, Spitzer WJ, Bender E. Grenzen der knöchernen Rekonstruktion des Unterkiefers mit autogener Spongiosa, Hydroxylapatitgranulat und Titangitter. *Fortschr Kiefer Gesichtschir* 1994;39:93–95

Dupuytren JF. Traité théoretique et pratique des blessures par armes de guerre. Vol 1. Paris: Baillière; 1834:66–67

Dwyer CM, Kerr RE. Contact allergy to aluminium in 2 brothers. *Contact Dermatitis* 1993;29:36–38

Eckelt U, Gerber S. Zugschraubenosteosynthese bei Unterkiefergelenkfortsatzfrakturen mit einem neuartigen Osteosynthesebesteck. *Dtsch Zahn Mund Kieferheilkd.* 1981;69:485–490

Eckelt U, Hlawitschka M. Clinical and radiological evaluation following surgical treatment of condylar neck fractures with lag screws. *J Craniomaxillofac Surg* 1999;27:235–242

Eckelt U. Zur funktionsstabilen Osteosynthese bei Unterkiefergelenkfortsatzfrakturen. Habilitationsschrift. Dresden: Medizinische Akademie Carl Gustav Carus; 1984

Eckelt U. Zugschraubenosteosynthese bei Unterkiefergelenkfortsatzfrakturen. *Dtsch Z Mund Kiefer Gesichtschir* 1991;15: 51–57

Eckelt U, Schneider M, Rasse M, et al. Open versus closed treatment of fractures of the mandibular condylar process—a prospective randomized multicenter study. *J Craniomaxillofac Surg* 2006;34:306–314

Eckelt U, Nitsche M, Müller A, et al. Ultrasound aided pin fixation of biodegradable osteosynthetic materials in cranioplasty for infants with craniosynostosis. *J Craniomaxillofac Surg* 2007a; 35:218–221

Eckelt U, Mai R, Pilling E, et al. The application of SonicWeld© osteosynthesis techniques in Craniofacial Surgery. *Indian J Oral Maxillofac Surg* 2007b;6:22–25

Edel J, Marafante E, Sabbioni E. Retention and tissue binding of titanium in the rat. *Hum Toxicol* 1985;4:177–185

Elagli K, Vérnon C, Hildebrand HF. Titanium-induced enzyme activation on murine peritoneal macrophages in primary culture. *Biomaterials* 1995;16:1345–1351

Ellis EIII, Moos KF, el-Attar A. Ten years of mandibular fractures: an analysis of 2137 cases. *Oral Surg Oral Med Oral Pathol* 1985;59:120–129

Ellis E, Reynolds ST, Park HS. A method to rigidly fix high condylar fractures. *Oral Surg Oral Med Oral Pathol* 1989;68: 369–374

Ellis E, Dean J. Rigid fixation of mandibular condyle fractures. *Oral Surg Oral Med Oral Pathol* 1993;76:6–15

Ellis E, Ghali GE. Lag screw fixation in anterior mandibular fractures. *J Oral Maxillofac Surg* 1991;49:13–21

Ellis E, Walker L. Treatment of mandibular angle fractures using two noncompression miniplates. *J Oral Maxillofac Surg* 1994;52:1032–1036

Ellis E, Walker L. Treatment of mandibular angle fractures using two noncompression miniplates. *J Oral Maxillofac Surg* 1996;54:846–871

Ellis EIII, Simon P, Throckmorton GS. Occlusal results after open or closed treatment of fractures of the mandibular condylar process. *J Oral Maxillofac Surg* 2000;58:260–268

Ellis E, Throckmorton GS. Treatment of mandibular condylar process fractures: biological considerations. *J Oral Maxillofac Surg* 2005;63:115–134

Ellis E, Throckmorton GS. Bite forces after open or closed treatment of mandibular condylar process fractures. *J Oral Maxillofac Surg* 2001;59:389–395

Epker BN. Modifications of the sagittal osteotomy of the mandible. *J Oral Surg* 1977;35:157–159

Eppley BL, Sparks C, Herman E, et al. Effects of skeletal fixation on craniofacial imaging. *J Craniofac Surg* 1993;4:67–73

Erbe M, Stoelinga PJW, Leenen RJ. Long-term results of segmental repositioning of the maxilla in cleft palate patients without previously grafted alveolo-palatal clefts. *J Craniomaxillofac Surg* 1996;24:109–117

Ewers R, Reuter E, Stoll W. Die parodontale Situation des Zahnes im Bruchspalt. *Dtsch Zahnarztl Z* 1976;31:251–253

Ewers R. Periorbitale Knochenstukturen und ihre Bedeutung für die Osteosynthese. *Fortschr Kiefer Gesichtschir* 1977;22: 45–46

Ewers R, Härle F. Osteotomieheilung im Unterkiefer nach Kontakt- und Spaltheilung sowie nach kortiko-kortikaler Heilung. *Dtsch Zahnarztl Z* 1983;38:361–362

Ewers R, Härle F. Biomechanics of the midface and mandibular fractures: Is a stable fixation necessary? In: Hjørting-Hansen E, ed. Oral and maxillofacial surgery. Chicago: Quintessence; 1985a:207–211

Ewers R, Härle F. Experimental and clinical results of new advances in the treatment of facial trauma. *Plast Reconstr Surg* 1985b;75:25–31

Exley C, Burgess E, Day JP, et al. Aluminum toxicokinetics. *J Toxicol Environ Health* 1996;48:569–584

Fairbanks GA, Hallock GG. Facial reconstruction using a combined flap of the subscapular axis simultaneously including separate medial and lateral scapular vascularized bone grafts. *Ann Plast Surg* 2002;49:104–108; discussion 108

Farmand M. 3-D-osteosynthesis in craniofacial surgery. *J Cranio-maxillofac Surg* 1991;19:299–305

Farmand M. The three-dimensional plate fixation of fractures and osteotomies. *Facial Plast Surg* 1995;3:39–42

Ferrari OJ, Zappettini DJ, Patetta LA, et al. Haematomas of the floor of the mouth caused by fracture of the lower jaw. Emergency tracheotomy. *Dia Med* 1962;34:380–382

Ferre JC, Barbois JY, Helary JL, Lumineau JP. Le système de suspension de la mandibule. Approche bioméchanique. *Orthod (Fr)* 1983;54:589–604

Fiala TGS, Novelline RA, Yaremchuk MJ. Comparison of CT imaging artifacts from craniomaxillofacial internal fixation devices. *Plast Reconstr Surg* 1993;92:1227–1232

Fiala TGS, Paige KT, Davis TL, et al. Comparison of artifacts from craniomaxillofacial internal fixation devices: Magnetic resonance imaging. *Plast Reconstr Surg* 1994;93:725–731

Fraedrich G, Kracht J, Scheld HH, et al. Sarcoma of the lung in a pacemaker pocket—simple coincidence or oncotaxis. *Thorac Cardiovasc Surg* 1984;32:67–69

Frankel VH, Burstein AH. The biomechanics of refracture of bone. *Clin Orthop Relat Res* 1968;60:221–225

Freihofer M, Peter H. Experience with transnasal canthopexy. *J Maxillofac Surg* 1980;8:119–124

Friedman KE, Vernon SE. Squamous cell carcinoma developing in conjunction with a mandibular staple bone plate. *J Oral Maxillofac Surg* 1983;41:265–266

Fritzemeier CU, Bechthold H. Die Osteosynthese von Unterkiefergelenkfortsatzfrakturen mit alleinigem Zugang von intraoral. *Dtsch Z Mund Kiefer Gesichtschir* 1993;17:66–68

Fuhr J, Setz D. Nachuntersuchungen von Zähnen, die zum Bruchspalt in Beziehung stehen. *Dtsch Zahnarztl Z* 1963;18:638–640

Galante JO, Lemons J, Spector M, Wilson PD, Wright TM. The biologic effects of implant materials. *J Orthop Res* 1991; 9:760–775

Gassner R, Tuli T, Hächl O, et al. Cranio-maxillofacial trauma: a 10 year review of 9543 cases with 21 067 injuries. *J Craniomaxillofac Surg* 2003;31:51–61

Gastelo L. Effects of mandibular osteosynthesis on teeth and dental occlusion. In: Champy M, ed. Course on miniplate osteosynthesis in facial and cranial surgery. Strasbourg: Service Stomatology, Faculté Médecine; 1978:46–48

Gbara A, Darwich K, Li L, Schmelzle R, Blake F. Long-term results of jaw reconstruction with microsurgical fibula grafts and dental implants. *J Oral Maxillofac Surg* 2007;65:1005–1009

Gerber JC. Les ostéosyntheses mandibulaires par la méthode de Michelet. Strasbourg: Thèse Faculté de Médecine; 1975

Gerlach KL, Pape H-D, Tuncer M. Funktionsanalytische Untersuchungen nach der Miniplattenosteosynthese von Unterkieferfrakturen. *Dtsch Z Mund Kiefer Gesichtschir* 1982;6:57–60

Gerlach KL, Khouri M, Pape H-D, Champy M. The Strasbourg miniplate osteosynthesis. Results of mandibular fracture treatment in Cologne and Strasbourg. In: Hjørting-Hansen E, ed. Oral and maxillofacial surgery. Chicago: Quintessence; 1985:138–140

Gerlach KL, Pape H-D. Untersuchungen zur Antibiotikaprophylaxe bei der operativen Behandlung von Unterkieferfrakturen. *Dtsch Z Mund Kiefer Gesichtschir* 1988;12:497–500

Gerlach KL, Mokros S, Erle A. Miniplate osteosyntheses of low subcondylar fractures of the mandible by intraoral approach. Indications, method, results. *J Craniomaxillofac Surg* 1996; 24(Suppl 1):47

Gerlach KL. Resorbierbare Polymere als Osteosynthesematerialien. *Mund Kiefer Gesichtschir* 2000;4:91–102

Gerstorfer J, Weber H. Corrosion resistance of the implant materials contimet 35 (titanium 99.6% pure) and Vitallium in artificial physiologic fluids. *Int J Oral Maxillofac Surg* 1988;3: 135–140

Gilbert A. Vascularized transfer of the fibula shaft. *Int J Microsurg.* 1979;1:100–102

Gillies H, Harrison SH. Operative correction by osteotomy of recessed maxillary compound in the case of oxycephaly. *Br J Plast Surg* 1950;3:123–138

Gillies HD, Kilner TP, Stone D. Fractures of the malarzygomatic compound with description of a new X-ray position. *Br J Surg* 1927;14:651–657

Giridhar G, Myrvik QN, Gristina AG. Biomaterial-induced dysfunction in the capacity of rabbit alveolar macrophages to kill Staphylococcus epidermidis RP12. *J Biomed Mater Res* 1995;29:1179–1183

Goh CL. Prevalence of contact allergy by sex, race and age. *Contact Dermatitis* 1986;14:237–240

Goodfellow J. Editorial: Malignancy and joint replacement. *J Bone Joint Surg Br* 1992;74:645

Gropp H, Wangerin K, Paello F, et al. Skeletal stability following distraction osteogenesis of the mandible with transorally applied distraction devices. *J Craniomaxillofac Surg* 1998;26(Suppl. 1):64

Gruss JS, Mackinnon SE. Complex maxillary fractures: role of buttress reconstruction and immediate bone grafts. *Plast Reconstr Surg* 1986;78:9–22

Gruss JS. Rigid fixation of nasoethmoid-orbital fractures. In: Yaremchuck MJ, Gruss JS, Manson PN, eds. Rigid fixation of the craniomaxillofacial skeleton. Boston: Butterworth-Heinemann; 1992:283–301

Guerrero C, Bell WH, Flores A, et al. Distracciòn osteogénica mandibular intraoral. *Revista Venezolana Ortodontia* 1995; 11:116–132

Gullane PJ. Primary mandibular reconstruction: Analysis of 64 cases and evaluation of interface radiation dosimetry on bridging plates. *Laryngoscope* 1991;101:1–24

Günther K, Gundlach KKH, Schwipper V. Der Zahn im Bruchspalt. *Dtsch Zahnarztl Z* 1983;38:346–348

Haers PE, van Straaten W, Stoelinga PJ, et alReconstruction of the severely resorbed mandible prior to vestibuloplasty or placement of endosseous implants. *Int J Oral Maxillofac Surg* 1991;20:149–154

Haers PE, Sailer HF. Self-reinforced poly-L-DL-lactide osteosynthesis in bimaxillary surgery: A prospective study on material related failures and skeletal stability (one year). *J Oral Maxillofac Surg* 1999;28(Suppl I):12–13

Härle F, Lange G. Operationstechnik zur Vermeidung des postoperativen Telekanthus bei Nasoethmoidalfrakturen. *Fortschr Kiefer Gesichtschir* 1975;19:147–148

Härle F. Die Lage des Mandibularkanals im zahnlosen Kiefer. *Dtsch Zahnarztl Z* 1977;32:275–276

Härle F. Strukturanalyse des Kieferköpfchens. *Fortschr Kiefer Gesichtschir* 1980;25:62–63

Hasund A. Clinical cephalometry for the Bergen Technique. Bergen, Norway: University of Bergen, Dental Institute; 1974

Hauenstein H, Steinhäuser EW. Erfahrungen mit dem Titangitter als temporäres Fremdimplantat zur Wiederherstellung bei Unterkieferdefekten. *Dtsch Zahnarztl Z* 1977;32: 523–528

Haug RH. Retention of asymptomatic bone plates used for orthognathic surgery and facial fractures. *J Oral Maxillofac Surg* 1996;54:611–617

Haug RH, Assael LA. Outcomes of open versus closed treatment of mandibular subcondylar fractures. *J Oral Maxillofac Surg* 2001;59:370–375

Hausamen J-E, Neukam FW. Resection of tumors in tongue, floor of the mouth and mandible: Possibilities of primary reconstruction. In: Pape H-D, Ganzer U, Schmitt G, eds. Carcinoma of the oral cavity and oropharynx. Berlin: Springer; 1994:25–35

Haynes DR, Rogers SD, Hay S, et al. The differences in toxicity and release of bone-resorbing mediators induced by titanium and cobalt-chromium-alloy wear particles. [see comments] *J Bone Joint Surg Am* 1993;75:825–834

Hayter JP, Cawood JI. Oral rehabilitation with endosteal implants and free flaps. *Int J Oral Maxillofac Surg* 1996;25:3–12

Hayward JR, Scott RF. Fractures of the mandibular condyle. *J Oral Maxillofac Surg* 1993;51:57–61

Heidemann W, Gerlach KL, Gröbel KH, Köllner HG. DFS—A new form of osteosynthesis screw. *J Craniomaxillofac Surg* 1996; 24(Suppl. 1):52

Heidemann W, Gerlach KL, Gröbel KH, Köllner HG. Drill-Free-Screws: a new form of osteosynthesis screw. *J Craniomaxillofac Surg* 1998a;26:163–168

Heidemann W, Gerlach KL, Gröbel KH, Köllner HG. Influence of different pilot hole sizes on torque measurements and pullout analysis of osteosynthesis screws. *J Craniomaxillofac Surg* 1998b;26:50–55

Heidemann W, Gerlach KL. Klinische Anwendung von Drill-Free-Schrauben. In: Hübner H, ed. Plastisch-rekonstruktive Chirurgie. Reinbeck:Einhorn; 1998:228–232

Heidemann W, Gerlach KL, Fischer JH, et al. Tissue reaction to implantation of poly(D,L)lactide with or without addition of calciumphosphates in rats. *Biomed Tech (Berl)* 1996;41: 408–409

Heidemann W, Jeschkeit-Schubbert S, Ruffieux K, et al. pH-Stabilization of predegraded PDLLA by an admixture of water-soluble sodiumhydrogenphosphate—results of an in vitro- and in vivo-study. *Biomaterials* 2002 a;23:3567–3574

Heidemann W, Gerlach KL. Anwendung eines resorbierbaren Osteosynthesesystems aus Poly(D,L)laktid in der Mund-, Kiefer- und Gesichtschirurgie. *Dtsch Zahnarztl Z* 2002 b;57:50–53

Heidemann W, Gerlach KL. Imaging of biodegradable osteosynthesis materials by ultrasound. *Dentomaxillofac Radiol* 2002c; 31:155–158

Heidemann W, Ruffieux K, Fischer JH, et al. The effect of an admixture of sodium hydrogen phosphate or heparin-coating to poly(D,L)lactide—results of an animal study. *Biomed Tech (Berl)* 2003a;48:262–268

Heidemann W, Fischer JH, Koebke J, et al. In vivo study of degradation of poly(D,L)lactide and poly(L-lactide-co-glycolide) osteosynthesis material. *Mund Kiefer Gesichtschir* 2003b;7: 283–288

Henderson D, Jackson IT. Nasomaxillary hypoplasia—Le Fort II osteotomy. *Br J Oral Surg* 1973;11:77–82

Hernández Altemir F. The submental route for endotracheal intubation: a new technique. *J Maxillofac Surg* 1986;14: 64–65

Hidalgo DA. Fibula free flap: A new method of mandible reconstruction. *Plast Reconstr Surg* 1989;84:71–82

Hidalgo DA. Aesthetic improvements in free flap mandible reconstruction. *Plast Reconstr Surg* 1991;88:574–585

Hidalgo DA. Fibula free flap mandibular reconstruction. *Clin Plast Surg* 1994;21:25–35

Hidalgo DA, Rekow A. A review of 60 consecutive fibula free flap mandible reconstructions. *Plast Reconstr Surg* 1995;96: 585–596

Hidalgo DA, Pusic AL. Free-flap mandibular reconstruction: a 10-year follow-up study. *Plast Reconstr Surg* 2002;110: 438–448

Hidding J, Wolf R, Pingel D. Surgical versus non surgical treatment of fractures of the articular process of the mandible. *J Craniomaxillofac Surg* 1992;20:345–347

Hidding J, Breier M. Distraction-osteogenesis of the maxilla. *Int J Oral Maxillofac Surg* 1997;26(Suppl 1):76

Hidding J, Zöller JE, Lazar F. Micro- and macrodistraction of the jaw. A sure method of adding new bone. *Mund Kiefer Gesichtschir* 2000;4(Suppl 2):432–437

Hildebrand HF, Champy M. Biocompatibility of Co-Cr-Ni Alloys. NATO-ASI Series A: Life Sciences Vol 158. New York: Plenum; 1987:369–371

Hillmann G, Donath K. Licht- und elektronenmikroskopische Untersuchungen zur Biostabilität dentaler Titanimplantate. *Zahnärztl Implantol.* 1991;7:170–177

Hlawitschka M, Loukota R, Eckelt U. Functional and radiological results of open and closed treatment of intracapsular (diacapitular) condylar fractures of the mandible. *Int J Oral Maxillofac Surg* 2005;34:597–604

Hochban W, Ellers M, Umstadt HE, Juchems KI. Zur operativen Reposition und Fixation von Unterkiefergelenkfortsatzfrakturen von enoral. *Fortschr Kiefer Gesichtschir* 1996;41: 80–85

Hofer O. Die operative Behandlung der alveolären Retraktion des Unterkiefers und ihre Anwendungsmöglichkeit für Prognathie und Mikrogenie. *Zahn Mund Kieferheilkd.* 1942;9:121–132

Hoffmeister B. Die parodontale Reaktion im Bruchspalt stehender Zähne bei Unterkieferfrakturen. *Dtsch Zahnarztl Z* 1985;40: 32–36

Hoffmeister B, Kreusch Th. Indikation zur Anwendung unterschiedlicher Osteosynthesematerialien bei der Behandlung der Mittelgesichtsfrakturen. *Fortschr Kiefer Gesichtschir* 1991;36:62–65

Hoffmeister B, Wangerin K. Skelettale Stabilität nach bimaxillärer Chirurgie. *Fortschr Kiefer Gesichtschir* 1995;40:57–65

Hoffmeister B, Marcks CH, Wolff K. The floating bone conception in intraoral mandibular destraction. . *J Craniomaxillofac Surg* 1998;26(Suppl 1):76

Hofmann H. Lid- und Bulbusschäden bei Gesichtsverletzungen. *Fortschr Kiefer Gesichtschir* 1966;11:59–62

Holgers KM, Roupe G, Tjellstrom A, Bjursten LM. Clinical, immunological and bacteriological evaluation of adverse reactions to skin-penetrating titanium implants in the head and neck region. *Contact Dermatitis* 1992;27:1–7

Hönig JF, Merten HA, Luhr HG. Passive and active intracranial translocation of osteosynthesis plates in adolescent minipigs. *J Craniofac Surg* 1995;6:292–298

Hoppenreijs TJM, Nijdam ES, Freihofer HPM. The chin as a donor site in early secondary osteoplasty: a retrospective clinical and radiological evaluation. *J Craniomaxillofac Surg* 1992;20: 119–124

Horch HH, Gerlach KL, Pape H-D. Indikation und Grenzen der intraoralen Miniplattenosteosynthese bei Frakturen des aufsteigenden Unterkieferastes. *Dtsch Zahnarztl Z* 1983; 38:447–450

Hori M, Nakada Y, Matsunaga S, et al. Use of two miniplates for intermaxillary skeletal fixation in the treatment of jaw deformity and fracture. *J Nihon Univ Sch Dent* 1992;34: 224–229

Huckel B. L'ostéosynthèse mandibulaire par plaques vissées miniaturisées: évolution des idées. Thèse Médecine Strasbourg 1996, No. 74.

Hunsuck EE. A modified intra-oral sagittal splitting technique for correction of mandibular prognathism. *J Oral Surg* 1968; 26:250–253

Iatrou I, Kolbe F, Champy M, et al. Behandlungskonzept und Ergebnisse der Jochbeinimpressionsfrakturen der Kölner und Straßburger Klinik von 1975–1988. *Fortschr Kiefer Gesichtschir* 1991;36:100–102

Iizuka T, Lindqvist C, Hallikainen D, et al. Severe bone resorption and osteoarthrosis after miniplate fixation of high condylar fractures. *Oral Surg Oral Med Oral Pathol* 1991;72: 400–407

Ikarashi Y, Momma J, Tsuchiya T, Nakamura A. Evaluation of skin sensitization potential of nickel, chromium, titanium and zirconium salts using guinea-pigs and mice. *Biomaterials* 1996;17:2103–2108

Ikemura K, Kouno J, Shibata H, Yamasaki K. Biomechanical study on monocortical osteosynthesis for the fracture of the mandible. *Int J Oral Surg* 1984;13:307–312

Ilizarov GA. The tension-stress effect on the genesis and growth of tissues: part I. The influence of stability of fixation and soft tissue preservation. *Clin Orthop Relat Res* 1989a;238: 249–281

Ilizarov GA. The tension-stress effect on the genesis and growth of tissues: part II. The influence of the rate and frequency of distraction. *Clin Orthop Relat Res* 1989b;239:263–285

Ilizarov GA. The principles of the Ilizarov method. *Bull Hosp Jt Dis* 1997;56:49–53

Illi OE, Sailer HF, Stauffer U. Résultats préliminaires de l'osteosynthèse biodegradable en chirurgie craniofaciale chez l'enfant. *Chir Pediatr* 1989;30:284

Isaacs RS, Sykes JM. Maxillomandibular fixation with intraoral cortical bone screws. *Laryngoscope* 1995;105:109

Ito M, Handa Y, Okutomi T, et al. Application of Otten intermaxillary immobilisation for infant condylar fracture. *J Jpn Stomatol Soc* 1988;37:773–778

Ito A, Okazaki Y, Tateishi T, Ito Y. In vitro biocompatibility, mechanical properties, and corrosion resistance of Ti-Zr-Nb-Ta-Pd and Ti-Sn-Nb-Ta-Pd alloys. *J Biomed Mater Res* 1995;29: 893–899

Ivy RH. Observation of fractures of the mandible. *J Am Med Assoc* 1922;79:295–298

Jacobovicz J, Lee C, Trabulsy P. Endoscopic repair of mandibular subcondylar fractures. *Plast Reconstr Surg* 1998;101: 437–441

Jacobs JJ, Skipor AJ, Black J, et al. Release and excretion of metal in patients who have a total hip replacement component made of titanium base alloy. *J Bone Joint Surg Am* 1991;73: 1475–1486

Jacobsson M, Tjellstrom A, Thomsen P, Albrektsson T. Soft tissue infection around a skin penetrating osseointegrated implant. *Scand J Plast Reconstr Surg Hand Surg* 1987;21: 225–228

Jaeger JH. Biomechanical principles applied to osteosynthesis. In: Champy M, ed. Course on miniplate osteosynthesis in facial and cranial surgery. Strasbourg: Service Stomatologie, Faculté Médecine; 1978:1–6

Jensen OT. Maxillo-mandibular fixation with screws. *Oral Surg Oral Med Oral Pathol* 1997;83:418

Jeter TS, van Sickels JE, Nishioka GJ. Intraoral open reduction with rigid internal fixation of mandibular subcondylar fractures. *J Oral Maxillofac Surg* 1988;46:1113–1116

Jeter TS, Hackney FL. Open reduction and rigid fixation of subcondylar fractures. In: Yaremchuk MJ, Fruss JS, Manson PN, eds. Rigid fixation of the craniomaxillofacial skeleton. Boston: Butterworth-Heinemann; 1992:209–216

Jones DC. Transalveolar screw. *Oral Surg Oral Med Oral Pathol* 1997;84:458–459

Joos U. An adjustable bone fixation system for sagittal split ramus osteotomy: preliminary report. *Br J Oral Maxillofac Surg* 1999;37: 99–103

Jovanovic SA, Spiekermann H. Bone regeneration on titanium dental implants with dehisced defect sites. *Int J Oral Maxillofac Implants* 1992;7:233–239

Julka D, Gill KD. Altered calcium homeostasis: a possible mechanism of aluminium-induced neurotoxicity. *Biochim Biophys Acta* 1996;1315:47–54

Kahn JL, Khouri M. Champy's System. In: Yaremchuk MJ, Gruss JS, Manson PN, eds. Rigid fixation of the craniomaxillofacial skeleton. Boston: Butterworth-Heinemann; 1992:116–123

Kakoschke D, Mohr C, Schettler D. Langzeitergebnisse nach intraoraler Miniplattenosteosynthese bei Kieferwinkelfrakturen. *Fortschr Kiefer Gesichtschir* 1996;41:91–94

Kanno T, Mitsuge M, Furuki Y, et al. Overcorrection in vertical alveolar distraction osteogenesis for dental implants. *Int J Oral Maxillofac Surg* 2007;36:398–402

Katou F, Andoh N, Motegi K, Nagura H. Immuno-inflammatory responses in the tissue adjacent to titanium miniplates used in the treatment of mandibular fractures. *J Craniomaxillofac Surg* 1996;24:155–162

Keen WW. Surgery, its principles and practice. Philadelphia: Saunders; 1909

Kellmann RM. Endoscopic approach to subcondylar mandible fractures. *Facial Plast Surg* 2004;20:239–247

Kellmann RM, Marenette LJ. Atlas of craniomaxillofacial fixation. New York: Raven; 1995:126–127

Kelly KJ, Manson PN, Vander Kolk CA, et al. Sequencing Le Fort fracture treatment. *J Craniofac Surg* 1990;1:168–178

Kennady MC, Tucker MR, Lester GE, Buckley MJ. Stress shielding effect of rigid internal fixation plates on mandibular bone grafts. A photon absorption dpensitometry and quantitative computerized tomographic evaluation. *Int J Oral Maxillofac Surg* 1989;18:307–310

Kerscher A, Soofizadeh A, Kreusch Th. Marginal gingival incision as surgical approach to Le Fort I-Osteotomy. *Int Dent J* 1995;45:328–331

Kermer Ch, Undt G, Rasse M. Surgical reduction and fixation of intracapsular condylar fractures. A follow up study. *Int J Oral Maxillofac Surg* 1998;27:191–194

Kessler P, Neukam FW, Wiltfang J. Effects of distraction forces and frequency of distraction on bony regeneration. *Br J Oral Maxillofac Surg* 2005;43:392–398

Khoury M, Champy M. Resultats des osteosyntheses mandibulaires par miniplaques. 800 fractures traitées en 10 ans. *Ann Chir Plast Esthet* 1987;32:262–266

Kim YK, Yeo HH, Lim SC. Tissue response to titanium plates: a transmitted electron microscopic study. *J Oral Maxillofac Surg* 1997;55:322–326

Kitayama S. A new method of intra-oral reduction using a screw applied through the mandibular crest in condylar fractures. *J Craniomaxillofac Surg* 1989;17:16–23

Kleier C, Kleinheinz J, Joos U. Prospektive Funktionsanalyse und Achsiographie bei Patienten mit sagittaler Ramusosteotomie. *Dtsch Zahnarztl Z* 1998;53:476–480

Klesper B, Wahn J, Koebke J. Comparison of bone volumes and densities relating to osseointegrated implants in microvascularreconstructed mandibles: a study of cadaveric rdius and fibula bones. *J Craniomaxillofac Surg* 2000;28:110–115

Klotch DW, Gilliland R. Internal fixation versus conventional therapy in midface fractures. *J Trauma* 1987;27:1136–1145

Koberg WR, Momma W-G. Treatment of fractures of the articular process by functional stable osteosynthesis using miniaturized dynamic compression plates. *Int J Oral Surg* 1978;7: 256–262

Kocher Th. Chirurgische Operationslehre. Jena: Fischer; 1892: 26–27

Kraissl CJ. The selection of appropriate lines for elective surgical incisions. *Plast Reconstr Surg* 1951;8:1–28

Krause H-R, Bremerich A, Kreidler J. Technik und Ergebnisse der operativen Behandlung von 400 lateralen Mittelgesichtsfrakturen. *Fortschr Kiefer Gesichtschir* 1991;36:109–111

Krenkel C, Grunert I. Der Zahn im Bruchspalt bei Unterkieferfrakturen, versorgt mit Silcadraht-Klebeschienen. *Dtsch Z Mund Kiefer Gesichtschir* 1987;11:208–210

Krenkel C, Lixl G. Axial lag screws with double-contoured washers. 9th Congress European Association for Cranio-Maxillofacial Surgery; Athens, Greece; 5th–9th September 1988

Krenkel C. Axial "anchor" screw (lag screw with biconcave washer) or "slanted screw" plate for osteosynthesis of fractures of the mandibular condylar process. *J Craniomaxillofac Surg* 1992;20:348–353

Krenkel C. Biomechanics and osteosynthesis of condylar neck fractures of the mandible. Chicago: Quintessence; 1994: 73–115

Krenkel Ch, Holzner K, Poisel S. Mundbodenhämatome nach oralchirurgischen Eingriffen und ihre anatomischen Besonderheiten. *Dtsch Z Mund Kiefer Gesichtschir* 1985;9: 448–451

Krenkel Ch, Holzner K. Die linguale Knochenperforation als Kausalfaktor einer bedrohlichen Mundbodenblutung bei einem Einzelzahnimplantat der Eckzahnregion. *Quintessenz* 1986; 37:1003–1008

Krenkel Ch, Grunert I. Endodistraction doubles the height of severely atrophic mandibles, EAO 2002, 11th Annual Scientific Congress, Sept. 12–14th, Poster 67, Brussels, Belgium

Krenkel Ch, Goriwoda W, Moser G, Plenk HJr. Distraction Bone-Engineering in Atrophic Edentulous Mandibles prior to Dental Implant Insertion. *Eur Cell Mater* 2007;14(Suppl. 1):72

Kretschmer W, Wangerin K. Transantral maxillary distraction—first results. Book of Abstracts: 4. International Symposium on Orthognathic Surgery and Distraction, Stuttgart; 2006:103

Kreusch Th, Fleiner B, Steinmann H. Der Zahnfleischrandschnitt als operativer Zugang bei der Kieferspaltosteoplastik. *Fortschr Kiefer Gesichtschir* 1993;38:43–44

Kroon FHM, Mathisson M, Cordey JR, et al. The use of miniplates in mandibular fractures. *J Craniomaxillofac Surg* 1991;19: 199–204

Krüger E. Indikation und Technik der operativen Kieferbruchbehandlung. *Dtsch Zahnarztl Z* 1964;19:1057–1072

Kuder J. Vertical distraction in patients with unilateral hemifacial microsomia-Long term results. Book of Abstracts: 4. International Symposium on Orthognathic Surgery and Distraction, Stuttgart; 2006:66.

Kufner J. Nove metody chirurgickeho leceni otevreneho skusu. *Cs Stomatol.* 1960;60:387–394

Kulkarni RK, Moore EG, Hegyeli AF, Leonhard F. Biodegradable poly(lactic acid) polymers. *J Biomed Mater Res* 1971;5: 169–181

Kung DS, Kaban LB. Supratarsal fold incision for approach to the superior lateral orbit. *Oral Surg Oral Med Oral Pathol* 1996;81:522–525

Küppers K. Analyse der funktionellen Struktur des menschlichen Unterkiefers. Berlin: Springer; 1971:7–91

Kusiak JF, Zins JE, Whitaker LA. The early revascularization of membranous bone. *Plast Reconstr Surg* 1985;76: 510–516

Kuttner P. Untersuchungen zur physikalischen Dynamik von Zugund Tandemschrauben mit bikonkaven Unterlegscheiben am Unterkiefer [Dissertation]. Innsbruck; 1989

Lachner J, Clanton JT, Waite PD. Open reduction and internal rigid fixation of subcondylar fractures via an intraoral approach. *Oral Surg Oral Med Oral Pathol* 1991;71:257–261

Lalor PA, Gray AB, Wright S, et al. Contact sensitivity to titanium in a hip prosthesis? *Contact Dermatitis* 1990;23:193–194

Lalor PA, Revell PA, Gray AB, et al. Sensitivity to titanium. A cause of implant failure? *J Bone Joint Surg Br* 1991;73:25–28

Lambotte A. Chirurgie operatoire des fractures. Paris: Masson; 1913:122–126

Langer K. Zur Anatomie und Physiologie der Haut. Über die Spaltbarkeit der Cutis. *S B Akad Wiss Wien* 1861;44:19–46

Lauer G, Haim D, Profft P, et al. Plate osteosynthesis of the mandibular condyle. *Ann Anat* 2007;189:412–417

Lauer G, Haim D, Profft P, et al. Biomechanical evaluation of osteosynthesis at the condylar neck using different plate designs. *Ann Anat* 2007;189:412–417

Lauer G, Schmelzeisen R. Endoscope-assisted fixation of mandibular condylar process fractures. *J Oral Maxillofac Surg* 1999;57:36–39

Lauer G, Pradel W, Schneider M, Eckelt U. A new 3-dimensional plate for transoral endoscopic-assisted osteosynthesis of condylar neck fractures. *J Oral Maxillofac Surg* 2007;65: 964–971

Lazar FC, Klesper B, Carls P, et al. Callusmassage. A new treatment modality for non-unions of the irradiated mandible. *Int J Oral Maxillofac Surg* 2005;34:202–207

Lee C, Mueller RV, Lee K, Mathes SJ. Endoscopic subcondylar fracture repair: functional, aesthetic and radiographic outcomes. *Plast Reconstr Surg* 1998;102:1434–1443

Leipziger LS, Manson PN. Nasoethmoid orbital fractures. *Clin Plast Surg* 1992;19:167–193

Levy FE, Smith RW, Odland RM, Marentette LJ. Monocortical miniplate fixation of mandibular angle fractures. *Arch Otolaryngol Head Neck Surg* 1991;117:149–154

Lindahl L. Condylar fractures of the mandible. IV. Function of the masticatory system. *Int J Oral Surg* 1977;6:195–203

Lindorf HH. Chirurgische-schädelbezügliche Einstellung des Gebisses (Doppelsplintmethode). *Dtsch Zahnarztl Z* 1977;32: 260–261

Lindquist CC, Obeid G. Complications of genioplasty done alone or in combination with sagittal split-ramus osteotomy. *Oral Surg Oral Med Oral Pathol* 1988;66:13–16

Llewelyn J, Sugar A. Lag screws in sagittal split osteotomies: should they be removed? *Br J Oral Maxillofac Surg* 1992; 30:83–85

Lodde JP, Champy M. Justification biomécanique d'un nouveau matériel d'ostéosynthèse en chirurgie faciale. *Ann Chir Plast* 1976;21:115–121

Lopez S, Pelaez A, Navarro LA, et al. Aluminium allergy in patients hyposensitized with aluminium-precipitated antigen extracts. *Contact Dermatitis* 1994;31:37–40

Loukota RA, Eckelt U, De Bont L, Rasse M. Subclassification of fractures of the condylar process of the mandible. *Br J Oral Maxillofac Surg* 2005;43:72–73

Luhr H-G. Zur stabilen Osteosynthese bei Unterkieferfrakturen. *Dtsch Zahnarztl Z* 1968;23:754

Luhr H-G. Ein Plattensystem zur Unterkieferrekonstruktion einschließlich des Gelenks. *Dtsch Zahnarztl Z* 1976;31: 747–748

Luhr H-G. Basic research, surgical technique and results of fracture treatment with the Luhr-Mandibular-Compression-Screw System (MCS System). In: Hjørting-Hansen E, ed. Oral and maxillofacial surgery. Berlin: Quintessence; 1985:124–132

Luhr HG, Jäger A. Indikation, Technik und Ergebnisse der bimaxillären Chirurgie. *Fortschr Kiefer Gesichtschir* 1995;40:20–32

MacLennan WD. Consideration of 180 cases of typical fractures of the mandibular condylar process. *Br J Plast Surg* 1952;5: 122–128

Macleod SP, Bainton R. Extrusion of a microplate: an unusual complication of osteosynthesis. *J Craniomaxillofac Surg* 1992;20:303–304

Mai R, Lauer G, Pilling E, et al. Bone welding—a histological evaluation in the jaw. *Ann Anat* 2007;189:350–355

Malgaigne JF. Traité des fractures et des luxations. Tome I, Des fractures. Paris 1847, with atlas

Manson PN, Hooper JE, Su CT. Structural pillars of the facial skeleton: An approach to the management of Le Fort fractures. *Plast Reconstr Surg* 1980;66:54–57

Manson PN. Some thoughts on the classification and treatment of Le Fort fractures. *Ann Plast Surg* 1986;17:356–364

Manson PN, Clark N, Robertson B, Crawley WA. Comprehensive management of pan-facial fractures. *J Craniomaxillofac Trauma* 1995;1:43–56

Marchac D, Cophignan J, van der Meulen J, Bouchta M. A propos des ostéotomies d'avancement du crane et de la face. *Ann Chir Plast* 1974;19:311–323

Mariano A. Choice of osteosynthesis areas according to bone solidity. In: Champy M, ed. Course on miniplate osteosynthesis in facial and cranial surgery. Strasbourg: Service Stomatologie, Faculté Médecine; 1978:10–11

Markowitz BL, Manson PN, Sargent LA, et al. Management of the medial canthal tendon in nasoethmoid orbital fractures: The importance of the central fragment in classification and treatment. *Plast Reconstr Surg* 1991;87:843–853

Maurer AM, Merritt K, Brown SA. Cellular uptake of titanium and vanadium from addition of salts or fretting corrosion in vitro. *J Biomed Mater Res* 1994;28:241–246

Mazzonetto R, Allais M, Maurette PE, Moreira RW. A retrospective study of the potential complications during alveolar distraction osteogenesis in 55 patients. *Int J Oral Maxillofac Surg* 2007;36:6–10

McCarthy JG, Schreiber J, Karp N, et al. Lengthening the human mandible by gradual distraction. *Plast Reconstr Surg* 1992;89: 1–10

McKay GC, Macnair R, MacDonald C, Grant MH. Interactions of orthopaedic metals with an immortalized rat osteoblast cell line. *Biomaterials* 1996;17:1339–1344

Mehta RP, Deschler DG. Mandibular reconstruction in 2004: an analysis of different techniques. *Curr Opin Otolaryngol Head Neck Surg* 2004;12:288–293

Merckx D, Lodde JP. Clinical tolerance of the material in mandibular tissues. Postoperative Infection. Management of infectious complications. In: Champy M, ed. Course on miniplates osteosynthesis in facial and cranial surgery. Strasbourg: Service Stomatologie, Faculté Médecine; 1978:31–41

Merritt K, Margevicius RW, Brown SA. Storage and elimination of titanium, aluminum, and vanadium salts, in vivo. *J Biomed Mater Res* 1992;26:1503–1515

Merritt K, Rodrigo JJ. Immune response to synthetic materials. Sensitization of patients receiving orthopaedic implants. *Clin Orthop Relat Res* 1996;326:71–79

Merville L. Multiple dislocations of the facial skeleton. *J Maxillofac Surg* 1974;2:187–200

Meyer C. Biomechanics of the temporo-mandibular joint. In: Kleinheinz J, Meyer C, eds. Treatment of condylar fractures of the mandible. Berlin: Quintessence; 2009a; in press.

Meyer C. The TCP® platting technique. In: Kleinheinz J, Meyer C, eds. Treatment of condylar fractures of the mandible. Berlin: Quintessence 2009b; in press.

Meyer C, Kahn JL, Boutemi P, Wilk A. Determination of the external forces applied to the mandible during various static chewing tasks. *J Craniomaxillofac Surg* 1998;26:331–341

Meyer C, Kahn JL, Boutemi P, Wilk A. Photoelastic analysis of bone deformation in the region of the mandibular condyle during mastication. *J Craniomaxillofac Surg* 2002;30:160–169

Meyer C, Martin E, Kahn JL, Zink S. Development and biomechanical testing of a new osteosynthesis plate (TCP) designed to stabilize mandibular condyle fractures. *J Craniomaxillofac Surg* 2007;35:84–90

Meyer C, Serhir L, Boutemi P. Experimental evaluation of three osteosynthesis devices used for stabilizing condylar fractures of the mandible. *J Craniomaxillofac Surg* 2006;34: 173–181

Michelet FX, Moll A. Traitements chirurgicaux des fractures du corps mandibulaire sans blocage par plaques vissées insérées par voie endo-buccale. *Rev Odontostomatol Midi Fr* 1971; 29:87–93

Michelet FX, Deymes J, Dessus B. Osteosynthesis with miniaturized screwed plates in maxillofacial surgery. *J Maxillofac Surg* 1973;1:79–84

Mikkonen P, Lindqvist C, Pihakari A, et al. Osteotomy–osteosynthesis in displaced condylar fractures. *Int J Oral Maxillofac Surg* 1989;18:267–270

Misch CM. Enhance maxillary implant sites through symphysis bone graft. *Dent Implantol Update* 1991;2:101–104

Moberg LE, Nordenram A, Kjellmaru O. Metal release from plates used in jaw fracture treatment: a pilot study. *Int J Oral Maxillofac Surg* 1989;18:311–314

Moenning JE, Graham LL. Elimination of mandibular labial undercut with autogenous bone grafts from a maxillary tuberosity. *J Prosthet Dent* 1986;56:211–214

Mokros St, Erle A. Die transorale Miniplattenosteosynthese von Gelenkfortsatzfrakturen–Optimierung der operativen Methode. *Fortschr Kiefer Gesichtschir* 1996;41:136–138

Montague A, Merritt K, Brown S, Payer J. Effects of Ca and H_2O_2 added to RPMI on the fretting corrosion of Ti6Al4V. *J Biomed Mater Res* 1996;32:519–526

Moran CA, Mullick FG, Ishak KG, et al. Identification of titanium in human tissues: probable role in pathologic processes. [see comments] *Hum Pathol* 1991;22:450–454

Morris CM, Candy JM, Kerwin JM, Edwardson JA. Transferrin receptors in the normal human hippocampus and in Alzheimer's disease. *Neuropathol Appl Neurobiol.* 1994;20:473–477

Motolese A, Truzzi M, Giannini A, Seidenari S. Contact dermatitis and contact sensitization among enamellers and decorators in the ceramics industry. *Contact Dermatitis* 1993;28: 59–62

Motsch A. Besitzt der menschliche Unterkiefer eine trajektonelle Struktur? *Dtsch Zahnarztl Z* 1968;23:1381–1387

Mühlbauer W, Anderl H, Ramatschi P, et al. Radical treatment of craniofacial anomalies in infancy and the use of miniplates in craniofacial surgery. *Clin Plast Surg* 1987;14:101–111

Müller ME, Allgöwer M, Willenegger H. Manual der Osteosynthese. Berlin: Springer; 1969:29

Müller ME, Allgöwer M, Schneider R, Willenegger H. Manual of internal fixation. 3 rd ed. Heidelberg: Springer; 1991:193

Muster D, Champy M, Schmuckler S, et al. Behaviour of the interface bone–metal. Approach by the method of the physics of the surfaces. In: Hildebrand HF, Champy M, eds. Biocompatibility of Co-Cr-Ni alloys. NATO ASI Series A: Life Sciences, Vol 158. New York: Plenum; 1987:25–26

Nakamura S, Takenoshita Y, Masuichiro O. Complications of miniplate osteosynthesis for mandibular fractures. *J Oral Maxillofac Surg* 1994;52:233–238

Neff A, Kolk A, Meschke F, Deppe H, Horch HH. Small fragment screws vs. plate osteosynthesis in condylar head fractures. *Mund Kiefer Gesichtschir* 2005;9:80–88

Neff A, Kolk A, Neff F, Horch HH. Surgical vs. conservative therapy of diacapitular and high condylar fractures with dislocation. A comparison between MRI and axiography. *Mund Kiefer Gesichtschir* 2002;6:66–73

Neff A, Kolk A, Horch HH. Position and mobility of the articular disk after surgical management of diacapitular and high condylar dislocation fractures of the temporomandibular joint. *Mund Kiefer Gesichtschir* 2000;4:111–117

Neff A, Mühlberger G, Karoglan M, et al. Stabilität der Osteosynthese bei Gelenkwalzenfrakturen in Klinik und biomechanischer Simulation. *Mund Kiefer Gesichtschir* 2004;8:63–74

Nehse G, Maerker R. Indikationsstellung verschiedener Rekonstruktions- und Osteosyntheseverfahren bei der operativen Versorgung von subkondylaren Frakturen des Unterkiefers. *Fortschr Kiefer Gesichtschir* 1996;41:120–123

Neubert J, Bitter K, Somsiri S. Refined intraoperative repositioning of the osteotomized maxilla in relation to the skull and TMJ. *J Craniomaxillofac Surg* 1988;16:8–12

Neukam FW, Schmelzeisen R, Schliephake H. Oromandibular reconstruction with vascularized bone grafts in combination with implants. *Oral Maxillofac Surg Clin North Am.* 1994; 2:717–738

Niederdellmann H, Schilli W, Düker J, Akuamoa-Boateng E. Osteosynthesis of mandibular fractures using lag screws. *Int J Oral Surg* 1976;5:117–121

Niederdellmann H, Shetty V. Solitary lag screw osteosynthesis in the treatment of fractures of the angle of the mandible: a retrospective study. *Plast Reconstr Surg* 1987;80: 68–74

Obwegeser H. Über eine einfache Methode der freihändigen Drahtschienung von Kieferbereichen. *Osterr Z Stomatol* 1952;49: 652–655

Obwegeser H. Eingriffe am Oberkiefer zur Korrektur des progenen Zustandbildes. *Schweiz Monatsschr Zahnmed* 1965;75:365–374

Obwegeser HL. Surgical correction of the small and retrodisplaced maxillae. *Plast Reconstr Surg* 1969;43:351–359

Obwegeser H. Die einzeitige Vorbewegung des Oberkiefers und Rückbewegung des Unterkiefers zur Korrektur der extremen '. *Schweiz Monatsschr Zahnheilk* 1970;80:547–556

Obwegeser HL, Weber G, Freihofer HP, Sailer HF. Facial duplications–The unique case of Antonio. *J Maxillofac Surg* 1978;6: 179–198

Oikarinen KS, Raustia AM, Lahti J. Signs and symptoms of TMJ dysfunction in patients with mandibular condyle fractures. *J Craniomandibular Pract* 1991;9:58–62

Oikarinen K, Ignatius E, Silvennoinen U. Treatment of mandibular fractures in the 1980 s. *J Craniomaxillofac Surg* 1993;21: 245–250

Onishi K, Maruyama Y. Simple intermaxillary fixation for maxillomandibular osteosynthesis. *J Craniofac Surg* 1996;7: 170–172

Onodera K, Ooya K, Kawamura H. Titanium lymph node pigmentation in the reconstruction plate system of a mandibular bone defect. *Oral Surg Oral Med Oral Pathol* 1993;75: 495–499

Otten JE. Modifizierte Methode zur intermaxillären Immobilisation. *Dtsch Zahnarztl Z* 1981;36:91–92

Paoli JR, Lauwers F, Boutault F. Technique rapide de fixation. *Rev Stomatol Chir Maxillofac* 1996;97:89–91

Pape H-D, Hauenstein H, Gerlach KL. Chirurgische Versorgung der Gelenkfortsatzfrakturen mit Miniplatten. Indikation–Technik-erste Ergebnisse und Grenzen. *Fortschr Kiefer Gesichtschir* 1980;25:81–89

Pape H-D, Gerlach KL, Rehm KE, Schippers Ch. Zur Rekonstruktion des Unterkiefers: Entwicklung und Techniken in mehreren Jahrzehnten. *Langenbecks Arch Chir Suppl Kongressbd* 1993;110:757–759

Pape H-D, Gerlach KL, Schippers Ch. Ergebnisse der Unterkieferrekonstruktion mit autogenen freien Knochentransplantaten. *Fortschr Kiefer Gesichtschir* 1994;39:79–81

Pape H-D, Schippers CG, Gerlach KL, Walz C. Die Funktionsstabilität der Miniplattenosteosynthese nach Champy bei Kieferwinkelfrakturen. *Fortschr Kiefer Gesichtschir* 1996;41: 94–96

Pape H-D. Microplate osteosynthesis of the midface–5 years of clinical use of a new technique. *Int J Oral Maxillofac Surg* 1997;26(Suppl 1):65

Pauwels F. Grundriss einer Biomechanik der Frakturheilung. *Verh Dtsch Orthop Ges.* 1940;34:62–108

Peled M, Abu El-Naaj I, Lipin Y, Ardekian L. The use of free fibular flap for functional mandibular reconstruction. *J Oral Maxillofac Surg* 2005;63:220–224

Peoc'h M, Pasquier D, Ducros V, et al. Reactions granulomateuses systemiques et prothese de hanche. Deux observations anatomocliniques. *Rev Chir Orthop Reparatrice Appar Mot* 1996;82:564–567

Perdijk FB, Meijer GJ, Strijen PJ, Koole R. Complications in alveolar distraction osteogenesis of the atrophic mandible. *Int J Oral Maxillofac Surg* 2007;36:916–921

Peri G, Vaillant JM, Jourde J, Meues R. L'osteosynthese corticale externe mandibulaire par voie intra-buccale de principe. *Ann Chir Plast* 1972;17:184–190

Perthes G. Über Frakturen und Luxationsfrakturen des Kieferköpfchens und ihre operative Behandlung. Verh dtsch Ges Chir. 1924; 418–433

Peters MS, Schroeder AL, van Hale HM, Broadbent JC. Pacemaker contact sensitivity. *Contact Dermatitis* 1984;11: 214–218

Petzel JR. Die chirurgische Behandlung des frakturierten Collum mandibulae durch funktionsstabile Zugschraubenosteosynthese. *Fortschr Kiefer Gesichtschir* 1980;25:84–91

Petzel JR. Functionally stable traction-screw osteosynthesis of condylar fractures. *J Oral Maxillofac Surg* 1982;40: 108–110

Philipps JH, Rahn BA. Bone healing. In: Yaremchuk MJ, Gruss JS, Manson PN, eds. Rigid fixation in the craniomaxillofacial skeleton. Boston: Butterworth-Heinemann; 1992:3–6

Pilling E, Mai R, Theissig F, et al. An experimental in vivo analysis of the resorption to ultrasound activated pins (Sonic weld®) and standard biodegradable screws (ResorbX®) in sheep. *Br J Oral Maxillofac Surg* 2007a;45:447–450

Pilling E, Meissner H, Jung R, et al. An experimental study of the biomechanical stability of ultrasound-activated pinned (Sonic-Weld Rx®+Resorb-X®) and screw-fixed (Resorb-X®) resorbable materials for osteosynthesis in the treatment of simulated craniosynostosis in sheep. *Br J Oral Maxillofac Surg* 2007b;45:451–456

Rae T. Comparative laboratory studies on the production of soluble and particulate metal by total joint prostheses. *Arch Orthop Trauma Surg* 1979;95:71–79

Rae T. The biological response to titanium and titanium-aluminim-vanadium alloy particles. I–tissue culture studies. *Biomaterials* 1986a;7:30–36

Rae T. The biological response to titanium and titanium-aluminim-vanadium alloy particles. II–long term animal studies. *Biomaterials* 1986b;7:37–40

Rahn BA. Knochenheilung unter Osteosynthesebedingungen. *Dtsch Zahnarztl Z* 1983;38:294–297

Rasse M, Fialka V, Paternostro T. Modifikationen des Zuganges zum Kiefergelenk und Ramus mandibulae. *Acta Chir Austr* 1993;1:49–54

Rasse M. Diakapituläre Frakturen der Mandibula.Eine neue Operationsmethode und erste Ergebnisse. *Z Stomatol.* 1993;90: 413–428

Rasse M, Koch A, Traxler H, Mallek R. Der Frakturverlauf von diakapitulären Frakturen der Mandibula-eine klinische Studie mit anatomischer Korrelation. *Z Stomatol.* 1993;90:119–125

Rasse M. Recent developments in therapy of condylar fractures of the mandible. *Mund Kiefer Gesichtschir* 2000;4: 69–87

Rasse M, Moser D, Zahl C, et al. Osteosynthessis of condylar neck fractures with resorbable poly(DL)lactide plates and screws. An animal experiment. *Br J Oral Maxillofac Surg* 2007;45: 35–40

Rasse M, Schober C, Piehslinger E, et al. Intra- und extrakapsuläre Kondylusfrakturen im Wachstumsalter. *Dtsch Zahnarztl Z* 1991;46:49–51

Raveh Y, Stich H, Sutter F, Greiner R. New concepts in the reconstruction of mandibular defects following tumor resection. *J Oral Maxillofac Surg* 1983;41:3–16

Raveh J, Vuillemin T, Lädrach K. Open reduction of the dislocated fractured condylar process. Indications and surgical procedures. *J Oral Maxillofac Surg* 1989;47:120–126

Raveh J. Lower jaw reconstruction with the THORP System for bridging of lower jaw. In: Fee WE, Goepfert H, Johns M, et al., eds. Head and neck cancer. Vol. 2. Toronto: Decker; 1990: 344–349

Raveh J, Ladrach K, Vuillemin TH, Zingg M. Indications for open reduction of the dislocated, fractured condylar process: evaluation and management of conservatively treated cases. In: Worthington P, Evans J, eds. Controversies in oral and maxillofacial surgery. Philadelphia: Saunders; 1994:174–183

Reichenbach E. Leitfaden der Kieferbruchbehandlung. Leipzig: JA Barth; 1938

Reichenbach E, Schönberger A. 50 Jahre Verwendung freier Knochentransplantate als Unterkieferersatz–Rückblick und Ausblick. *Dtsch Zahn Mund Kieferheilkd.* 1957;26:436–445

Reinhart E, Reuther J, Michel C, et al. Behandlungsergebnisse und Komplikationen bei operativ und konservativ versorgten Unterkieferfrakturen. *Fortschr Kiefer Gesichtschir* 1996;41: 64–67

Remmert S, Mohadjer C, Siems T, Weerda H. Vergleichende Untersuchung zwischen Killianscher Schnittführung und modifiziertem Schnitt entsprechend den RSTL. *Laryngorhinootologie* 1994;73:268–269

Reuther JF. Druckplattenosteosynthese und freie Unterkieferrekonstruktion. Berlin: Quintessenz; 1979

Reuter E, Koper L. Die Platte zur intermaxillären Fixation. Eine Alternative im zahnlosen Kiefer. *Dtsch Z Mund Kiefer Gesichtschir* 1985;9:249–250

Richardson D, Cawood JI. Anterior maxillary osteoplasty to broaden the narrow maxillary ridge. *Int J Oral Maxillofac Surg* 1991;20:342–348

Robinson M. Prognathism corrected by open vertical condylotomy. *J S California Dent Ass.* 1956;24:22–26

Robinson M, Yoon C. New onlay–inlay metal splint for immobilization of mandibular subcondylar fractures. *Am J Surg* 1960;100:845–849

Rosenberg A, Gratz KW, Sailer HF. Should titanium miniplates be removed after bone healing is complete? *Int J Oral Maxillofac Surg* 1993;22:185–188

Rosengren B, Wulff L, Carlsson E, et al. Backscatter radiation at tissue–titanium interfaces. Biological effects from diagnostic 65 kV X-rays. *Acta Oncol* 1993;32:73–77

Rousseau D, Segard C. Reconstruction mandibulaire par plaques miniaturisées vissées pour différents cas de pertes de substance interruptrices. Strasbourg: Ecole Nationale Supérieure des Arts et Industrie, Filière Génie Mécanique; 1994

Rudderman RH, Mullen RL. Biomechanics of the facial skeleton. *Clin Plast Surg* 1992;19:11–29

Rudner EJ, Clendenning WE, Epstein E. The frequence of contact dermatitis in North America 1972–1974. *Contact Dermatitis* 1975;1:277–280

Sailer HF. Osteosynthesis of orbital margin fractures via the transconjunctival approach using staples. A preliminary report. *J Maxillofac Surg* 1977;5:184–186

Sailer HF. Erfahrungen mit dem transkonjunktivalen Zugang. *Fortschr Kiefer Gesichtschir* 1978;22:39–40

Sailer HF. Transplantation of lyophilized cartilage in maxillofacial surgery. Experimental foundations and clinical success. Basel: Karger; 1983:43–58

Sailer HF, Obwegeser HL. Langzeitergebnisse nach Korrektur von kraniofazialen Anomalien. In: Mühlbauer W, Anderl H, eds. Kraniofaziale Fehlbildungen und ihre operative Behandlung. Stuttgart: Thieme; 1983:144–155

Sailer HF. Insuffiziente Ergebnisse nach Le Fort III-Osteotomie und deren Vermeidung durch die doppelstufige Mittelgesichtsbewegung. *Fortschr Kiefer Gesichtschir* 1985;30:102–104

Sailer HF, Landolt AM. A new method for the correction of hypertelorism with preservation of the olfactory nerve filaments. *J Maxillofac Surg* 1987a;15:122–124

Sailer HF, Landolt AM. Hypertelorism with herniation of brain and pituitary gland into the oronasal cavity. In: Marchac D, ed. Craniofacial surgery. Berlin: Springer; 1987b:197–204

Sailer HF. A new method of inserting endosseous implants in totally atrophic maxillae. *J Craniomaxillofac Surg* 1989;17:299–305

Sailer HF, Landolt AM. Treatment concepts for craniosynostosis and hypertelorism. In: Pfeifer G, ed. Craniofacial abnormalities and clefts of the lip, alveolus and palate. Stuttgart: Thieme; 1991:85–91

Sailer HF. Longterm results after implantation of different lyophilized bones and cartilage for reconstruction in craniofacial surgery. In: Montoya AG, ed. Craniofacial surgery. Bologna: Monduzzi; 1992:69–72

Sailer HF, Grätz KW. Surgical treatment of hypertelorism. In: Turvey AT, Vig KWL, Fonseca RJ, eds. Facial clefts and craniosynostosis: principles and management. Philadelphia: Saunders; 1995:686–713

Sailer HF, Grätz KW, Oechslin C, et al. Occipitale Korrektur bei Scapho- und Plagiocephalie. *Mund Kiefer Gesichtschir* 1998;2(Suppl 1):79–80

Sailer HF, Haers PE, Suuronen R, Lindqvist C. Biodegradable self reinforced polylactide osteosynthesis in maxillofacial traumatology. *J Craniomaxillofac Surg* 1998;26(Suppl 1):150

Sailer HF, Haers PE. Is resorbable osteosynthesis material 'state of the art' in paediatric craniofacial surgery? *J Craniomaxillofac Surg* 2000;28(Suppl 3):90

Sakurai H. Vanadium distribution in rats and DNA cleavage by vanadyl complex: implication for vanadium toxicity and biological effects. *Environ Health Perspect* 1994;102(Suppl 3):35–36

Sandor GKB, Stoelinga PJW, Tideman H. The mandibular intra-oral step osteotomy a re-appraisal). *J Oral Maxillofac Surg* 1982;40:78–91

Sarmiento A, Latta LL, Tarr RR. The effects of function in fracture healing and stability. *Instr Course Lect* 1984;33:83–106

Sarmiento A, Sobol PA, Sew Hoy AL, et al. Prefabricated functional braces for the treatment of fractures of the tibial diaphysis. *J Bone Joint Surg* 1984;66:1328–1339

Scales JT. Black staining around titanium alloy prostheses–an orthopaedic enigma. *J Bone Joint Surg Br* 1991;73:534–536

Schenk R, Willenegger H. Zum histologischen Bild der sogenannten Primärheilung der Knochenkompakta nach experimentellen Osteotomien am Hund. *Experientia* 1963;19:593–595

Schenk R, Willenegger H. Zur Histologie der primären Knochenheilung. *Langenbecks Arch Klin Chir Ver Dtsch Z Chir.* 1964;308:440–452

Schenk R. Biology of fracture repair. In: Browner BD, Jupiter JB, Levine AM, Trafton PG, eds. Skeletal trauma. Philadelphia: Saunders; 1992:31–75

Schilli W. Behandlungsmöglichkeiten bei Frakturen. *Therapie* 1969;41:2008–2014

Schliephake H, Lehmann H, Kunz U, et al. Ultrastructural findings in soft tissues adjacent to titanium plates used in jaw fracture treatment. *Int J Oral Maxillofac Surg* 1993;22:20–27

Schliephake H. Entnahmetechniken autogener Knochentransplantate. Teil I: Spenderareale innerhalb des Kopf-Hals-Bereiches. *Implantol* 1994;2:317–327

Schliephake H. Entnahmetechniken autogener Knochentransplantate. Teil II: Spenderareale außerhalb des Kopf-Hals-Bereiches. *Implantol* 1995;3:39–45

Schmelzeisen R, Neukam FW, Hausamen J-E. Atlas der Mikrochirurgie im Kopf-Halsbereich. Munich: Hanser; 1996

Schmelzeisen R, Neukam FW, Shirota T, et al. Postoperative function after implant insertion in vascularized bone grafts in maxilla and mandible. *Plast Reconstr Surg* 1996;97:719–725

Schmid W, Pape H-D. Vergleichende experimentelle Untersuchungen von Minirekonstruktionsplatten. *Dtsch Z Mund Kiefer Gesichtschir* 1991;15:271–274

Schmitz R, Höltje W, Cordes V. Vergleichende Untersuchungen über die Regeneration des parodontalen Gewebes nach Unfallverletzungen und Osteotomien des Alveolarfortsatzes. *Dtsch Zahnarztl Z* 1973;28:219–223

Schmoker R, Von Allmen G, Tschopp HM. Application of functionally stable fixation in maxillofacial surgery according to the ASIF principles. *J Oral Maxillofac Surg* 1982;40:457–461

Schneider A, Schulze J, Eckelt U, Laniado M. Lag screw osteosynthesis of fractures of the mandibular condyle: potential benefit of preoperative planning using multiplanar CT reconstruction. *Oral Surg Oral Med Oral Pathol Oral Radiol Endod* 2005;99:142–147

Schön R, Fakler O, Gellrich NC, Schmelzeisen R. Five-year experience with the transoral endoscopically assisted treatment of displaced condylar mandible fractures. *Plast Reconstr Surg* 2005;116:44–50

Schönberger A. Behandlung der Zähne im Bruchspalt. *Fortschr Kiefer Gesichtschir* 1956;2:108–111

Schroeder HE, Page RC. The normal periodontium. In: Schluger S, Yuodelis RA, Page RC, eds. Periodontal disease. Philadelphia: Lea-Febiger; 1977:8–55

Schultes G, Gaggl A, Karcher H. Stability of dental implants in microvascular osseous transplants. *Plast Reconstr Surg* 2002;109:916–921 discussion 922–914

Schwimmer A. Management of mandibular fractures. In: Nussbaum M, ed. Modern techniques in surgery. Head and neck surgery. Philadelphia: Futura; 1988:17–23

Schwimmer A. Lag screw technique and advanced applications. In: Greenberg AM, ed. Craniofacial fractures. New York: Springer; 1993:69–76

Semlitsch M. Titanium alloys for hip joint replacements. *Clin Mater* 1987;2:1–13

Shanbhag AS, Jacobs JJ, Black J, et al. Human monocyte response to particulate biomaterials generated in vivo and in vitro. *J Orthop Res* 1995;13:792–801

Shaw RJ, Sutton AF, Cawood JI, et al. Oral rehabilitation after treatment for head & neck malignancy. *Head Neck* 2005; 27: 459–470

Shepherd DE, Ward Booth RP, Moos KF. The morbidity of bicoronal flaps in maxillofacial surgery. *Br J Oral Maxillofac Surg* 1985; 23:1–8

Shetty V, Niederdellmann H. Maxillomandibular fixation with minihooks: a clinical evaluation. *Oral Surg Oral Med Oral Pathol* 1987;64:677–679

Shetty V, Brearty D, Fournay M, Caputo A. Fracture line stability as a function of the internal fixation system: an in vitro comparison using a mandibular angle fracture model. *J Oral Maxillofac Surg* 1995;53:791–802

Sicher H, Tandler J. Anatomie für Zahnärzte. Vienna: Springer; 1928:298–307

Silvennoinen U, Iizuka T, Lindqvist C, Oikarinen K. Different patterns of condylar fractures: an analysis of 382 patients in a 3-year period. *J Oral Maxillofac Surg* 1992;50:1032–1037

Silvennoinen U, Iizuka T, Oikarinen K, Lindqvist C. Analysis of possible factors leading problems after nonsurgical treatment of condylar fractures. *J Oral Maxillofac Surg* 1994;52: 793–799

Silverberg B, Banis JCJr, Acland RD. Mandibular reconstruction with microvascular bone transfer. Series of 10 patients. *Am J Surg* 1985;150:440–446

Silverman S. A new operation for displaced fractures at the neck of the mandibular condyle. *Dental Cosmos* 1925;67:876–877

Smith JD, Abramson M. Membranous versus endochondral bone autografts. *Arch Otolaryngol* 1974;99:203–205

Smith RB, Henstrom DK, Karnell LH, et al. Scapula osteocutaneous free flap reconstruction of the head and neck: impact of flap choice on surgical and medical complications. *Head Neck* 2007;29:446–452

Snell JA, Dott WA. Internal fixation of certain fractures of the mandible by bone plating. *Plast Reconstr Surg* 1969;43(3): 281–286

Snyder CC, Levine GA, Swanson HM. Mandibular lengthening by gradual distraction: preliminary report. *Plast Reconstr Surg* 1973;51:506–508

Solar RJ, Pollak SR, Korostoff E. In vitro corrosion testing of titanium surgical implant alloys: an approach to understanding titanium release from implants. *J Biomed Mater Res* 1979;13:217–221

Speculand B, Jackson M. A halo-caliper-guidance system for bimaxillary dual-arch orthognathic surgery. *J Maxillofac Surg* 1984;12:167–173

Spiessl B. Erfahrungen mit dem AO-Besteck bei Kieferbruchbehandlungen. *Schweiz Mschr Zahnmed.* 1969;79:112–113

Spiessl B. Grundsätzlich Zur Knochentransplantation. *Fortschr Kiefer Gesichtschir* 1976;20:14–17

Spiessl B. Internal fixation of the mandible. A manual of AO/ASIF principles. Berlin: Springer; 1989

Spiessl B, Schroll K. Gesichtsschädel. In: Nigst H. Spezielle Frakturen- und Luxationslehre. 4th ed.Stuttgart: Thieme; 1972

Stegenga B, de Bont LGm, de Leeuw R, Boering G. Assessment of mandibular function impairment associated with temporomandibular joint osteoarthrosis and internal derangement. *J Orofac Pain* 1993;7:183–195

Steinemann SG. Implants for stable fixation of fractures. In: Rubin LR, ed. Biomaterials in reconstructive surgery. St. Louis: Mosby; 1983:283–311

Steinemann S. Titanium as an implant material. In: Prein J, ed. AO-ASIF maxillofacial course. Rigid fixation with plates and screws in cranio-maxillofacial trauma. Davos: Syllabus; 1993:14

Steinhäuser E. Eingriffe am Processus articularis auf dem oralen Weg. *Dtsch Zahnärztl Z* 1964;19:694–700

Steinhäuser EW. Die Anwendung des Titanium-Mesh-Systems bei der Unterkieferrekonstruktion. In: Scheunemann H, Schmidseder R, eds. Plastische und Wiederherstellungs-chirurgie bei bösartigen Tumoren. Berlin: Springer; 1982:128–132

Stephenson KL, Graham WC. The use of the Kirschner pin in fractures of the condyle. *Plast Reconstr Surg* 1952;10:19–23

Stoelinga PJW. van de Vijver HRM, Leenen RJ, Blijdorp PA, Schoenaers JHA. The prevention of relapse after maxillary osteotomies in cleft palate patients. *J Craniomaxillofac Surg* 1987;15:326–331

Stoelinga PJW, Leenen RJ. Combined mandibular vertical ramus and body step osteotomies for correction of exceptional skeletal and occlusal anomalies. *J Craniomaxillofac Surg* 1992; 20:233–243

Stoelinga PJW, Brouns JJA. The quadrangular Kufner osteotomy revised. *J Craniomaxillofac Surg* 1996;24(Suppl I):110

Stoelinga PJ, Slagter AP, Brouns JJ. Rehabilitation of patients with severe (Class VI) maxillary resorption using Le Fort 1 osteotomy, interposed bone grafts and endosteal implants: 1-8 years follow-up in a two-stage procedure. *Int J Oral Maxillofac Surg* 2000;29:188–193

Stoll P, Niederdellmann H, Sauter R. Zahnbeteiligung bei Unterkieferfrakturen. *Dtsch Zahnärztl Z* 1983;38:349–351

Stout RA. Intermaxillary wiring and intermaxillary elastic traction and fixation. In: Ivy HR, David JS, Ebi JD, et al., eds. Military surgical manuals. Practice of plastic and maxillofacial surgery. Philadelphia: Saunders; 1942:272–280

Stromeyer L. Handbuch der Chirurgie. Vol 1. Freiburg: Herder; 1844:703

Sunderman FWJr. Carcinogenicity of metal alloys in orthopedic prostheses: clinical and experimental studies. *Fundam Appl Toxicol* 1989;13:205–210

Sustrac B, Villebrun JP. Biomechanique des osteosyntheses par plaques vissées miniaturisées des fractures du corps de la mandibule. Etude. Strasbourg: Ecole Nat. Sup. Art. Ind.; 1976:134

Sutton DN, Lewis BR, Patel M, Cawood JI. Changes in facial form relative to progressive atrophy of the edentulous jaws. *Int J Oral Maxillofac Surg* 2004;33:676–682

Swanson KS, Laskin DM, Campbell RL. Auriculotemporal syndrome following the preauricular approach to temporomandibular joint surgery. *J Oral Maxillofac Surg* 1991;49: 680–682

Swartz WM, Banis JC, Newton ED, et al. The osteocutaneous scapular flap for mandibular and maxillary reconstruction. *Plast Reconstr Surg* 1986;77:530–545

Takamura K, Hayashi K, Ishinishi N, et al. Evaluation of carcinogenicity and chronic toxity associated with orthopedic implants in mice. *J Biomed Mater Res* 1994;28:583–592

Takenoshita Y, Oka M, Tashiro H. Surgical treatment of fractures of the mandibular condylar neck. *J Craniomaxillofac Surg* 1989;17:119–124

Takenoshita Y, Ishibashi H, Oka M. Comparison of functional recovery after nonsurgical and surgical treatment of condylar fractures. *J Oral Maxillofac Surg* 1990;48:1191–1195

Tallgren A. The continuing resorption of the residual alveolar ridges in complete denture wearers: a mixed longitudinal study covering 25 years. *J Prosthet Dent* 1972;27: 120–132

Tasanen A, Lamberg MA. Transosseous wiring in the treatment of condylar fractures of the mandible. *J Maxillofac Surg* 1976;4:200–206

Teichgraeber JF, Rappaport NH, Harris JHJr. The radiology of upper airway obstruction in maxillofacial trauma. *Ann Plast Surg* 1991;27:103–109

ten Bruggenkate CM, Kraaijenhagen HA, van der Kwast WA, Krekeler G, Oosterbeek HS. Autogenous maxillary bone grafts in conjunction with placement of I.T.I. endosseous implants. A preliminary report. *Int J Oral Maxillofac Surg* 1992;21:81–84

Tengvall P, Hornsten EG, Elwing H, Lundstrom I. Bactericidal properties of a titanium-peroxy gel obtained from metallic titanium and hydrogen peroxide. *J Biomed Mater Res* 1990;24: 319–330

Terheyden H. Self adaptic spheric washer for lag screw application. Poster AG Kieferchirurgie, Bad Homburg: 21–23 May 1998

Terheyden H, Ludwig K, Feldmann H, Härle F. The self adapting washer for lag screw osteosynthesis of mandibular fractures. Finite elemente analysis and preclinical results. *J Craniomaxillofac Surg* 1999;27:58–67

Tessier P. Ostéotomies totales de la face: syndrome de Crouzon, syndrome d'Apert, oxycéphalies, scaphocéphalies, turricéphalies. *Ann Chir Plast* 1967;12:273–285

Tessier P, Guiot G, Rougerie J, et al. Osteotomies cranio-naso-orbital-faciales. Hypertelorisme. *Ann Chir Plast* 1967;12:103–118

Tessier P. Orbital hypertelorism. *Scand J Plast Reconstr Surg* 1972;6:135–143

Thacker JG, Jachetta FA, Allaire PE, et al. Biomechanical properties—their influence on planning surgical excisions. In: Krizek TJ, Hoopes PE, eds. Symposium on basic science in plastic surgery. Vol 15. St. Louis: Mosby; 1975:72–79

Thoma KH. Treatment of condylar fractures. *J Oral Surg (Chic)* 1954;12:112–120

Thompson GJ, Puleo DA. Ti-6Al-4V ion solution inhibition of osteogenic cell phenotype as a function of differentiation time-course in vitro. *Biomaterials* 1996;17:1949–1954

Tideman H, Stoelinga P, Gallia L. Le Fort I advancement with segmental palatal osteotomies in patients with cleft palates. *J Oral Surg* 1980;38:196–199

Tillmann B, Härle F, Schleicher A. Biomechanik des Unterkiefers. *Dtsch Zahnarztl Z* 1983;38:285–293

Timmel R. Die Osteosynthese von Luxationsfrakturen des Kiefergelenkes mittels Kirschner Drahtung. *Dtsch Z Mund Kiefer Gesichtschir* 1981;5:243–254

Torgersen S, Gilhuus-Moe OT, Gjerdet NR. Immune response to nickel and some clinical observations after stainless steel miniplate osteosynthesis. *Int J Oral Maxillofac Surg* 1993;22:246–250

Torgersen S, Gjerdet NR, Erichsen ES, et al. Metal particles and tissue changes adjacent to miniplates. A retrieval study. *Acta Odontol Scand* 1995;53:65–71

Torgersen S, Moe G, Jonsson R. Immunocompetent cells adjacent to stainless steel and titanium miniplates and screws. *Eur J Oral Sci* 1995;103:46–54

Toth-Bagi Z, Ujpal M, Gyenes V. Tapasztalataink az Otten-fele mandibulomaxillaris rogzitessel. *Fogorv Sz* 1994;87: 71–73

Trauner R, Obwegeser HL. The surgical correction of mandibular prognathism and retrognathia with consideration of genioplasty. Part I. Surgical procedures to correct mandibular prognathism and reshaping of chin. *Oral Surg Oral Med Oral Pathol* 1957a;10:677–689

Trauner R, Obwegeser HL. The surgical correction of mandibular prognathism and retrognathia with consideration of genioplasty. Part II. Operating methods for micrognathia and distocclusion. *Oral Surg Oral Med Oral Pathol* 1957b;10: 899–909

Triaca A, Minoretti R, McGurk M, et al. A new system for multidirectional intraoral distraction—rationale and application to ten patients. In: Diner PA, Vazquez MP, eds. 2. International Congress of Cranial and Facial Bone Distraction Processes. Bologna: Moduzzi; 1999:297–304

Trinchi V, Nobis M, Cecchele D. Emission spectrophotometric analysis of titanium, aluminium, and vanadium levels in the blood, urine, and hair of patients with total hip arthroplasties. *Ital J Orthop Traumatol.* 1992;18:331–339

Tsusaki T. Anatomie der Mundhöhle. 7th ed. Kyoto und Tokio: Nagasue-Shoten; 1955:9

Tuovinen V, Norhold SE, Sindet-Petersen SS, Jensen JJ. A retrospective analysis of 279 patients with isolated mandibular fractures treated with titanium miniplates. *J Oral Maxillofac Surg* 1994;52:931–936

Upton LG. Management of injuries to the temporomandibular joint region. In: Fonseca RJ, Walker RV, eds. Oral and maxillofacial trauma. Philadelphia: Saunders; 1991:418–434

Uhthoff HK, Boisvert D, Finnegan M. Cortical porosis under plates. Reaction to unloading or to necrosis? *J Bone Joint Surg Am* 1994;76:1507–1512

Verbov J. Pacemaker contact sensitivity. *Contact Dermatitis* 1985;12:173

Vincente J, Stoelinga PJW. Toepassing van bottransplantaten uit het corpus mandibulae voor preimplantologische chirurgie. *Ned Tijdschr Tandheelkd* 2005;112:211–215

Visuri T, Koskenvuo M. Cancer risk after Mc Kee-Farrar total hip replacement. *Orthopedics* 1991;14:137–142

Wackerbauer R. Zur operativen Behandlung von Kiefergelenkköpfchenfrakturen–Untersuchung am Krankengut von 1948–1960 [dissertation]. Munich, 1962

Wagner A, Krach W, Schicho K, et al. A 3-dimensional finite-element analysis investigating the biomechanical behavior of the mandible and plate osteosynthesis in cases of fractures of the condylar process. *Oral Surg Oral Med Oral Pathol Oral Radiol Endod.* 2002;94:678

Walz C, Pape D, Lenz M. Miniplattenosteosynthesen der Unterkieferfraktur in Lokalanästhesie. Indikation und Ergebnisse bei 316 Patienten. *Fortschr Kiefer Gesichtschir* 1996;41: 133–135

Wang JY, Wicklund BH, Gustilo RB, Tsukayama DT. Titanium, chromium and cobalt ions modulate the release of bone-associated cytokines by human monocytes/macrophages in vitro. *Biomaterials* 1996a;17:2233–2240

Wang JY, Tsukayama DT, Wicklund BH, Gustilo RB. Inhibition of T and B cell proliferation by titanium, cobalt, and chromium: role of IL-2 and IL-6. *J Biomed Mater Res* 1996b;32: 655–661

Wangerin K. Einzeitige bimaxilläre Korrektur extremer Fehlbisse – Vorbehandlung, Planung und Operationsmethode mit funktionsstabiler Fixierung im Ober- und Unterkiefer. *Dtsch Z Mund Kiefer Gesichtschir* 1990;14:424–431

Wangerin K. Adjunctive aesthetic procedures in orthognathic surgery. Book of Abstracts. 4. International Symposium on Orthognathic Surgery and Distraction, Stuttgart, 2006:106

Wangerin K. Our concept of intraoral distraction. *Stomatologie* 2005;102(2):59–66

Wangerin K. Simultaneous repositioning of maxilla and both mandibular condyles by positioning plates and three interocclusal splints during bimaxillary surgery. *Asian J Oral Max Fac Surg* 1994;6:71–81

Wangerin K, Gropp H. Die enorale Distraktionsosteotomie des mikrogenen Unterkiefers zur Beseitigung der Atemwegsobstruktion. *Dtsch Z Mund Kiefer Gesichtschir* 1994;18:236

Wangerin K, Gropp H. Der enorale Zugang bei der Ilizarov-Kallusdistraktion am Unterkiefer. *Dtsch Z Mund Kiefer Gesichtschir* 1995;19:303–307

Wangerin K, Gropp H, Kreusch Th, Hammer B. The multidirectional enoral callus distraction on the mandible. *J Craniomaxillofac Surg* 1996;24(Suppl 1):123

Wangerin K, Gropp H. Multidimensional intraoral distraction osteogenesis of the mandible—4 years of clinical experience. *Int J Oral Maxillofac Surg* 1997;26(Suppl 1):14

Wangerin K, Kretschmer W, Fassnacht J, Zoder W. Step by step treatment of severe midface deficiencies including enoral maxillary distraction. Book of Abstracts: 5th International Congress of Maxillofacial and Craniofacial Distraction, Paris 2006.

Warnekros L. Allgemeines über Schienenbehandlung bei Kieferbrüchen und die Befestigung von Goldschienen unter dem losgelösten Periost mit und ohne Verwendung eines Transplantates. In: Soerensen I, Warnekros L, eds. Chirurg und Zahnarzt. Berlin: Springer; 1917:25–69

Warren SM, Borud LJ, Brecht LE, et al. Microvascular reconstruction of the pediatric mandible. *Plast Reconstr Surg* 2007;119: 649–661

Wassmund M. Frakturen und Luxationen des Gesichtsschädels. Leipzig: Meusser; 1927:307

Wassmund M. Lehrbuch der praktischen Chirurgie des Mundes und der Kiefer. Vol I. Leipzig: Meusser; 1935:293–298

Watt DM, MacGregor AR. Designing complete dentures. Philadelphia: Saunders; 1976:4–14

Weber W, Reuther J, Michel C, Muhling J. Erfahrungen bei der Versorgung von Gesichtsschädelfrakturen mit dem Würzburger Titan-Miniplattensystem. *Dtsch Z Mund Kiefer Gesichtschir* 1990;14:46–52

Weber WD. Treatment of mandibular angle fractures. *Atlas Oral Maxillofac Surg Clin North Am* 1997;5:77–125

Weigele B. Ein Versuch am Bau des Unterkiefers die Gesetze der Mechanik und Statik aufzufinden. *Korresp Bl Zahnärzte.* 1921;47(4):3–19

Weinberg MJ, Merx P, Antonyshyn O, Farb R. Facial nerve palsy after mandibular fracture. *Ann Plast Surg* 1995;34:546–549

Weingart D, Steinemann S, Schilli W. Titanium deposition in regional lymph nodes after insertion of titanium screw implants in maxillofacial region. *Int J Oral Maxillofac Surg* 1994;23:450–452

West RA, Epker BN. Posterior maxillary surgery: its place in the treatment of dentofacial deformities. *J Oral Surg* 1972;30:562–575

Whitley SP, Sandhu S, Cardozo A. Preoperative vascular assessment of the lower limb for harvest of a fibular flap: the views of vascular surgeons in the United Kingdom. *Br J Oral Maxillofac Surg* 2004;42:307–310

Wilk A, Biotchane J, Rosenstiel M, et al. Osteosynthèse des fractures sous-condyliennes par une plaque rectangulaire de stabilisation tridimensionelle. *Rev Stomatol Chir Maxillofac* 1997;98:40–44

Williams JG, Cawood JI. Effects of intermaxillary fixation on pulmonary function. *Int J Oral Maxillofac Surg* 1990;19: 76–78

Win KK, Handa Y, Ichihara H, et al. Intermaxillary fixation using screws. Report of a technique. *Int J Oral Maxillofac Surg* 1991;20:283–284

Winkler R. Der funktionelle Bau des menschlichen Kieferapparates. *Dtsch Zahnheilkd.* 1922;55:84–155

Wolfe SA, Lovaas M, McCafferty LR. Use of miniplate to provide intermaxillary fixation in the edentulous patient. *J Craniomaxillofac Surg* 1989;17:31–33

Wolff KD, Ervens J, Herzog K, Hoffmeister B. Experience with the osteocutaneous fibula flap: an analysis of 24 consecutive reconstructions of composite mandibular defects. *J Craniomaxillofac Surg* 1996;24:330–338

Woodman JL, Jacobs JJ, Galante JO, Urban RM. Metal ion release from titanium-based prosthetic segmental replacements of long bones in baboons: a long-term study. *J Orthop Res* 1984;1:421–430

Wooley PH, Nasser S, Fitzgerald RHJr. The immune response to implant materials in humans. *Clin Orthop Relat Res* 1996;326:63–70

Worsaae N, Thorn JJ. Surgical versus non-surgical treatment of unilateral dislocated low subcondylar fractures: a clinical study of 52 cases. *J Oral Maxillofac Surg* 1994;52: 353–361

Wunderer S. Die Prognathieoperation mittels frontal gestieltem Maxillafragment. *Oest Z Stomatol* 1962;59:98–102

Yamamoto H, Sawaki Y, Ohbuko H, Ueda M. Maxillary advancement by distraction osteogenesis using osseointegrated implants. *J Craniomaxillofac Surg* 1997;25:186–191

Yaremchuk MJ, Fiala TG, Barker F, Ragland R. The effects of rigid fixation on craniofacial growth of rhesus monkeys. *Plast Reconstr Surg* 1994;93:1–10

Yaremchuk MJ, Posnick JC. Symposium: Resolving controversies related to plate and screw fixation in the growing cranio-facial skeleton. *J Craniofac Surg* 1995;6:525–527

Yeung RWK, Samman N, Cheung LK, et al. Stereomodel-assisted fibula flap harvest and mandibular reconstruction. *J Oral Maxillofac Surg* 2007;65:1128–1134

Ziccardi VB, Schneider RE, Kummer FJ. Würzburg lag screw plate versus four-hole miniplate for the treatment of condylar process fractures. *J Oral Maxillofac Surg* 1997;55:602–607

Zide MF, Kent JN. Indications for open reduction of mandibular condyle fractures. *J Oral Maxillofac Surg* 1983;41: 89–98

Zide MF. Outcomes of open versus closed treatment of mandibular subcondylar fractures. *J Oral Maxillofac Surg* 2001;59: 375

Zingg M, Chowdhury K, Lädrach K, et al. Treatment of 813 zygoma-lateral orbital complex fractures. *Arch Otolaryngol Head Neck Surg* 1991;117:611–620

Zins JE, Whitaker LA. Membranous versus endochondral bone: implications for craniofacial reconstruction. *Plast Reconstr Surg* 1983;72:778–785

Zitter H, Plenk HJr. The electrochemical behaviour of metallic implants as an indicator for their biocompatibility. *J Biomed Mater Res* 1987;21:881–896

Zöller JE. Techniken und Fehler der vertikalen Alveolarfortsatz-Distraktion—Distraction versus Augmentation, Grosses AKH-Symposium, 8–9 March 2002, Universitätskliniken AKH, Vienna

Zou ZJ, Wu WT, Sun QX, et al. Remodeling of the temporomandibular joint after conservative treatment of condylar fractures. *Dentomaxillofac Radiol* 1987;16:91–98

Index

Page numbers in *italics* refer to illustrations or tables